ACP American College of Physicians®
Internal Medicine | *Doctors for Adults*

MKSAP® 16

Medical Knowledge Self-Assessment Program®

Endocrinology and Metabolism

Welcome to the Endocrinology and Metabolism Section of MKSAP 16!

Here, you will find updated information on diabetes mellitus, disorders of the pituitary gland, disorders of the thyroid gland, disorders of the adrenal glands, reproductive disorders, and calcium and bone disorders. All of these topics are uniquely focused on the needs of generalists and subspecialists *outside* of endocrinology and metabolism.

The publication of the 16th edition of Medical Knowledge Self-Assessment Program heralds a significant event, culminating 2 years of effort by dozens of leading subspecialists across the United States. Our authoring committees have strived to help internists succeed in Maintenance of Certification, right up to preparing for the MOC examination, and to get residents ready for the certifying examination. MKSAP 16 also helps you update your medical knowledge and elevates standards of self-learning by allowing you to assess your knowledge with 1,200 all-new multiple-choice questions, including 84 in Endocrinology and Metabolism.

MKSAP began more than 40 years ago. The American Board of Internal Medicine's examination blueprint and gaps between actual and preferred practices inform creation of the content. The questions, refined through rigorous face-to-face meetings, are among the best in medicine. A psychometric analysis of the items sharpens our educational focus on weaknesses in practice. To meet diverse learning styles, we offer MKSAP 16 online and in downloadable apps for PCs, tablets, laptops, and smartphones. We are also introducing the following:

High-Value Care Recommendations: The Endocrinology and Metabolism section starts with several recommendations based on the important concept of health care value (balancing clinical benefit with costs and harms) to address the needs of trainees, practicing physicians, and patients. These recommendations are part of a major initiative that has been undertaken by the American College of Physicians, in collaboration with other organizations.

Content for Hospitalists: This material, highlighted in blue and labeled with the familiar hospital icon (H), directly addresses the learning needs of the increasing number of physicians who work in the hospital setting. MKSAP 16 Digital will allow you to customize quizzes based on hospitalist-only questions to help you prepare for the Hospital Medicine Maintenance of Certification Examination.

We hope you enjoy and benefit from MKSAP 16. Please feel free to send us any comments to mksap_editors@acponline.org or visit us at the MKSAP Resource Site (mksap.acponline.org) to find out how we can help you study, earn CME, accumulate MOC points, and stay up to date. I know I speak on behalf of ACP staff members and our authoring committees when I say we are honored to have attracted your interest and participation.

Sincerely,

Patrick Alguire

Patrick Alguire, MD, FACP
Editor-in-Chief
Senior Vice President
Medical Education Division
American College of Physicians

Endocrinology and Metabolism

Committee

Silvio E. Inzucchi, MD, FACP, Editor[2]
Professor of Medicine
Clinical Chief, Section of Endocrinology
Yale University School of Medicine
Director, Yale Diabetes Center
Yale-New Haven Hospital
New Haven, Connecticut

Howard H. Weitz, MD, FACP, Associate Editor[1]
Professor of Medicine
Director, Jefferson Heart Institute
Director, Division of Cardiology
Jefferson Medical College of Thomas Jefferson University
Philadelphia, Pennsylvania

Baha M. Arafah, MD, FACP[1]
Professor of Medicine
Chief, Division of Endocrinology
Case Western Reserve University
Case Medical Center
Cleveland, Ohio

Kenneth D. Burman, MD, MACP[2]
Chief, Endocrine Section
Washington Hospital Center
Professor, Department of Medicine
Georgetown University
Washington, DC

Elizabeth Holt, MD, PhD[2]
Assistant Professor of Medicine
Department of Internal Medicine, Section of Endocrinology
Yale University School of Medicine
New Haven, Connecticut

Laurence Katznelson, MD[2]
Professor of Medicine and Neurosurgery
Stanford University School of Medicine
Medical Director, Pituitary Center
Stanford Hospital and Clinics
Stanford, California

David K. McCulloch, MD[2]
Clinical Professor of Medicine
Department of Endocrinology and Metabolism
University of Washington
And Diabetologist and Medical Director of Clinical Improvement
Group Health Cooperative
Seattle, Washington

Maria A. Yialamas, MD, FACP[1]
Associate Program Director, Internal Medicine Residency
Department of Medicine
Brigham and Women's Hospital
Boston, Massachusetts

Editor-in-Chief

Patrick C. Alguire, MD, FACP[1]
Senior Vice President, Medical Education
American College of Physicians
Philadelphia, Pennsylvania

Deputy Editor-in-Chief

Philip A. Masters, MD, FACP[1]
Senior Medical Associate for Content Development
American College of Physicians
Philadelphia, Pennsylvania

Senior Medical Associate for Content Development

Cynthia D. Smith, MD, FACP[2]
American College of Physicians
Philadelphia, Pennsylvania

Endocrinology and Metabolism Clinical Editor

Cynthia A. Burns, MD, FACP[1]

Endocrinology and Metabolism Reviewers

Amindra S. Arora, MD[1]
Arnold A. Asp, MD, FACP[1]
Lee R. Berkowitz, MD, FACP[1]
Lara Hume, MD[1]
Lia Logio, MD, FACP[1]

Endocrinology and Metabolism Reviewers Representing the American Society for Clinical Pharmacology & Therapeutics

Linda A. Hershey, MD, PhD[2]
L. Amy Sun, MD, PhD[1]

Endocrinology and Metabolism ACP Editorial Staff

Ellen McDonald, PhD[1], Senior Staff Editor
Sean McKinney[1], Director, Self-Assessment Programs
Margaret Wells[1], Managing Editor
Linnea Donnarumma[1], Assistant Editor

ACP Principal Staff

Patrick C. Alguire, MD, FACP[1]
Senior Vice President, Medical Education

D. Theresa Kanya, MBA[1]
Vice President, Medical Education

Sean McKinney[1]
Director, Self-Assessment Programs

Margaret Wells[1]
Managing Editor

Valerie Dangovetsky[1]
Program Administrator

Becky Krumm[1]
Senior Staff Editor

Ellen McDonald, PhD[1]
Senior Staff Editor

Katie Idell[1]
Senior Staff Editor

Randy Hendrickson[1]
Production Administrator/Editor

Megan Zborowski[1]
Staff Editor

Linnea Donnarumma[1]
Assistant Editor

John Haefele[1]
Assistant Editor

Developed by the American College of Physicians

---

1. Has no relationships with any entity producing, marketing, re-selling, or distributing health care goods or services consumed by, or used on, patients.

2. Has disclosed relationships with entities producing, marketing, re-selling, or distributing health care goods or services consumed by, or used on, patients. See below.

Conflicts of Interest

The following committee members, reviewers, and ACP staff members have disclosed relationships with commercial companies:

Kenneth D. Burman, MD, MACP
Research Grants/Contracts
Pfizer, Amgen, Exelixis, Innovative Technologies
Board Member
American Thyroid Association; FDA, Endocrine Advisory Committee
Other
UpToDate, Medscape, Endocrine Society

Linda A. Hershey, MD, PhD
Research Grants/Contracts
Reviewer for AAAS Research Competitiveness Program
Honoraria
Medlink Neurology
Speakers Bureau
Medical Education Speakers Network

Elizabeth Holt, MD, PhD
Consultantship
Merck

Silvio E. Inzucchi, MD, FACP
Consultantship
Takeda, Merck, Amylin, Medtronic, Boehringer Ingelheim
Honoraria
NovoNordisk
Research Grants/Contracts
Boehringer Ingelheim, Eli Lilly
Other
Endocrine Society, UpToDate

Laurence Katznelson, MD
Research Grants/Contracts
Novartis, Ipsen, Pfizer, Genentech
Consultantship
Pfizer
Speakers Bureau
Ipsen

David K. McCulloch, MD
Royalties
UpToDate

Cynthia D. Smith, MD, FACP
Stock Options/Holdings
Merck and Company

Acknowledgments

The American College of Physicians (ACP) gratefully acknowledges the special contributions to the development and production of the 16th edition of the Medical

Knowledge Self-Assessment Program® (MKSAP® 16) made by the following people:

Graphic Services: Michael Ripca (Technical Administrator/Graphic Designer) and Willie-Fetchko Graphic Design (Graphic Designer).

Production/Systems: Dan Hoffmann (Director, Web Services & Systems Development), Neil Kohl (Senior Architect), and Scott Hurd (Senior Systems Analyst/Developer).

MKSAP 16 Digital: Under the direction of Steven Spadt, Vice President, ACP Digital Products & Services, the digital version of MKSAP 16 was developed within the ACP's Digital Product Development Department, led by Brian Sweigard (Director). Other members of the team included Sean O'Donnell (Senior Architect), Dan Barron (Senior Systems Analyst/Developer), Chris Forrest (Senior Software Developer/Design Lead), Jon Laing (Senior Web Application Developer), Brad Lord (Senior Web Developer), John McKnight (Senior Web Developer), and Nate Pershall (Senior Web Developer).

The College also wishes to acknowledge that many other persons, too numerous to mention, have contributed to the production of this program. Without their dedicated efforts, this program would not have been possible.

Introducing the MKSAP Resource Site (mksap.acponline.org)

The MKSAP Resource Site (mksap.acponline.org) is a continually updated site that provides links to MKSAP 16 online answer sheets for print subscribers; access to MKSAP 16 Digital, Board Basics® 3, and MKSAP 16 Updates; the latest details on Continuing Medical Education (CME) and Maintenance of Certification (MOC) in the United States, Canada, and Australia; errata; and other new information.

ABIM Maintenance of Certification

Check the MKSAP Resource Site (mksap.acponline.org) for the latest information on how MKSAP tests can be used to apply to the American Board of Internal Medicine for Maintenance of Certification (MOC) points.

RCPSC Maintenance of Certification

In Canada, MKSAP 16 is an Accredited Self-Assessment Program (Section 3) as defined by the Maintenance of Certification Program of The Royal College of Physicians and Surgeons of Canada (RCPSC) and approved by the Canadian Society of Internal Medicine on December 9, 2011. Approval of Part A sections of MKSAP 16 extends from July 31, 2012, until July 31, 2015. Approval of Part B sections of MKSAP 16 extends from December 31, 2012, to December 31, 2015. Fellows of the Royal College may earn three credits per hour for participating in MKSAP 16 under Section 3. MKSAP 16 will enable Fellows to earn up to 75% of their required 400 credits during the 5-year MOC cycle. A Fellow can achieve this 75% level by earning 100 of the maximum of 174 *AMA PRA Category 1 Credits*™ available in MKSAP 16. MKSAP 16 also meets multiple CanMEDS Roles for RCPSC MOC, including that of Medical Expert, Communicator, Collaborator, Manager, Health Advocate, Scholar, and Professional. For information on how to apply MKSAP 16 CME credits to RCPSC MOC, visit the MKSAP Resource Site at mksap.acponline.org.

The Royal Australasian College of Physicians CPD Program

In Australia, MKSAP 16 is a Category 3 program that may be used by Fellows of The Royal Australasian College of Physicians (RACP) to meet mandatory CPD points. Two CPD credits are awarded for each of the 174 *AMA PRA Category 1 Credits*™ available in MKSAP 16. More information about using MKSAP 16 for this purpose is available at the MKSAP Resource Site at mksap.acponline.org and at www.racp.edu.au. CPD credits earned through MKSAP 16 should be reported at the MyCPD site at www.racp.edu.au/mycpd.

Continuing Medical Education

The American College of Physicians is accredited by the Accreditation Council for Continuing Medical Education (ACCME) to provide continuing medical education for physicians.

The American College of Physicians designates this enduring material, MKSAP 16, for a maximum of 174 *AMA PRA Category 1 Credits*™. Physicians should claim only the credit commensurate with the extent of their participation in the activity.

Up to 12 *AMA PRA Category 1 Credits*™ are available from December 31, 2012, to December 31, 2015, for the MKSAP 16 Endocrinology and Metabolism section.

Learning Objectives

The learning objectives of MKSAP 16 are to:

- Close gaps between actual care in your practice and preferred standards of care, based on best evidence
- Diagnose disease states that are less common and sometimes overlooked and confusing
- Improve management of comorbid conditions that can complicate patient care
- Determine when to refer patients for surgery or care by subspecialists

- Pass the ABIM Certification Examination
- Pass the ABIM Maintenance of Certification Examination

Target Audience

- General internists and primary care physicians
- Subspecialists who need to remain up-to-date in internal medicine
- Residents preparing for the certifying examination in internal medicine
- Physicians preparing for maintenance of certification in internal medicine (recertification)

Earn "Same-Day" CME Credits Online

For the first time, print subscribers can enter their answers online to earn CME credits in 24 hours or less. You can submit your answers using online answer sheets that are provided at mksap.acponline.org, where a record of your MKSAP 16 credits will be available. To earn CME credits, you need to answer all of the questions in a test and earn a score of at least 50% correct (number of correct answers divided by the total number of questions). Take any of the following approaches:

1. Use the printed answer sheet at the back of this book to record your answers. Go to mksap.acponline.org, access the appropriate online answer sheet, transcribe your answers, and submit your test for same-day CME credits. There is no additional fee for this service.

2. Go to mksap.acponline.org, access the appropriate online answer sheet, directly enter your answers, and submit your test for same-day CME credits. There is no additional fee for this service.

3. Pay a $10 processing fee per answer sheet and submit the printed answer sheet at the back of this book by mail or fax, as instructed on the answer sheet. Make sure you calculate your score and fax the answer sheet to 215-351-2799 or mail the answer sheet to Member and Customer Service, American College of Physicians, 190 N. Independence Mall West, Philadelphia, PA 19106-1572, using the courtesy envelope provided in your MKSAP 16 slipcase. You will need your 10-digit order number and 8-digit ACP ID number, which are printed on your packing slip. Please allow 4 to 6 weeks for your score report to be emailed back to you. Be sure to include your email address for a response.

If you do not have a 10-digit order number and 8-digit ACP ID number or if you need help creating a username and password to access the MKSAP 16 online answer sheets, go to mksap.acponline.org or email custserv@acponline.org.

Disclosure Policy

It is the policy of the American College of Physicians (ACP) to ensure balance, independence, objectivity, and scientific rigor in all of its educational activities. To this end, and consistent with the policies of the ACP and the Accreditation Council for Continuing Medical Education (ACCME), contributors to all ACP continuing medical education activities are required to disclose all relevant financial relationships with any entity producing, marketing, re-selling, or distributing health care goods or services consumed by, or used on, patients. Contributors are required to use generic names in the discussion of therapeutic options and are required to identify any unapproved, off-label, or investigative use of commercial products or devices. Where a trade name is used, all available trade names for the same product type are also included. If trade-name products manufactured by companies with whom contributors have relationships are discussed, contributors are asked to provide evidence-based citations in support of the discussion. The information is reviewed by the committee responsible for producing this text. If necessary, adjustments to topics or contributors' roles in content development are made to balance the discussion. Further, all readers of this text are asked to evaluate the content for evidence of commercial bias and send any relevant comments to mksap_editors@acponline.org so that future decisions about content and contributors can be made in light of this information.

Resolution of Conflicts

To resolve all conflicts of interest and influences of vested interests, the ACP precluded members of the content-creation committee from deciding on any content issues that involved generic or trade-name products associated with proprietary entities with which these committee members had relationships. In addition, content was based on best evidence and updated clinical care guidelines, when such evidence and guidelines were available. Contributors' disclosure information can be found with the list of contributors' names and those of ACP principal staff listed in the beginning of this book.

Hospital-Based Medicine

For the convenience of subscribers who provide care in hospital settings, content that is specific to the hospital setting has been highlighted in blue. Hospital icons (H) highlight where the hospital-only content begins, continues over more than one page, and ends.

Educational Disclaimer

The editors and publisher of MKSAP 16 recognize that the development of new material offers many opportunities for error. Despite our best efforts, some errors may persist in print. Drug dosage schedules are, we believe, accurate and in accordance with current standards. Readers are advised, however, to ensure that the recommended dosages in MKSAP 16 concur with the information provided in the product information material. This is especially important in cases of new, infrequently used, or highly toxic drugs. Application of the information in MKSAP 16 remains the professional responsibility of the practitioner.

The primary purpose of MKSAP 16 is educational. Information presented, as well as publications, technologies, products, and/or services discussed, is intended to inform subscribers about the knowledge, techniques, and experiences of the contributors. A diversity of professional opinion exists, and the views of the contributors are their own and not those of the ACP. Inclusion of any material in the program does not constitute endorsement or recommendation by the ACP. The ACP does not warrant the safety, reliability, accuracy, completeness, or usefulness of and disclaims any and all liability for damages and claims that may result from the use of information, publications, technologies, products, and/or services discussed in this program.

Publisher's Information

Unauthorized Use of This Book Is Against the Law

MKSAP 16 ISBN: 978-1-938245-00-8
(Endocrinology and Metabolism) ISBN: 978-1-938245-07-7

Printed in the United States of America.

For order information in the U.S. or Canada call 800-523-1546, extension 2600. All other countries call 215-351-2600. Fax inquiries to 215-351-2799 or email to custserv@acponline.org.

Errata and Norm Tables

Errata for MKSAP 16 will be available through the MKSAP Resource Site at mksap.acponline.org as new information becomes known to the editors.

MKSAP 16 Performance Interpretation Guidelines with Norm Tables, available July 31, 2013, will reflect the knowledge of physicians who have completed the self-assessment tests before the program was published. These physicians took the tests without being able to refer to the syllabus, answers, and critiques. For your convenience, the tables are available in a printable PDF file through the MKSAP Resource Site at mksap.acponline.org.

Table of Contents

Diabetes Mellitus

Disorders of the Pituitary Gland

Disorders of the Thyroid Gland

Disorders of the Adrenal Glands

Endocrinology and Metabolism High-Value Care Recommendations

The American College of Physicians, in collaboration with multiple other organizations, is embarking on a national initiative to promote awareness about the importance of stewardship of health care resources. The goals are to improve health care outcomes by providing care of proven benefit and reducing costs by avoiding unnecessary and even harmful interventions. The initiative comprises several programs that integrate the important concept of health care value (balancing clinical benefit with costs and harms) for a given intervention into various educational materials to address the needs of trainees, practicing physicians, and patients.

To integrate discussion of high-value, cost-conscious care into MKSAP 16, we have created recommendations based on the medical knowledge content that we feel meet the below definition of high-value care and bring us closer to our goal of improving patient outcomes while conserving finite resources.

High-Value Care Recommendation: A recommendation to choose diagnostic and management strategies for patients in specific clinical situations that balances clinical benefit with cost and harms with the goal of improving patient outcomes.

Below are the High-Value Care Recommendations for the Endocrinology and Metabolism section of MKSAP 16.

- The older diabetic agents, such as insulin, the sulfonylureas, and metformin, have proven long-term glycemic control and cost effectiveness (see Item 35).
- For most patients with type 2 diabetes mellitus, lifestyle modifications and metformin therapy are the best initial treatments (see Item 11).
- Cost concerns are a factor in determining which pharmacologic agents for diabetes mellitus are used because the newer insulin preparations (insulin glargine, detemir, aspart, lispro, and glulisine) are far more expensive than regular insulin or neutral protamine Hagedorn (NPH) insulin (see Item 35).
- Repeated or serial measurements of antithyroid antibody titers are not recommended in the management of thyroid disorders in most persons because the degree of a titer's elevation does not indicate a need for treatment; only an abnormal TSH level does.
- A thyroid scan and radioactive iodine uptake test are not useful in the evaluation of patients with hypothyroidism.
- Ultrasonography is recommended for imaging thyroid nodules, with fine-needle aspiration biopsy reserved for nodules larger than 1 cm in diameter.
- Patients with asymptomatic stable simple goiters can be serially monitored clinically; serial ultrasonography is not recommended for these goiters.
- The best initial test for male hypogonadism is a morning (8 AM) measurement of the total testosterone level; if this level is normal, then hypogonadism is excluded (see Item 21 and Item 51).
- Screening woman for osteoporosis with bone mineral density measurements (using dual-energy x-ray absorptiometry [DEXA]) should not begin before age 65 years unless the patient has a particularly high risk for osteoporosis (risk factors such as a previous fracture, glucocorticoid use, a family history of hip fracture, current tobacco use, alcoholism, or secondary osteoporosis).
- Do not screen women who are premenopausal for osteoporosis.
- Do not repeat bone mineral density testing before 10 years in patients with normal or low normal values on previous testing.
- No clear benefit of newer bisphosphonate drugs has been demonstrated compared with older agents, which are available in generic form and may be more cost-effective for long-term therapy.

Endocrinology and Metabolism

Diabetes Mellitus

Classification and Diagnosis of Diabetes

Overview

Diabetes mellitus occurs when inadequate glycemic control results in elevated blood glucose levels. An inadequate production of the hormone insulin, resistance to the actions of insulin, or some combination of both mechanisms can cause this state. Patients with diabetes have a significantly increased risk of developing macrovascular disease (coronary artery, cerebrovascular, and peripheral vascular disorders) and microvascular disease (retinopathy, nephropathy, and neuropathy).

The two major forms of diabetes are type 1 and type 2 (**Table 1**). Diabetes not only can develop from autoimmunity or genetic predisposition, but also can result from use of drugs that damage the pancreas or cause resistance to the actions of insulin. Drug-induced diabetes is becoming more common because of the increasing use of immunosuppressive drugs (such as cyclosporine and tacrolimus) that can inhibit insulin secretion and of HIV protease inhibitors and atypical antipsychotic drugs (such as clozapine and olanzapine) that can induce weight gain, central obesity, elevated triglyceride levels, and insulin resistance.

KEY POINT

- Patients with diabetes mellitus have a significantly increased risk of developing macrovascular disease (coronary artery, cerebrovascular, and peripheral vascular disorders) and microvascular disease (retinopathy, nephropathy, and neuropathy).

Insulin Resistance

When the body becomes resistant to the effects of insulin, the pancreas compensates by secreting more insulin. Because the pancreas secretes one C-peptide molecule with each insulin

TABLE 1. Classification of Diabetes Mellitus

Type 1 Diabetes[a]
Immune mediated
Idiopathic (seronegative)
Type 2 Diabetes[b]
Ketosis Prone[c]
Gestational Diabetes
Other Types
Genetic defects in beta-cell function (including six distinct MODY syndromes)
Genetic defects in insulin action
Diseases of the exocrine pancreas (pancreatitis, trauma/pancreatectomy, neoplasia, cystic fibrosis, hemochromatosis, fibrocalculous pancreatopathy)
Endocrinopathies (acromegaly, Cushing syndrome, glucagonoma, pheochromocytoma, hyperthyroidism)
Drug related (glucocorticoids, thiazides, β-blockers, diazoxide, tacrolimus, cyclosporine, niacin, HIV protease inhibitors, atypical antipsychotics [clozapine, olanzapine])
Infections (congenital rubella, cytomegalovirus)
Rare forms of immune-mediated diabetes ("stiff man" syndrome, anti–insulin receptor autoantibodies)
Genetic syndromes (Down, Klinefelter, Turner, Wolfram [DIDMOAD], and Prader-Willi syndromes; myotonic dystrophy)

DIDMOAD = diabetes insipidus, diabetes mellitus, optic atrophy, and deafness; MODY = maturity-onset diabetes of the young.

[a]Beta-cell destruction usually leading to absolute insulin deficiency.

[b]Insulin resistance with progressive relative insulin deficiency.

[c]More common in nonwhite patients who present with diabetic ketoacidosis but become non–insulin dependent over time.

molecule, endogenous insulin production can be determined by measuring the amount of insulin or C-peptide in the blood. Although this method may be useful in diagnosing causes of hypoglycemia in persons without diabetes, it may not help determine the degree of insulin resistance or reliably distinguish between type 1 and type 2 diabetes. In the early stages of both types of diabetes, obese persons secrete high levels of insulin and C-peptide. Therefore, the most useful test in determining whether obese patients have type 1 or type 2 diabetes is to determine whether they have pancreatic autoantibodies (such as islet cell antibodies or glutamic acid decarboxylase antibodies) in their blood. This determination is essential because in patients with type 1 diabetes, treatment with insulin should begin as soon as possible.

Screening for Diabetes

After reviewing the available literature, the U.S. Preventive Services Task Force has found no direct evidence of future health benefits from mass screening and treatment of diabetes mellitus in asymptomatic individuals. Screening is recommended in asymptomatic adults who have treated or untreated sustained blood pressure greater than 135/80 mm Hg. In contrast, the American Diabetes Association (ADA) suggests a more comprehensive recommendation for screening that focuses on asymptomatic adults who either are at increased risk for developing diabetes or are age 45 years or older (**Table 2**).

Diagnostic Criteria for Diabetes

The diagnosis of diabetes is usually based on elevated (in the diabetes range) hemoglobin A_{1c} values, fasting or random plasma glucose levels, or oral glucose tolerance test results on two separate occasions or on a single random plasma glucose level of 200 mg/dL (11.1 mmol/L) or greater while a patient is experiencing classic symptoms of hyperglycemia, such as polyuria, polydipsia, or blurred vision (**Table 3**). Patients whose results on these tests are above normal but less than the diabetes range are considered to be at increased risk for diabetes.

Type 1 Diabetes

Type 1 diabetes usually presents dramatically with severe hyperglycemic symptoms, such as fatigue, polyuria, polydipsia, polyphagia, visual blurring, weight loss, nausea, vomiting, and dehydration. This type, which comprises approximately 5% of all diabetes, most commonly results from slow autoimmune destruction of insulin-producing pancreatic beta cells by autoantibodies in persons with particular *HLA* susceptibility genes in the DQA and DQB regions of chromosome 6. Age of onset and rate of beta-cell destruction depend on the particular combination of susceptibility and protective genes a person has and on exposure to one or more environmental triggers (possibly viral). Left untreated, patients with type 1 diabetes may rapidly develop diabetic ketoacidosis (DKA), which has a high morbidity and mortality (see later discussion).

Although most common in children and lean young adults, type 1 diabetes can present less dramatically in obese persons and in older adults. At the time of disease presentation, 60% to 80% of the affected person's pancreatic beta cells are already destroyed, and the remaining beta cells are not functioning well because of the hyperglycemia and metabolic dysfunction associated with the untreated disease. After insulin therapy (and fluid and electrolyte replacement, if needed) has begun, the residual beta-cell function may

TABLE 2. American Diabetes Association Screening Guidelines for Diabetes Mellitus

Overweight persons (BMI ≥25) with one (or more) additional risk factor(s):
Physical inactivity
First-degree relative with diabetes
High-risk ethnicity (black, Latin American, American Indian, Asian American, Pacific Islander)
Delivered an infant weighing >4500 g (158.7 oz) (women)
Gestational diabetes (women)
Hypertension
HDL cholesterol level <35 mg/dL (0.90 mmol/L) and/or triglyceride level >250 mg/dL (2.82 mmol/L)
Polycystic ovary syndrome (women)
Hemoglobin A_{1c} value ≥5.7% and IGT or IFG on previous testing
Acanthosis nigricans
History of cardiovascular disease
In the absence of the above criteria, anyone age 45 years or older
If results are normal, repeat testing every 3 years

IFG = impaired fasting glucose; IGT = impaired glucose tolerance.

Adapted with permission of American Diabetes Association, from Standards of Medical Care in Diabetes—2011. Diabetes Care. 2011;34(Suppl 1):S14. [PMID: 21193625]; permission conveyed through Copyright Clearance Center, Inc.

TABLE 3. Diagnostic Criteria for Diabetes Mellitus[a]

Criteria No.	Test	Normal Range	Increased Risk for Diabetes	Diabetes
1	—	—	—	Classic hyperglycemic symptoms plus a random plasma glucose ≥200 mg/dL (11.1 mmol/L)
2	Fasting plasma glucose	<100 mg/dL (5.6 mmol/L)	100-125 mg/dL (5.6-6.9 mmol/L)	≥126 mmol/L (7.0 mmol/L)
3	Random plasma glucose or during a 2-hour 75-g OGTT	<140 mg/dL (7.8 mmol/L)	140-199 mg/dL (7.8-11.0 mmol/L)	≥200 mg/dL (11.1 mmol/L)
4	Hemoglobin A_{1c}	<5.7%	5.7%-6.4%	≥6.5%

OGTT = oral glucose tolerance test.

[a]In the absence of hyperglycemic symptoms, criteria 2 through 4 should be confirmed by repeat testing. If two tests are performed and only one has abnormal results, the American Diabetes Association recommends repeating the test with abnormal results.

Data from American Diabetes Association. Standards of Medical Care in Diabetes—2011. Diabetes Care. 2011;34(Suppl 1):S13. [PMID: 21193625]

improve sufficiently for the insulin dosage to be reduced. This "honeymoon" period may persist for several weeks to months. Although insulin was routinely discontinued during this period in the past, the standard practice now is continuous insulin therapy after diagnosis to preserve endogenous insulin secretion for many months (or years) longer. This makes the goal of maintaining good glycemic control much more attainable.

Although DKA is usually considered a hallmark of type 1 diabetes, certain patients (most often nonwhite patients) with DKA at presentation who are initially treated with insulin and fluid replacement can stop taking insulin and be treated with lifestyle changes and oral hypoglycemic agents for many years. They do not have autoantibodies or the characteristic *HLA* gene associations of typical type 1 diabetes.

KEY POINT

- Left untreated, patients with type 1 diabetes may rapidly develop diabetic ketoacidosis.

Type 2 Diabetes

Type 2 diabetes (approximately 90% of all diabetes) occurs because of a slow decline in pancreatic beta-cell function. This process results in decreasing insulin secretion over decades, although most patients continue to produce some insulin throughout their lives. Besides progressive insulin deficiency, patients with type 2 diabetes develop varying degrees of insulin resistance. The severity of the insulin resistance and insulin deficiency determines when in life frank hyperglycemia develops to a degree that the patient meets diagnostic criteria for diabetes. Although type 2 diabetes most often affects middle-aged and older patients, the disorder can occur much earlier in life, especially in an era of increasing obesity and inactivity among children and adolescents.

Although the genetic association of type 2 diabetes is much stronger than that of type 1 and the penetrance of type 2 diabetes in families is high, the specific genes involved have not yet been identified. Because some insulin secretion continues in type 2 diabetes, lipolysis is suppressed, DKA is rare, and the presenting symptoms usually are much less dramatic. Because the onset can be so insidious, some patients already have evidence of microvascular complications at the time of diagnosis, which suggests the presence of hyperglycemia for many years before diagnosis.

In addition to abnormal glucose metabolism and insulin resistance, many patients with type 2 diabetes have central obesity, hypertension, and hyperlipidemia, features often collectively called "the metabolic syndrome." Although these features individually confer additional cardiovascular risk, it is unknown if their combination does so. Consensus is lacking about the exact way to diagnose the metabolic syndrome and whether doing so is clinically valuable.

Prediction and Prevention of Type 2 Diabetes

Many features listed in Table 2 identify persons with a high risk of developing type 2 diabetes. Several studies have randomized persons at high risk (for example, those with impaired glucose tolerance or women who have had gestational diabetes) to interventions aimed at preventing them from later developing diabetes (**Table 4**). Whether diabetes has been prevented or simply delayed for a few years is still unclear. No long-term studies have shown whether early treatment prolongs life or delays long-term complications. However, counseling persons to eat a healthier diet, exercise more, maintain normal weight, and stop smoking—all of which help prevent type 2 diabetes—should be a public health imperative in the twenty-first century.

TABLE 4. Strategies to Prevent or Delay Onset of Type 2 Diabetes Mellitus

Intervention	Effectiveness
Diet and exercise	Sustained weight loss of 7%, with at least 150 minutes of moderate exercise per week, shown to delay onset of diabetes by up to 3 years
Smoking cessation	Modestly effective as long as it does not cause weight gain
Bariatric surgery	Effective if used in obese persons (BMI >40)
Metformin	Shown to delay onset of diabetes by up to 3 years
Lipase inhibitors (orlistat)	Shown to delay onset of diabetes by up to 3 years
α-Glucosidase inhibitors (acarbose, voglibose)	Shown to delay onset of diabetes by up to 3 years
Thiazolidinediones (troglitazone, rosiglitazone, pioglitazone)	Shown to delay onset of diabetes by up to 3 years
Insulin and insulin secretagogues (sulfonylureas, meglitinides)	Ineffective
ACE-inhibitors (such as ramipril) and angiotensin receptor blockers (such as valsartan)	Ineffective
Estrogen-progestin	Modest effect only

KEY POINTS

- In addition to abnormal glucose metabolism and insulin resistance, patients with type 2 diabetes also often have central obesity, hypertension, and hyperlipidemia, features that often are collectively called "the metabolic syndrome."
- Counseling persons to eat a healthier diet, exercise more, maintain a normal weight, and stop smoking can help delay or prevent onset of type 2 diabetes.

Gestational Diabetes

Gestational diabetes occurs when a woman's pancreas cannot increase insulin secretion enough to overcome the acute insulin resistance of pregnancy. This condition affects at least 7% of pregnancies in the United States; this number may be higher when women with overt diabetes at their first prenatal visit are included. Untreated gestational diabetes is associated with large babies (macrosomia); premature delivery; an increased risk of preeclampsia, stillbirth, and more complex delivery (including cesarean section); and neonatal respiratory compromise, jaundice, hypoglycemia, and hypocalcemia. The International Association of Diabetes and Pregnancy Study Group (IADPSG) recommends screening women for previously undiagnosed diabetes at the first obstetric visit using the criteria in Table 3. If a woman does not have diabetes by these criteria, then screening for gestational diabetes is recommended at 24 to 28 weeks of gestation by performing a 75-g oral glucose tolerance test (**Table 5**). Women at low risk for gestational diabetes (age <25 years, thin body habitus, no family history of diabetes, white race) can be excluded from this screening. Screening should be considered earlier than 24 weeks in women at increased risk for gestational diabetes (BMI >30, history of previous gestational diabetes or polycystic ovary syndrome, previous newborn with excessive birth weight [>4500 g {158.7 oz}], family history of diabetes, or high-risk race/ethnicity [black, Hispanic, American Indian, South Asian, Pacific Islander]).

The mainstays of gestational diabetes treatment are diet and exercise to maintain fasting and premeal plasma glucose levels less than 95 mg/dL (5.3 mmol/L) and 1-hour postprandial values less than 130 to 140 mg/dL (7.2-7.8 mmol/L). Most women can meet these goals with lifestyle changes alone. If they cannot, then insulin should be started. Although glyburide and metformin have been used successfully in pregnancy and are options for women who refuse to take insulin, their safety in pregnancy relative to insulin has not been definitively established.

Although gestational diabetes usually resolves after delivery, it is likely to recur in future pregnancies. Women with a history of gestational diabetes are at high risk for type 2 diabetes in the decade after pregnancy. Therefore, they should be

TABLE 5. Screening for Gestational Diabetes

When to Screen[a]	Test	Result[b]
At 24-28 weeks' gestation (after a minimum 8-hour fast)	Oral glucose tolerance test using a 75-g glucose load followed by plasma glucose measurement 1 and 2 hours after the glucose load	Fasting, ≥92 mg/dL (5.1 mmol/L) At 1 h, ≥180 mg/dL (10 mmol/L) At 2 h, ≥153 mg/dL (8.5 mmol/L)

[a]It is reasonable to exclude women at low risk from screening and to screen earlier in women at high risk.

[b]Gestational diabetes is diagnosed if one or more of these values is equaled or exceeded.

advised to lose weight (if BMI is >25), continue healthy diet and exercise patterns, and undergo annual screening for diabetes (see Table 3). It has been recently recognized that the offspring of mothers with prepregnancy obesity who develop gestational diabetes during pregnancy are at increased risk for childhood obesity. The reason for this is not clear but may involve a combination of genetic factors and maternal imprinting of genes during intrauterine life.

KEY POINT

- Gestational diabetes, which occurs when a woman's pancreas cannot increase insulin secretion enough to overcome the acute insulin resistance of pregnancy, develops in approximately 7% of pregnancies in the United States.

Other Types of Diabetes

Rare genetic forms of type 2 diabetes caused by defects in beta-cell function are grouped together as maturity-onset diabetes of the young (*MODY* genes 1-6) or as genetic defects in insulin action (such as type A insulin resistance). Diseases of the exocrine pancreas, such as pancreatitis and cystic fibrosis, can lead to diabetes if enough of the pancreas is destroyed or removed. Similarly, endocrine conditions in which excessive amounts of hormones antagonistic to insulin action are secreted (acromegaly, Cushing syndrome, and glucagonoma) can lead to diabetes (see Table 1).

Management of Diabetes

Glycemic Monitoring

Chronic hyperglycemia causes significant microvascular and macrovascular damage, and strategies to lower blood glucose levels remain the mainstay of diabetes management, with the exact target level individualized for each patient. The effectiveness of self-monitoring in patients with type 2 diabetes who take only oral medications that do not predispose to hypoglycemia is not clear. Self-monitoring of eating and exercise habits and blood glucose levels is crucial for patients taking multiple injections of insulin or using continuous infusion insulin pumps and for those taking medications that increase the risk of hypoglycemia, such as sulfonylureas. This step not only gives all patients with diabetes a tool with which to understand how their lifestyle choices and responses to different life situations can affect their blood glucose level, but also provides physicians with a tool with which to discuss a patient's status and recommend changes to his or her diabetes regimen.

Testing blood glucose levels 1 or 2 hours after meals can show the different effects of portion size and type of food being consumed and is necessary for a complete picture of a patient's glycemic status. Testing before, during, and after exercise can show the impact of exercise on glycemic control. Testing blood glucose levels at times when a patient experiences symptoms possibly due to a high or low level (such as sweating, nausea, or anxiety) provides useful insights into a patient's daily glycemic control, whether the finding is hypoglycemia, hyperglycemia, or euglycemia. The most common cause of day-to-day variability of blood glucose levels is variability in a patient's eating and exercise habits. Finally, testing in the middle of the night can identify nocturnal hypoglycemia.

Erythrocytes circulate for approximately 120 days before being destroyed, and glucose attaches to hemoglobin during periods of sustained hyperglycemia. The percentage of hemoglobin that has been glycosylated (the hemoglobin A_{1c} value) is thus a surrogate indicator of the average blood glucose level during the previous 3 months. The hemoglobin A_{1c} value should thus be obtained at regular intervals, with patients whose diabetes treatment is being adjusted tested at 3-month intervals and patients at goal receiving a stable treatment regimen tested every 6 months. In patients receiving hemodialysis, those with hemolytic anemia or certain hemoglobinopathies, or those with recent blood transfusions, hemoglobin A_{1c} values may be falsely lowered because of the presence of erythrocytes less than 120 days old in the sample.

The findings from the Diabetes Control and Complications Trial (DCCT) led to the creation of a table showing the estimated average plasma glucose level for any given hemoglobin A_{1c} level (**Table 6**). A hemoglobin A_{1c} goal of less than 7.0% is appropriate for many nonpregnant adults with a long life expectancy, no cardiovascular disease, and a short duration of diabetes because studies have shown reductions in microvascular and neuropathic complications and long-term macrovascular disease in such patients who reached this goal. For patients with a long duration of diabetes, known cardiovascular disease, multiple comorbid conditions, or a history of severe hypoglycemia, hemoglobin A_{1c} goals

TABLE 6. Comparison of Hemoglobin A_{1c} Value and Estimated Average Plasma Glucose Level

Hemoglobin A_{1c} Value	Estimated Average Plasma Glucose Level	
	mg/dL	mmol/L
5.0	97	5.0
6.0	126	6.0
7.0	154	7.0
8.0	183	8.0
9.0	212	9.0
10.0	240	10.0
11.0	269	14.9
12.0	298	16.5

Adapted with permission of American Diabetes Association, from Translating the A1C assay into estimated average glucose values. Nathan DM, Kuenen J, Borg R, Zheng H, Schoenfeld D, Heine RJ; A1C-derived average glucose study group. [erratum in Diabetes Care. 2009;32(1):207]. Diabetes Care. 2008;31(8):1476. [PMID: 18540046]; permission conveyed through Copyright Clearance Center, Inc.

should be less stringent because of the risk of hypoglycemia and because studies of intensive hemoglobin A_{1c}–lowering regimens have shown no correlation with reduction in macrovascular outcomes in these patients.

Many blood glucose monitors have a memory function that provides the average reading for the past 7, 14, or 30 days, and this meter average can be compared with the estimated average plasma glucose level. If the meter average is lower or higher than the estimated average plasma glucose level, hyperglycemia or hypoglycemia is likely occurring when the patient is not testing (such as postprandially or during sleep). Real-time continuous glucose monitoring is available and has the potential to improve glycemic control while decreasing the incidence of hypoglycemia. Thus far, however, clinical trials testing the efficacy of real-time continuous glucose monitoring systems have had mixed results.

KEY POINTS

- Because erythrocytes circulate for approximately 120 days before being destroyed and because glucose becomes attached to hemoglobin during periods of hyperglycemia, the hemoglobin A_{1c} value provides an estimate of the average blood glucose level during the previous 3 months.
- The hemoglobin A_{1c} value should be obtained at regular intervals, every 6 months for patients with diabetes receiving a stable treatment regimen whose previous values were at goal and every 3 months for those whose diabetes regimens are being adjusted because their previous values were not at goal.

Cardiovascular Risk

Because diabetes is associated with a significantly increased risk of macrovascular complications, especially atherosclerotic vascular disease, reducing future cardiovascular risk is a priority in diabetes management. Ten measures that should be considered for patients with diabetes appear below:

1. Stopping smoking
2. Maintaining a normal weight
3. Eating a healthy diet
4. Exercising moderately for at least 150 minutes per week
5. Using a statin
6. Using an ACE inhibitor or angiotensin receptor blocker (ARB)
7. Using aspirin
8. Maintaining an LDL cholesterol level of less than 100 mg/dL (2.59 mmol/L)
9. Maintaining a blood pressure of less than 130/80 mm Hg
10. Maintaining a hemoglobin A_{1c} level of less than 7.0%

The health benefits of smoking cessation and maintaining a normal weight are not controversial. However, what constitutes a healthy diet, how often to exercise, at what age to start medication, and what to recommend as blood pressure, hemoglobin A_{1c} level, and lipid level targets have been debated. Regarding statins, the Heart Protection Study showed significant benefit with simvastatin, 40 mg/d, in all patients with diabetes who were older than 40 years and had at least one other risk factor for heart disease, even for patients whose cholesterol level was not elevated at baseline. Regarding blood pressure medication, the Heart Outcomes Prevention Evaluation (HOPE) study found that ramipril was beneficial in patients with diabetes who were older than 55 years, even those who did not have hypertension. The ADA and American Heart Association recommend that LDL cholesterol levels be less than 100 mg/dL (2.59 mmol/L) for all persons with diabetes and that a target of less than 70 mg/dL (1.81 mmol/L) be considered for those who already have heart disease or macrovascular disease of any type, including stroke and peripheral vascular disease.

Whether all patients with diabetes should have a blood pressure less than 130/80 mm Hg is unclear. The ACCORD study group compared a conservative systolic blood pressure target (<140 mm Hg) with a more aggressive one (<120 mm Hg) in more than 4700 patients with type 2 diabetes (mean age, 62 years) who had evidence of preexisting cardiovascular disease. No difference in the annual rate of fatal and nonfatal cardiovascular disease events was found over 8 years of follow-up, although more adverse events related to drug side effects occurred in those trying to achieve the more aggressive target. Although treatment efforts have traditionally focused on achieving hemoglobin A_{1c} levels close to the normal range, recent evidence suggests that values approaching normal in older patients with preexisting cardiovascular disease may be associated with increased all-cause mortality. This information underscores the need to establish individualized treatment goals in this population.

KEY POINTS

- Because diabetes is associated with a significantly increased risk of macrovascular complications, especially atherosclerotic vascular disease, reducing future cardiovascular risk is a priority in diabetes management.
- Statins have significant benefit in patients with diabetes who are older than 40 years and have at least one other risk factor for heart disease.

Lowering Blood Glucose Levels in Type 2 Diabetes

Nonpharmacologic Approaches

Lifestyle changes (such as weight loss, increased exercise, and decreased carbohydrate intake) are the cornerstone of type 2 diabetes treatment and should be considered in every person with the disease. For patients with type 2 diabetes and obesity, a slow, steady weight loss—achieved by eating a diet with moderate amounts of complex high-fiber carbohydrates, protein, and fat and engaging in moderate exercise on a daily basis—should be a goal. Only approximately 5% to 10% of patients with type 2 diabetes will be able to control their blood glucose levels with lifestyle measures alone. Even if pharmacologic agents must be added later, these drugs will be much more effective and will require lower doses if patients also focus on lifestyle measures. Although exercise usually lowers the blood glucose level in patients with diabetes, this level may increase if exercise is attempted when the patient's insulin level is low, such as first thing in the morning before any insulin is taken, as a result of exercise-induced hepatic gluconeogenesis; in the absence of sufficient plasma insulin (hypoinsulinemia), the glucose cannot be absorbed by the muscles and other tissues, and the blood glucose level continues to increase.

For patients with diabetes and morbid obesity, various forms of weight-loss surgery (bariatric surgery) are available. Bariatric surgery causes weight loss by restriction, malabsorption, or a combination of the two and has resulted in a significant rate of remission of diabetes in some studies. For more information on bariatric surgery and its complications, see MKSAP 16 Gastroenterology and Hepatology and MKSAP 16 General Internal Medicine.

Pharmacologic Agents

At the time of diabetes diagnosis, lifestyle changes should be encouraged and a noninsulin agent started. In the past decade, agents to help lower blood glucose levels in patients with diabetes have proliferated, with no fewer than 12 different drug classes now available (**Table 7**). The available drugs vary markedly in cost, route and frequency of administration, effect on body weight, mechanism of action, adverse effect profile, and known effects on serious outcomes (microvascular and macrovascular events, morbidity, and mortality). Much is now known about older diabetes agents, such as insulin, the sulfonylureas, and metformin, that provide proven long-term glycemic control and cost effectiveness. Newer agents offer the potential advantage of targeting different metabolic pathways, and adding or combining these agents can lower blood glucose levels by different mechanisms. However, the long-term efficacy and safety of these drugs relative to older drugs are not as well established, and the newer drugs tend to be considerably more expensive.

The natural history of type 2 diabetes is of progressive loss of pancreatic beta-cell function in addition to underlying insulin resistance; as pancreatic beta-cell function continues to decline, postprandial blood glucose levels increase. Therefore, most patients will require more than one pharmacologic agent over time to maintain their plasma glucose level at goal. No consensus exists among experts about which combination of agents works best. Options are to add oral agents that help lower postprandial blood glucose levels (sulfonylureas, α-glucosidase inhibitors, meglitinides, or dipeptidyl peptidase-4 inhibitors), injectable agents that slow gastric emptying and suppress glucagon (pramlintide, exenatide, or liraglutide), or insulin. For most patients, metformin is the best agent to add to lifestyle modifications as an initial therapy.

The sulfonylureas vary mostly in dose and half-life. Those with long half-lives, such as chlorpropamide and glyburide, can cause profound, prolonged hypoglycemia, especially in older patients and patients with impaired kidney function. Therefore, these drugs should be avoided in these two populations. For the past 40 years, concern has existed that treatment with certain sulfonylureas increases myocardial damage after coronary artery occlusion because first- and second-generation sulfonylureas (such as glyburide) bind to myocardial and pancreatic adenosine triphosphate–sensitive potassium channels, thus blocking myocardial preconditioning mechanisms. Third-generation sulfonylureas (such as gliclazide and glimepiride) bind exclusively to pancreatic beta-cell potassium channels. One study showed that in-patient mortality of patients with diabetes who sustained acute ST-elevation and non–ST-elevation myocardial infarctions was significantly lower for those taking gliclazide or glimepiride (2.7%) than those taking glyburide (7.5%; $P<0.02$).

KEY POINT

- For most patients with type 2 diabetes, lifestyle modifications and metformin therapy are the best initial treatments; as their disease progresses, many will need to use additional pharmacologic agents.

Insulin Therapy for Diabetes

Basal insulin generally is used in type 2 diabetes if a patient is unable to achieve a target fasting plasma glucose level with lifestyle modification and oral hypoglycemic agents alone. Adding a longer-acting form of insulin (such as neutral protamine Hagedorn [NPH] insulin, insulin detemir, or insulin glargine) either at bedtime or first thing in the morning also can be effective. (Of note, insulin detemir and insulin glargine are two- to four-times more expensive than NPH insulin and, in randomized controlled trials, generally achieve the same hemoglobin A_{1c} values and only modestly less hypoglycemia than does NPH insulin.) A basal insulin usually is combined with an oral hypoglycemic agent (such as a long-acting insulin at bedtime combined with daytime metformin) to achieve adequate control.

Premixed insulins (**Table 8**), which combine different insulin types with differing pharmacokinetic profiles, can minimize the number of daily injections a patient takes. The size and timing of the peak insulin effect can be altered by using different proportions of a rapid-acting insulin analogue, short-acting regular insulin, and long-acting insulin (**Figure 1**). Although twice-daily premixed insulins can be used quite effectively in patients with type 2 diabetes who have stable daily routines of what and when they eat and how much they exercise, the day-to-day variability of insulin absorption means that

TABLE 7. Pharmacologic Agents Used to Lower Blood Glucose Levels in Type 2 Diabetes Mellitus

Class	Route of Administration	Mechanism of Action	Effect on Weight	Risks and Concerns	Long-Term Studies on Definitive Outcomes
Insulin	Injection	Decreases hepatic glucose production, increases peripheral glucose uptake, and supports anabolism	Increase	Hypoglycemia; insulin allergy (rare)	Decrease in both microvascular and macrovascular events
Sulfonylureas (tolbutamide, chlorpropamide, glipizide, glyburide, gliclazide, glimepiride)	Oral	Stimulate insulin secretion from pancreatic beta cells	Increase	Hypoglycemia (especially in drugs with long half-lives); weight gain; skin rashes (including photosensitivity)	Decrease in microvascular events but possible increase in macrovascular events with tolbutamide, chlorpropamide, glyburide, and glipizide; not seen with gliclazide or glimepiride
Biguanides (metformin)	Oral	Decrease hepatic glucose production, decrease free fatty acids, increase insulin-mediated uptake of glucose in muscles	Neutral	Diarrhea and abdominal discomfort; lactic acidosis (exceedingly rare); contraindicated in presence of progressive liver, kidney, or cardiac failure	Decrease in both microvascular and macrovascular events and decreased risk of cancer
α-Glucosidase inhibitors (acarbose, miglitol, voglibose)	Oral	Inhibit polysaccharide absorption	Neutral	Flatulence; abdominal discomfort	May reduce CVD events (acute MI and hypertension)
Thiazolidinediones (rosiglitazone, pioglitazone)	Oral	Activate nuclear PPARγ receptors to regulate gene expression in numerous tissues, increase peripheral uptake of glucose, decrease hepatic glucose production	Increase	Fluid retention; heart failure; macular edema; osteoporosis (possible increased risk of bladder cancer with pioglitazone)	Increase in CVD events (heart failure, acute MI) and mortality with rosiglitazone; unclear whether pioglitazone causes net harm or good
Meglitinides (repaglinide, nateglinide)	Oral	Stimulate insulin release from pancreatic beta cells	Increase	Hypoglycemia	None
Lipase inhibitors (orlistat)	Oral	Inhibit dietary fat absorption	Decrease	Flatulence; abdominal discomfort; oily feces; occasional fecal incontinence; reduced absorption of fat-soluble vitamins	None
Amylinomimetics (pramlintide)	Injection	Slow gastric emptying, suppress glucagon secretion, increase satiety	Decrease	Nausea; vomiting; increased hypoglycemic risk of insulin	None
GLP-1 mimetics (exenatide and liraglutide)	Injection	Slow gastric emptying, suppress glucagon secretion, increase satiety	Decrease	Hypoglycemia when used in combination with sulfonylureas; nausea and vomiting; possible increased risk of pancreatitis and chronic kidney disease	None

(continued on next page)

TABLE 7. Pharmacologic Agents Used to Lower Blood Glucose Levels in Type 2 Diabetes Mellitus (*continued*)

Class	Route of Administration	Mechanism of Action	Effect on Weight	Risks and Concerns	Long-Term Studies on Definitive Outcomes
DPP-4 inhibitors (sitagliptin, saxagliptin, vildagliptin)	Oral	Slow gastric emptying, suppress glucagon secretion	Neutral	Hypoglycemia when used in combination with sulfonylureas; nausea; skin rashes; increased risk of infections; possible increased risk of pancreatitis	None
Bile acid sequestrants (colesevelam)	Oral	Unclear	Neutral	Constipation; dyspepsia; increased triglyceride level; possible increase in LDL cholesterol level; reduced absorption of fat-soluble vitamins	None
Dopamine agonists (bromocriptine)	Oral	Unclear central nervous system effects	Neutral	Nausea; headache; orthostatic hypotension; inhibition of lactation; potential exacerbation of psychosis	None

CVD = cardiovascular disease; DPP-4 = dipeptidyl peptidase-4; GLP-1 = glucagon-like peptide-1; MI = myocardial infarction; PPARγ = peroxisome proliferator-activated receptor-γ.

TABLE 8. Pharmacokinetic Properties of Insulin Products[a]

Insulin Type	Onset	Peak	Duration
Rapid-acting (lispro, aspart, glulisine)	5-15 min	45-90 min	2-4 h
Short-acting (regular)	0.5-1 h	2-4 h	4-8 h
NPH insulin	1-3 h	4-10 h	10-18 h
Detemir	1-2 h	None[b]	12-24 h[c]
Glargine	2-3 h	None[b]	20-24+ h
Premixed insulins			
70% NPH/30% regular	0.5-1 h	2-10 h	10-18 h
50% NPH/50% regular	0.5-1 h	2-10 h[d]	10-18 h
75% NPL/25% lispro	10-20 min	1-6 h	10-18 h
50% NPL/50% lispro	10-20 min	1-6 h[d]	10-18 h
70% NPA/30% aspart	10-20 min	1-6 h	10-18 h

NPA = neutral protamine aspart; NPH = neutral protamine Hagedorn; NPL = neutral protamine lispro.

[a]The time course of each insulin varies significantly between persons and within the same person on different days. Therefore, the time periods listed should be considered general guidelines only.

[b]Both insulin detemir and insulin glargine can produce a peak effect in some persons, especially at higher doses.

[c]The duration of action for insulin detemir varies depending on the dose given.

[d]Premixed insulins containing a larger proportion of rapid- or short-acting insulin tend to have larger peaks occurring at an earlier time than mixtures containing smaller proportions of rapid- or short-acting insulin.

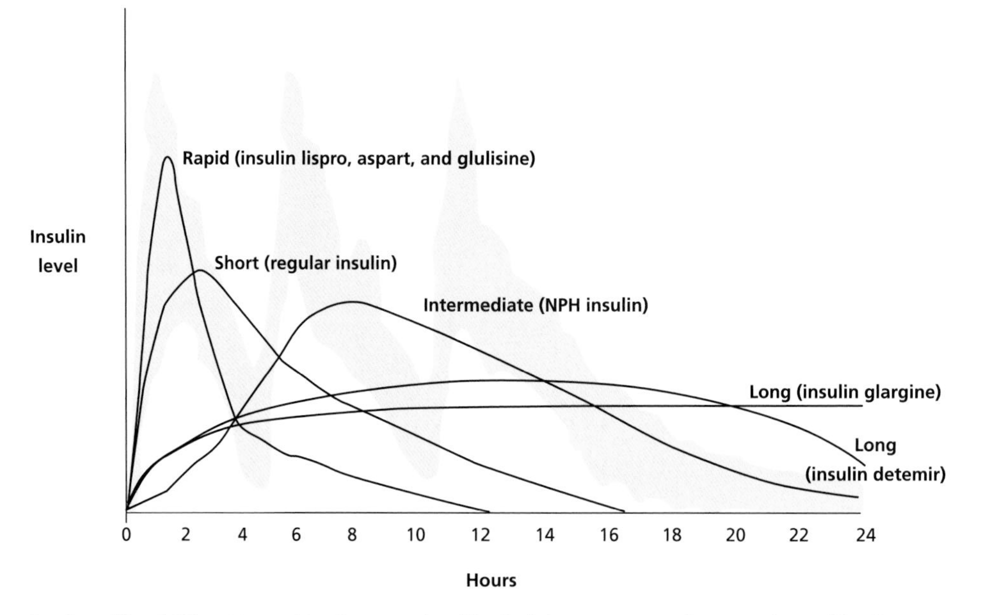

FIGURE 1. Plasma insulin profiles of different types of insulin preparations. The shaded areas represent the range of normal insulin responses to three meals in persons without diabetes. NPH = neutral protamine Hagedorn.

patients may experience unpredictable episodes of hypoglycemia during the middle of the day or night with these preparations. An alternative strategy is to use an intensified insulin regimen of basal and preprandial insulins, similar to approaches used by patients with type 1 diabetes. Cost concerns are a factor in determining which pharmacologic choices are made (see Table 8) because the newer insulin preparations (insulin glargine, detemir, aspart, lispro, and glulisine) are far more expensive than regular insulin and NPH insulin.

Insulin treatment is essential for all patients with type 1 diabetes and for many patients with type 2 diabetes who have significant insulin deficiency in addition to their underlying insulin resistance. The degree of complexity in the regimen should be decided collaboratively with each patient. Although once or twice daily regimens with long- or intermediate-acting or premixed insulins offer the convenience and lower cost of fewer injections and fewer blood glucose tests, concern has been raised that these agents may lead to higher plasma insulin levels throughout the day, which may cause unpredictable hypoglycemia and weight gain. Intensified insulin regimens with three to five insulin injections per day or a continuous subcutaneous insulin infusion, although more complicated, allow for more precise control of blood glucose levels between meals, overnight, after food intake or exercise, and with stress. This approach separates insulin delivery into basal and prandial components.

Most patients require 0.5 to 1.5 units/kg/d of insulin, although this may vary greatly depending on the patient's degree of insulin resistance or sensitivity. Most persons with type 1 diabetes are quite sensitive to insulin, and thus 0.5 units/kg/d is a good initial dose. In contrast, most persons with type 2 diabetes have significant insulin resistance and thus may require upward titration from this starting dose to 1 to 1.5 units/kg/d, depending on their individual response. Approximately half the daily dose is given as a basal insulin (one or two injections of NPH insulin, insulin glargine, or insulin detemir, or a continuous basal subcutaneous infusion from an insulin pump). Before each meal, a bolus of rapid-acting insulin is given, and these three injections account for the other half of the day's total insulin use. Ideally, the total bolus amount is determined by the amount of carbohydrates about to be consumed (typically, 1 unit for every 10 [or 15] grams of carbohydrate) plus a correction factor predicated on the preprandial blood glucose level. A typical correction factor for a patient with type 1 diabetes is 1 additional unit for every 40 (or 50) mg/dL (2.2 [or 2.8] mmol/L) above 100 mg/dL (5.6 mmol/L) the preprandial glucose level is; for patients with type 2 diabetes, the correction factor is 1 additional unit for every 25 mg/dL (1.4 mmol/L) above 100 mg/dL (5.6 mmol/L) the preprandial glucose level is. These preprandial bolus injections must be given as separate injections and not mixed with the basal insulin. When short-acting or rapid-acting insulin is mixed with longer-acting insulin, the pharmacokinetics change to cause a significantly delayed single peak (as seen with premixed insulins) (see Figure 1).

For patients trying to achieve hemoglobin A_{1c} levels less than 7.0%, fasting and premeal glucose targets usually are set at approximately 80 to 130 mg/dL (4.4-7.2 mmol/L). If these levels are not being attained or postprandial levels are consistently greater than 200 mg/dL (11.1 mmol/L) despite using these calculations, the formulae can be changed (for example, to take 1 unit for every 10 grams of carbohydrates consumed and 1 additional unit for every 30 mg/dL [1.7 mmol/L] above target the preprandial blood glucose level is).

KEY POINTS

- Although more convenient and less costly, once or twice daily regimens with intermediate-acting or premixed insulins can cause more frequent and unpredictable hypoglycemia and weight gain in patients with diabetes.
- Most patients with diabetes who take daily insulin receive an intensified regimen of basal and preprandial insulins, with the dosage of the latter varying depending on the amount of carbohydrates about to be consumed and on what the preprandial blood glucose level is.

Inpatient Management of Hyperglycemia and Diabetes

When patients with type 1 or type 2 diabetes are admitted to a hospital for treatment of diabetes or other conditions, glycemic control is likely to deteriorate. Additionally, when patients with previously undiagnosed diabetes are admitted to a hospital, their outcomes and length of stay are likely to be much worse if the diabetes remains undiagnosed or untreated. For these reasons, measurement of plasma glucose and hemoglobin A_{1c} levels should be routine when most adults are admitted.

The main goals for patients with diabetes during hospitalization are to (1) avoid hypoglycemia; (2) avoid severe hyperglycemia, volume depletion, and electrolyte abnormalities; (3) ensure adequate nutrition; (4) address diabetes education needs; and (5) facilitate smooth transition back to the ambulatory setting. Success and ease in achieving these goals depend on the type of diabetes and the severity of the underlying illness precipitating the admission. The key is to perform frequent blood glucose testing during hospitalization (either before meals and bedtime or every 6 hours if the patient is receiving nothing by mouth).

For patients with type 2 diabetes who follow dietary therapy and take oral agents, continuing their oral agents may be reasonable if they are still eating. If patients are not able or allowed to eat, then oral agents should be stopped. Oral agents should also be stopped in the presence of specific contraindications:

- Metformin should be stopped if intravenous contrast dye will be used or if the reason for admission could cause lactic acidosis.
- Thiazolidinediones (pioglitazone, rosiglitazone) should be stopped in patients admitted with prevalent or suspected cardiovascular disease, peripheral edema, heart failure, ventricular dysfunction, or osteoporosis.
- Both metformin and thiazolidinediones should be discontinued in patients with either acute or chronic liver dysfunction.
- Sulfonylureas and meglitinides, which increase the risk of hypoglycemia, should be stopped if food intake may be unpredictable.

A plasma glucose range of 140 to 180 mg/dL (7.8-10.0 mmol/L) is recommended for critically ill hospitalized patients with hyperglycemia. The glycemic targets for noncritically ill hospitalized patients have not been adequately determined by research trials, but current recommendations from a consensus statement by the ADA and the American Association of Clinical Endocrinologists are to maintain fasting and premeal glucose levels of less than 140 mg/dL (7.8 mmol/L) but no lower than 90 mg/dL (5.0 mmol/L) and random or postprandial levels of less than 180 mg/dL (10.0 mmol/L).

All patients with type 1 diabetes and many with type 2 will require insulin treatment while in the hospital. The use of sliding-scale insulin without basal insulin generally is discouraged. When sliding-scale regular or rapid-acting insulin is used without basal insulin, the likelihood of wide swings from hyperglycemia to hypoglycemia is much stronger. If the blood glucose level is at target and no insulin is given, then the glucose level is almost certain to be much higher when next checked; at that time, a large dose of rapid-acting insulin most likely will be given, which will result in hypoglycemia. A better approach is to give basal insulin subcutaneously and then add a preprandial rapid-acting insulin in a variable dose based on the amount of carbohydrate the patient is planning to eat, with an additional amount to correct for the degree of preprandial hyperglycemia. For patients who are more critically ill or whose blood glucose level cannot be maintained in the target range with subcutaneous insulin, an intravenous glucose infusion, which allows much more rapid adjustments, should be considered, provided adequate skilled staff is available for safe administration.

KEY POINTS

- A plasma glucose range of 140 to 180 mg/dL (7.8-10.0 mmol/L) is recommended for critically ill hospitalized patients with hyperglycemia.
- In noncritically ill hospitalized patients with hyperglycemia, a consensus statement recommends fasting and premeal glucose levels of less than 140 mg/dL (7.8 mmol/L) but no lower than 90 mg/dL (5.0 mmol/L) and random or postprandial levels of less than 180 mg/dL (10.0 mmol/L).

Acute Complications of Diabetes

Diabetic Ketoacidosis and Hyperglycemic Hyperosmolar Syndrome

Insulin-deficient states, whether absolute or relative, can result in DKA or hyperglycemic hyperosmolar syndrome (HHS), which are both serious and life-threatening conditions. The most common causes of DKA are new-onset type 1 diabetes,

H CONT.

inappropriate underdosing of insulin or missed insulin dosing (alone or in combination with infection or other serious illnesses), and myocardial ischemia. A spectrum of metabolic decompensation occurs in DKA (**Figure 2**). The degree of hyperglycemia and acidosis depends on several factors, including the severity of insulin deficiency, diet, kidney function, and any additional inciting factor. A patient with type 1 diabetes who has complete insulin deficiency can develop acidosis in a matter of hours, frequently with plasma glucose levels in excess of 400 to 500 mg/dL (22.2-27.8 mmol/L). In certain patients, however, only relatively mild hyperglycemia (200-250 mg/dL [11.1-13.9 mmol/L]) is seen. For example, if the patient is not eating or drinking, severe ketoacidosis may occur before the plasma glucose level has increased by very much. Alternatively, patients with impaired hepatic function or ongoing use of alcohol may have a relatively dampened degree of hepatic glucose production, which is the primary driver of hyperglycemia in DKA. In contrast, an older patient with only partial insulin deficiency might develop hyperglycemia and dehydration subacutely over days or even weeks. If the patient still produces enough endogenous insulin to prevent lipolysis, but not enough to control the plasma glucose level, he or she will remain nonketotic. However, if sugary liquids are consumed to quench thirst, if the patient has impaired renal clearance of glucose, or if a coexisting infection or other inciting factor is present, HHS—a severe hyperosmolar nonketotic hyperglycemia—can develop.

The earliest symptoms of severe hyperglycemia are polyuria, polydipsia, and weight loss. As hyperglycemia worsens, neurologic symptoms appear, including lethargy, drowsiness, focal deficits, and coma. As the acidosis and electrolyte disturbance worsen, patients experience nausea, vomiting, abdominal pain, and hyperventilation. Total-body loss of electrolytes, especially potassium, can be severe but may not be apparent initially because potassium leaks out of cells, which causes the serum potassium level to appear falsely "normal." After insulin is administered, the available potassium moves rapidly back inside the cells, which results in a precipitous decrease in the serum potassium level.

The initial evaluation of a patient with suspected DKA or HHS should include laboratory studies, such as measurement of plasma glucose, serum electrolyte, serum creatinine, and

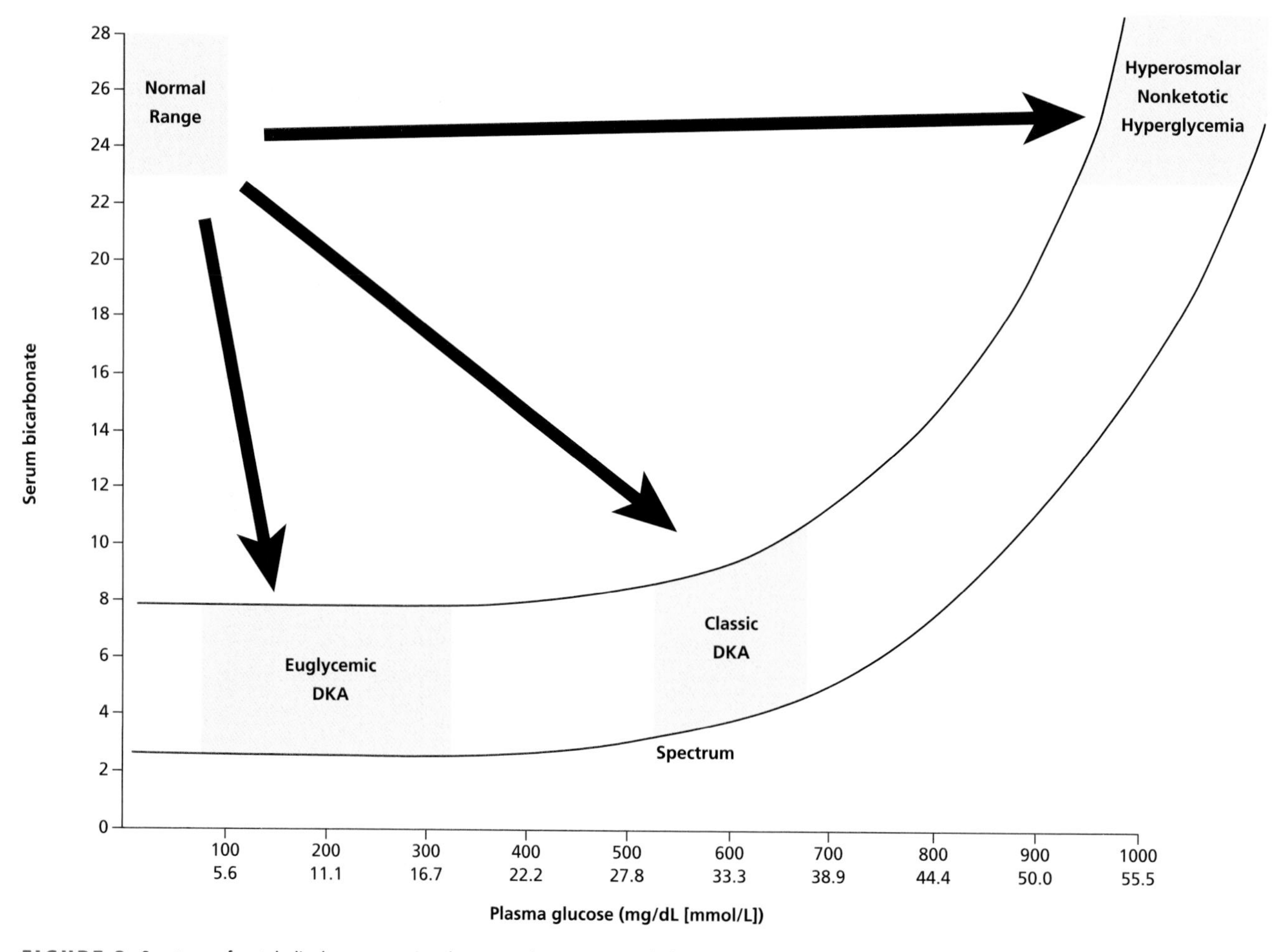

FIGURE 2. Spectrum of metabolic decompensation that occurs in DKA. DKA = diabetic ketoacidosis.

blood urea nitrogen levels; a complete blood count with leukocyte differential; urinalysis, including urine ketones; determination of plasma osmolality and the presence of serum ketones (if urine ketones are present); and an arterial blood gas analysis (if the serum bicarbonate level is substantially reduced). Electrocardiography is also recommended. The plasma glucose level should be measured every hour, whereas the other serum and plasma levels should be measured every 2 to 4 hours, depending on the severity of the acidosis and the clinical response. Unless profound acidemia is detected, repeat arterial blood gas measurement is usually unnecessary if the venous pH or serum bicarbonate level can be obtained every 2 to 4 hours.

DKA and HHS are best managed in an intensive care unit, especially if the patient has signs of clinical instability (such as hypotension, bradycardia, increased work of breathing, altered mental status, or a pH less than 7.0). Treatment includes careful replacement of fluids, electrolytes, and insulin (with intravenous infusion of regular insulin) and correction of acidosis, if present (**Table 9**). Although the appropriate additional testing to identify the underlying causes of the DKA or HHS will depend on clinical circumstances, a few points are worth noting. In the absence of infection, the leukocyte count may be greater than 20,000/microliter (20×10^9/L) in DKA because of ketoacidosis alone. Because metabolic decompensation also can suppress temperature, the lack of a fever does not rule out infection. Additionally, abdominal pain in the setting of diabetic ketoacidosis is typically generalized and usually seen when the serum bicarbonate level is substantially less than 15 meq/L (15 mmol/L); focal abdominal pain, especially if the acidosis is not severe (>15 meq/L [15 mmol/L]), more likely represents an intra-abdominal problem. Because metabolic decompensation also can cause an increased serum amylase level (to >1000 units/L), a high amylase level is not a reliable indicator of acute pancreatitis. H

KEY POINTS

- The initial evaluation of a patient with suspected diabetic ketoacidosis or hyperglycemic hyperosmolar syndrome should include frequent measurement of plasma glucose, serum electrolyte, serum creatinine, and blood urea nitrogen levels and plasma osmolality; a complete blood count; urinalysis; an arterial blood gas analysis (if the serum bicarbonate level is substantially reduced); and electrocardiography.
- Management of diabetic ketoacidosis and hyperglycemic hyperosmolar syndrome should include careful replacement of fluids, electrolytes, and insulin (with intravenous infusion of regular insulin) and correction of acidosis, preferably in an intensive care unit if the patient is unstable clinically.

Hypoglycemia

The brain uses glucose as its preferred fuel. When a person's plasma glucose level is less than 70 mg/dL (3.9 mmol/L), signals are sent from the brain to the pancreas, liver, and

TABLE 9. Management of Hyperglycemic Crisis (DKA and HHS)

Fluids	Insulin (Regular)	Potassium	Correction of Acidosis
Assess for volume status, then give 0.9% saline at 1 L/h initially in all patients, and continue if patient is severely hypovolemic. Switch to 0.45% normal saline at 250-500 mL/h if corrected serum sodium level becomes normal or high. When the plasma glucose level reaches 200 mg/dL (11.1 mmol/L) in patients with DKA or 300 mg/dL (16.7 mmol/L) in HHS, switch to 5% dextrose with 0.45% normal saline at 150-250 mL/h.	Give regular insulin, 0.1 unit/kg, as an intravenous bolus followed by 0.1 unit/kg/h as an intravenous infusion; if the plasma glucose level does not decrease by 10% in the first hour, give an additional bolus of 0.14 unit/kg and resume previous infusion rate; when the plasma glucose level reaches 200 mg/dL (11.1 mmol/L) in DKA and 300 mg/dL (16.7 mmol/L) in HHS, reduce to 0.02-0.05 unit/kg/h, and maintain the plasma glucose level between 150-200 mg/dL (8.3 mmol/L) until anion gap acidosis is resolved in DKA.	Assess for adequate kidney function, with adequate urine output (approximately 50 mL/h). If serum potassium is <3.3 meq/L (3.3 mmol/L), do not start insulin but instead give intravenous potassium chloride, 20-30 meq/h, through a central line catheter until the serum potassium level is >3.3 meq/L (3.3 mmol/L); then add 20-30 meq of potassium chloride to each liter of intravenous fluids to keep the serum potassium level in the 4.0-5.0 meq/L (4.0-5.0 mmol/L) range. If the serum potassium level is >5.2 meq/L (5.2 mmol/L), do not give potassium chloride but instead start insulin and intravenous fluids and check the serum potassium level every 2 hours.	If pH is <6.9, give sodium bicarbonate, 100 mmol in 400 mL of water, and potassium chloride, 20 meq, infused over 2 hours. If pH is 6.9 or greater, do not give sodium bicarbonate.

DKA = diabetic ketoacidosis; HHS = hyperglycemic hyperosmolar syndrome.

adrenal glands that collectively raise the plasma glucose level. The hormones involved are glucagon, epinephrine, norepinephrine, cortisol, and growth hormone; hepatic gluconeogenesis also occurs. Hyperadrenergic symptoms (sweating, rapid heartbeat, anxiety, hunger, and tremor) are usually experienced first. If the plasma glucose level continues to decline, brain function becomes impaired, and neuroglycopenic signs and symptoms (cognitive impairment, somnolence, dizziness, slurred speech, and change in personality) develop. If these signs and symptoms are not recognized and treated and the plasma glucose level continues to decrease, the patient may lose consciousness, develop focal neurologic signs (such as hemiparesis), or have seizures.

Although most common in type 1 diabetes, severe hypoglycemia also can occur in type 2 diabetes in patients who are taking insulin or drugs (such as sulfonylureas and meglitinides) that stimulate the release of insulin. The situations in which hypoglycemia most commonly develops involve patients taking too large a dose of insulin, delaying or skipping a meal, eating fewer carbohydrates than normally, or exercising more than usual. Older patients who take sulfonylureas with long half-lives or who develop heart failure or kidney impairment can have high drug levels in their blood due to decreased clearance, which results in profound and prolonged hypoglycemia. Prolonged exercise that is not followed by consumption of complex carbohydrates can lead to hypoglycemia several hours later as the muscles and the liver continue to remove glucose from the blood to replenish their glycogen stores. This is especially problematic if exercise occurs in the evening before bedtime. Excess alcohol consumption also can cause hypoglycemia by suppressing hepatic glucose production. Alcohol additionally may blunt a person's ability to recognize hypoglycemic symptoms (slurred speech, altered personality), and these symptoms may be wrongly attributed by others to his or her alcohol use.

Distinguishing between the following four hypoglycemic situations can be useful:

1. Severe hypoglycemia, which requires the assistance of another person to administer a carbohydrate (preferably glucose sublingually or intravenously) or subcutaneous glucagon
2. Documented symptomatic hypoglycemia, which occurs when a patient feels typical hyperadrenergic hypoglycemic symptoms and verifies that the blood glucose level is less than 70 mg/dL (3.9 mmol/L) before self-treating with 15 grams of a carbohydrate
3. Asymptomatic hypoglycemia (or hypoglycemic unawareness), in which a patient does not develop typical hyperadrenergic symptoms but has a measured plasma glucose level of less than 70 mg/dL (3.9 mmol/L); this situation occurs most often in type 1 diabetes in patients striving for excellent glycemic control (hemoglobin A_{1c} value <7.0%) who have chronic, frequent episodes of hypoglycemia. The body's ability to recognize hypoglycemia and secrete counterregulatory hormones in response to hypoglycemia deteriorates and leaves these patients vulnerable to further episodes of severe hypoglycemia. Treatment for this hypoglycemic unawareness is to reduce the insulin dosage and eat more carbohydrates both at meals and between meals to ensure a blood glucose level of 150 to 200 mg/dL (8.3-11.1 mmol/L) at all times for several weeks. This step allows the body to "reset" so that hypoglycemia is recognized and the counterregulatory response to hypoglycemia is improved.
4. Relative hypoglycemia, in which a patient experiences hyperadrenergic hypoglycemic symptoms but has a measured plasma glucose level greater than 70 mg/dL (3.9 mmol/L); this situation occurs most often in patients who have had months (or longer) of hyperglycemia (plasma glucose levels >200 mg/dL [11.1 mmol/L] at all times) whose plasma glucose levels are then lowered by medication or lifestyle changes closer to the normal range. Hyperadrenergic hypoglycemic symptoms can occur when the plasma glucose level in these patients is 120 mg/dL (6.7 mmol/L) or even higher. If these patients continue to keep their plasma glucose level substantially less than 200 mg/dL (11.1 mmol/L), the threshold at which they manifest hypoglycemic symptoms will fall to more typical levels (<70 mg/dL [3.9 mmol/L]).

Patients vary in how well they tolerate the hyperadrenergic symptoms of hypoglycemia psychologically. Fear of the symptoms and of the hypoglycemia itself is a common barrier to achieving hemoglobin A_{1c} goals. Although the human brain can tolerate recurrent episodes of hypoglycemia relatively well, cognitive deficits can be found among children and adults who have had years of repeated episodes of severe hypoglycemia. In older patients and those whose livelihood would be jeopardized by hypoglycemia (commercial vehicle drivers, persons who work with dangerous equipment), it is reasonable (and indeed preferable) to set hemoglobin A_{1c} targets at higher levels and to adjust treatment regimens to reduce the chance of hypoglycemia.

KEY POINTS

- Although most common in type 1 diabetes mellitus, hypoglycemia also occurs in patients with type 2 diabetes who are taking insulin or drugs that stimulate the release of insulin.
- In relative hypoglycemia, a patient experiences typical hypoglycemic symptoms but has a measured plasma glucose level greater than 70 mg/dL (3.9 mmol/L).

Chronic Complications of Diabetes

Diabetic Retinopathy

Because the retina is highly vascular and can be viewed directly through an ophthalmoscope, it gives the earliest indication of microvascular damage from hyperglycemia. Diabetic retinopathy generally develops and progresses slowly and predictably. Chronic hyperglycemia causes edema, hard exudates, and tiny hemorrhages in the retinal layers. Microaneurysms in the vessel wall may result in retinal infarcts (soft exudates or "cotton wool" spots). These features are collectively called background or nonproliferative diabetic retinopathy. As the retina becomes more ischemic, proliferative retinopathy can occur, in which blood vessels rupture and often cause extensive intraocular bleeding. Fibrosis and contraction follow, leading to retinal detachment. This severe proliferative retinopathy may thus result in a substantial loss of vision.

Management of diabetic retinopathy consists of regular retinal evaluation by direct visual examination through an ophthalmoscope or by high-quality retinal photographs. Screening guidelines are shown in **Table 10**. This screening does not need to be started until 5 years after diagnosis of type 1 diabetes because of the general lack of retinopathy seen in the early years of the disease. Because type 2 diabetes usually develops slowly, undetected hyperglycemia may be present for many years before diagnosis. Therefore, retinal screening should start immediately in patients with this type of diabetes; approximately 10% of these patients have evidence of diabetic retinopathy at diagnosis. In patients with background retinopathy and poor glycemic control, a rapid improvement in glycemic control can result in a temporary worsening of retinopathy (particularly retinal infarcts). This pattern also is seen in pregnant women with diabetes in whom diabetic retinopathy can appear suddenly and progress rapidly. Therefore, pregnant women with diabetes should be screened for retinopathy during the first trimester and in each trimester thereafter.

The risk of retinopathy can be reduced (or the progression slowed) by excellent glycemic control (hemoglobin A_{1c} value <7.0%), lowering blood pressure, smoking cessation, or use of ACE inhibitors. The mainstay of treatment for advanced diabetic retinopathy is laser photocoagulation. In patients with macular edema, focal laser therapy in the surrounding retina can reduce the edema and restore vision. When proliferative retinopathy develops, more widespread laser therapy (often several thousand tiny laser burns delivered to the periphery of the retina) is used. As these burns scar and become avascular, the total retinal area is reduced by approximately one third; the remaining retina thus receives more blood, and new vessels involute. As a result, the risk of major intraocular bleeding or retinal detachment is reduced and central vision is preserved, but at the expense of a loss of peripheral vision. After widespread (panretinal) laser photocoagulation, many patients notice a significant worsening of their peripheral vision while driving, which can be especially noticeable and troubling at night.

In addition to laser photocoagulation therapy, an alternative or complementary management of proliferative diabetic retinopathy is intraocular injections of inhibitors of vascular endothelial growth factors, such as bevacizumab or ranibizumab, every 4 to 8 weeks.

KEY POINT

- The mainstay of treatment of advanced diabetic retinopathy is laser photocoagulation.

Diabetic Nephropathy

Chronic hyperglycemia causes progressive damage to the glomerular basement membranes of the kidneys in patients with diabetes. The kidneys then begin to release excessive amounts of protein into the urine. This proteinuria is associated with an increased serum creatinine level, worsening hypertension, and progression to end-stage kidney disease requiring dialysis or kidney transplantation. Although diabetes remains the leading cause of chronic kidney failure in the United States and is the most common reason for dialysis and kidney transplantation, the overall incidence of diabetic nephropathy has declined significantly in the past two decades. Improved glycemic and blood pressure control, the use of ACE inhibitors or ARBs, and smoking cessation programs are largely responsible for this decrease. Some research

TABLE 10. Screening Recommendations for Diabetic Retinopathy

Clinical Situation	When to Start Screening	Screening Frequency
Type 1 diabetes	At 5 years after diagnosis	Annually[a]
Type 2 diabetes	At diagnosis	Annually[a]
In pregnant women with either type of diabetes	First trimester	Every trimester and then closely for 1 year postpartum
In women with either type of diabetes planning to conceive	During preconception planning	Same as recommendations for pregnant women once conception occurs

[a]It is reasonable to screen every 2 years if no diabetic retinopathy is present and to screen more often than annually if diabetic retinopathy is advanced or progressing rapidly.

evidence suggests that intensive glucose management may prevent or delay the onset and progression of diabetic nephropathy. Patients with type 1 diabetes who have no detectable proteinuria 20 years after diagnosis are unlikely to develop end-stage kidney disease. Although the incidence of diabetic nephropathy is somewhat lower in type 2 diabetes, significant genetic and ethnic variation exists.

Protein in the urine can be measured by determining the albumin-creatinine ratio. Values between 30 and 300 mg/g indicate microalbuminuria, and values greater than 300 mg/g indicate macroalbuminuria (or overt proteinuria). Patients with type 2 diabetes should be tested annually for microalbuminuria from the time of diagnosis, and patients with type 1 diabetes should begin annual testing 5 years after diagnosis. Persistent microalbuminuria suggests not only that a patient is at significantly increased risk of developing overt diabetic nephropathy in the future, but also that the risk of future cardiovascular disease is at least four times higher than that of age- and gender-matched patients with no microalbuminuria. Vigorous exercise, menstruation, illness, and acute hyperglycemia can cause false elevations in the urine albumin-creatinine ratio.

For more information on diabetic nephropathy, see MKSAP 16 Nephrology.

Diabetic Neuropathy

Nerve cells (sensory, motor, and autonomic) are vulnerable to damage from chronic hyperglycemia, and clinical manifestations of neuropathy tend to appear as a later complication of diabetes, particularly diabetes that is not optimally controlled. Also, an acute distal symmetric diabetic neuropathy may occur after an episode of severe hyperglycemia and cause segmental demyelination in a stocking-glove distribution. Peripheral diabetic neuropathy results in sharp, stabbing, or burning pain in the toes, feet, lower legs, and hands. Patients also may feel discomfort when the skin is touched (dysesthesia) and a heaviness and clumsiness in their feet and legs. Symptoms often are worse at night. Immediate relief often is obtained by topical application of capsaicin cream and relatively low oral doses of tricyclic antidepressants or partial serotonin and norepinephrine reuptake inhibitors. If this approach does not relieve symptoms, adding an antiseizure medication (gabapentin, pregabalin, carbamazepine, or phenytoin) may help, but opiates should be avoided. Patients also should be encouraged to try to reduce their hemoglobin A_{1c} levels to less than 7.0%, which may help remyelinate the nerves and reverse the neuropathy.

Acute ocular or truncal mononeuropathies can occur. No specific treatment for these mononeuropathies is effective, but they usually resolve spontaneously over a few months. Diabetic amyotrophy should be considered in patients with recently diagnosed or well-controlled diabetes who develop acute proximal leg pain or weakness and weight loss. The nerves of patients with diabetes are more vulnerable to entrapment neuropathies, including carpal tunnel syndrome or meralgia paresthetica.

The combination of nerve damage and impaired peripheral vascular circulation places patients with chronic diabetic neuropathy at high risk for foot ulcers and amputations. All patients with diabetes should have their feet examined at least annually to assess for decreased sensation and detect ulcers, calluses, foot deformities, pain, abnormal pressure sensation, and peripheral pulses. These patients should be strongly encouraged to inspect their feet daily and seek help at the earliest signs of ulceration or infection. Charcot foot deformity may develop over time in patients with seemingly minor foot trauma, axonal loss, and small muscle atrophy.

Damage to autonomic nerves elsewhere in the body can present as erectile dysfunction (present in 50% of men with diabetes who are older than 50 years), gastroparesis (see MKSAP 16 Gastroenterology and Hepatology), chronic diarrhea or constipation, orthostatic hypotension, resting sinus tachycardia, postprandial hypotension, abnormal hidrosis, and neurogenic bladder. Patients with manifestations of cardiovascular neuropathy are at increased risk of sudden cardiac death, and thus cardiac risk reduction should be strongly encouraged.

For more information on diabetic neuropathy, see MKSAP 16 Neurology.

KEY POINT

- All patients with diabetes should have their feet examined at least annually to assess for decreased sensation and detect ulcers, calluses, foot deformities, pain, abnormal pressure sensation, and peripheral pulses.

Hypoglycemia in Patients Without Diabetes

Hypoglycemia is rare in persons without diabetes because the healthy body has robust mechanisms for maintaining glucose homeostasis. As the plasma glucose falls to less than the normal range, the pancreatic islet cells turn off insulin secretion and hepatic glycogenolysis supplies glucose to maintain the plasma glucose level above 70 mg/dL (3.9 mmol/L). When this level is less than 70 mg/dL (3.9 mmol/L), glucagon and epinephrine secretion increases, and when it is less than 60 mg/dL (3.3 mmol/L), cortisol and growth hormone secretion increases. When hepatic glycogen stores are exhausted (in approximately 8 hours), hepatic gluconeogenesis becomes the sole source of glucose production. Hypoglycemia can occur when hepatic glycogen stores are depleted as a result of extreme starvation, sepsis, or hepatic dysfunction; when alcohol ingestion suppresses hepatic glucose production; and when cortisol is deficient (as in untreated Addison disease and adrenocorticotropic hormone deficiency [secondary glucocorticoid deficiency]).

In apparently healthy persons without diabetes, hypoglycemic symptoms usually occur either in the fasting or postprandial state.

Fasting Hypoglycemia

When hypoglycemic symptoms occur in the fasting state or at least not in the immediate postprandial period, the differential diagnosis includes the presence of an insulin-secreting tumor (insulinoma), which is exceedingly rare; the surreptitious injection of insulin; or the ingestion of a sulfonylurea or meglitinide (see Table 7). Because symptoms of hypoglycemia are nonspecific and can be caused by anxiety or stress, one must document that the plasma glucose level is actually low at the times when symptoms are experienced. Therefore, hypoglycemia is best diagnosed when three conditions coexist (Whipple triad): (1) hypoglycemic symptoms are present, (2) a low plasma glucose level is documented by a laboratory (because self–blood glucose monitors may be unreliable at low glucose levels), and (3) prompt resolution of symptoms occurs after glucose ingestion. When Whipple triad is observed, further evaluation for the cause of pathologic hypoglycemia should include an inpatient 72-hour fast with regular measurement of simultaneous plasma glucose, proinsulin, insulin, C-peptide (a measure of endogenous insulin secretion), β-hydroxybutyrate (a ketone body produced in the absence of insulin), and sulfonylurea levels (to rule out surreptitious ingestion) (**Table 11**). If the results are consistent with insulinoma, only then should CT imaging of the pancreas be performed to localize the tumor and direct its surgical resection by an endocrine surgeon. Because insulinomas are often small, further testing (with, for example, endoscopic ultrasonography) may be necessary for localization. If the results indicate exogenous injection of insulin or surreptitious ingestion of sulfonylureas, a psychiatric evaluation may be appropriate, especially in patients with a history of a mood or psychiatric disorder.

Postprandial Hypoglycemia

The occurrence of true postprandial hypoglycemia among persons without diabetes who have no history of gastric bypass surgery is extremely uncommon although frequently misdiagnosed. A patient may report feeling sleepy, shaky, or weak 1 to 3 hours after a large meal rich in simple carbohydrates, and a tentative diagnosis of hypoglycemia may be made. Using an oral glucose tolerance test to confirm the diagnosis should be avoided because of the high incidence of hypoglycemia in healthy persons given a 75-g glucose load.

A better way to establish the diagnosis is to observe the patient and measure the plasma glucose level when symptoms occur. Most of the time, euglycemia will be detected. Whether or not symptoms are due to hypoglycemia, the best treatment is to recommend smaller and more frequent meals.

Disorders of the Pituitary Gland

Hypothalamic Disease

The hypothalamus produces multiple hormones that control pituitary function, especially anterior pituitary gland function. These include corticotropin-releasing hormone, which stimulates the release of adrenocorticotropic hormone (ACTH); gonadotropin-releasing hormone (GnRH), which stimulates the release of luteinizing hormone (LH) and follicle-stimulating hormone (FSH); thyrotropin-releasing hormone, which stimulates the release of thyroid-stimulating hormone (TSH); and growth hormone (GH)–releasing hormone, which stimulates the release of GH. These hormones travel from the hypothalamus through the pituitary stalk and are then released into the pituitary gland. Pathologic disruption of the pituitary stalk may disrupt the flow of these hypothalamic hormones and thus cause a decrease in hormone secretion, which leads to a reduction in pituitary gland function. An exception to this process occurs with the hormone prolactin, an anterior pituitary gland hormone under the tonic inhibitory control of dopamine released from the pituitary stalk; disruption of dopamine delivery from the pituitary stalk causes the prolactin level to increase.

The posterior pituitary gland consists mainly of neuronal axons that extend from the supraoptic and paraventricular

TABLE 11. Differential Diagnosis of Spontaneous Fasting Hypoglycemia in a Person Without Diabetes

Diagnosis	Plasma Glucose Level	Serum Insulin Level	Plasma C-Peptide Level	Urine or Blood Metabolites of Sulfonylureas or Meglitinides
Insulinoma	↓	↑	↑	Negative
Surreptitious use of sulfonylureas or meglitinides	↓	↑	↑	Positive
Surreptitious use of insulin	↓	↑	↓	Negative

nuclei of the hypothalamus through the stalk. The two major hormones associated with the posterior pituitary gland are antidiuretic hormone and oxytocin.

Most causes of hypothalamic disorders are acquired, although rare genetic causes of hypothalamic dysfunction exist. Causes of acquired hypothalamic disease include trauma due to brain injury, neurosurgery, or cranial irradiation; infiltrative diseases, including sarcoidosis, Langerhans cell histiocytosis, lymphoma, and metastatic cancer (most commonly from breast and lung cancer); and compression by pituitary tumors with suprasellar extension, particularly tumors with a cystic composition or (rarely) associated with cancer. Acquired hypothalamic structural diseases (such as craniopharyngioma) present with signs and symptoms related to the anatomic location of the lesion and the rapidity of the increase in lesion size. Besides its role in pituitary function, the hypothalamus is involved in the regulation of various behaviors and functions, such as satiety and body temperature. Hypothalamic dysfunction may lead to excessive eating, profound hypothermia, hypersexuality, or somnolence. Hypothalamic lesions also often cause central diabetes insipidus by disrupting antidiuretic hormone production.

KEY POINT

- Hypothalamic lesions often cause diabetes insipidus by disrupting antidiuretic hormone production.

Hypopituitarism

Causes and General Management

Hypopituitarism results from disorders of the pituitary gland or hypothalamus that lead to decreased secretion of pituitary gland hormones (**Table 12**). Pituitary tumors and their treatment (surgery and radiation therapy) are the most common causes of hypopituitarism in adults (>75%), followed by extrapituitary lesions (<15%), such as a craniopharyngioma or Rathke cleft cyst. Other mass lesions that can lead to hypopituitarism include nonpituitary neoplasms (such as germinoma and meningioma), metastatic cancers, Langerhans cell histiocytosis, and lymphocytic hypophysitis (an autoimmune disorder characterized by symmetric enlargement of the sellar contents that occurs mostly during or after pregnancy and is commonly associated with ACTH deficiency). The presence of a sellar mass in the setting of diabetes insipidus suggests the presence of a lesion of nonpituitary origin. Neurosurgical removal or debulking of the tumor may reduce the pressure on the pituitary gland and thus result in improved pituitary function. However, neurosurgery performed on the pituitary gland also may result in resection of normal gland, which can lead to hypopituitarism.

H Pituitary tumor apoplexy, which denotes hemorrhagic infarction of the tumor, causes sudden onset of headache, possible diplopia (from compression of cranial nerves within the cavernous sinus[es]), and acute hypopituitarism. Pituitary tumor apoplexy is a neurosurgical emergency. In addition to neurosurgical decompression of the pituitary gland, urgent replacement of glucocorticoids may be necessary because of acute ACTH deficiency. Replacement of thyroid hormone, sex hormones, and GH is typically not urgent but may be necessary. Sheehan syndrome in pregnancy involves pituitary gland infarction in the setting of severe blood loss and hypotension at delivery and presents with subacute, progressive hypopituitarism, an inability to lactate because of prolactin deficiency, and amenorrhea. Central adrenal insufficiency is the primary cause of mortality in Sheehan syndrome. H

Cranial irradiation causes progressive hypopituitarism in approximately 40% of patients. Some degree of hypopituitarism also has been reported in approximately 25% of patients after severe traumatic brain injury, ischemic stroke, and subarachnoid hemorrhage. Hormonal deficiencies are typically noted acutely, although rarely they may be detected more than 1 year after injury. The more severe the injury, the more likely are hormone deficiencies. GH deficiency is the most commonly noted, is usually seen together with at least one other pituitary deficiency, and has been associated with reduced quality of life after injury.

Infiltrative lesions that can lead to hypopituitarism include hemochromatosis, lymphocytic hypophysitis, and granulomatous diseases (such as sarcoidosis). Hypopituitarism is managed with replacement of the hormones secreted directly from the pituitary gland (GH or vasopressin) or those normally secreted under pituitary control (hydrocortisone, levothyroxine, testosterone, or estrogen-progesterone), with adjustment of daily replacement doses determined clinically by whether the hormone has been over- or underreplaced (**Table 13**). Because ACTH deficiency can be life threatening in light of the associated cortisol deficiency, the hypothalamic-pituitary-adrenal axis should be assessed acutely in patients in whom hypopituitarism is suspected.

TABLE 12. Acquired Causes of Hypopituitarism
Tumors (pituitary adenomas, craniopharyngiomas, dysgerminomas, meningiomas, gliomas, metastatic tumors, Rathke cleft cysts)
Irradiation
Trauma (neurosurgery, external blunt trauma)
Infiltrative disease (sarcoidosis, Langerhans cell histiocytosis, tuberculosis)
Empty sella syndrome
Vascular (apoplexy, Sheehan syndrome, subarachnoid hemorrhage)
Lymphocytic hypophysitis
Metabolic causes (hemochromatosis, critical illness, malnutrition, anorexia nervosa, psychosocial deprivation)
Idiopathic causes

TABLE 13. Hormonal Replacement Therapy in Hypopituitarism

Hormone Deficiency	Therapeutic Replacement Regimen
TSH	Levothyroxine, 50-200 mg/d; adjust by measuring free T_4 levels; obtaining TSH levels is not indicated because these levels are uninterpretable in patients known to be TSH deficient.
ACTH	Hydrocortisone, 10-20 mg in AM and 5-10 mg in PM *or* prednisone, 2.5-5 mg in AM and 2.5 mg in PM; adjust clinically.
	Stress dosing for hydrocortisone, 50-100 mg IV every 8 hours.
LH/FSH	
Men	Testosterone: 1% gel, 1-2 packets (5-10 g) or 1.62% gel, 2-4 pumps (40.5-81 mg) daily; transdermal patch, 5 g daily; or testosterone enanthate or cypionate, 50-300 mg IM every 1-4 weeks. Adjust by measuring testosterone levels. Will need injectable gonadotropins (LH, FSH) or GnRH for spermatogenesis (if fertility is desired).
Women	Cyclic conjugated estrogens (0.3-0.625 mg) and medroxyprogesterone acetate (5-10 mg) *or* low-dose oral contraceptive pills. Estrogen patches also available. Will need injectable gonadotropins (LH, FSH) if fertility is desired.
GH	Adults start at 200-300 µg subcutaneously daily and increment by 100-200 µg at bimonthly intervals. Adjust to maintain IGF-1 levels in the midnormal range. Women receiving oral estrogens require higher doses.
Vasopressin	Desmopressin: metered nasal spray, 10-20 µg once or twice daily; or tablets, 0.1-0.4 mg every 8-12 h; or injected, 1-2 µg subcutaneously or IV, every 6-12 h

ACTH = adrenocorticotropic hormone; FSH = follicle-stimulating hormone; GH = growth hormone; GnRH = gonadotropin-releasing hormone; IGF-1 = insulin-like growth factor 1; IM = intramuscularly; IV = intravenously; LH = luteinizing hormone; µg = microgram(s); T_4 = thyroxine; TSH = thyroid-stimulating hormone.

KEY POINTS

- Pituitary tumors and their treatment are the most common causes of hypopituitarism in adults; neurosurgical removal or debulking of these tumors may reduce the pressure on the pituitary gland and result in improved pituitary function.
- Urgent glucocorticoid replacement is necessary in patients with pituitary tumor apoplexy.

Growth Hormone Deficiency

GH deficiency in adults may reflect either persistence of childhood-onset disease or newly acquired disease and typically occurs with other pituitary deficiencies. In children, GH deficiency causes short stature. In adults, however, acquired GH deficiency causes reduced lean muscle mass and increased fat mass, reduced strength and stamina, decreased bone mineral density, an increased cardiovascular risk profile, and a decreased quality of life. Adult-onset GH deficiency is the most common pituitary deficiency associated with a structural sellar or suprasellar lesion that has been treated with neurosurgical intervention and/or cranial irradiation.

Biochemical testing includes demonstration of a low serum insulin-like growth factor 1 (IGF-1) level and a test for GH reserve based on a stimulation test that uses insulin (to induce hypoglycemia), glucagon, arginine, or GH-releasing hormone. GH replacement therapy should be considered in patients with other pituitary deficiencies and in those with unequivocal evidence of deficiency, with resultant benefits in lean body and fat mass, improvement in lipid profiles, and improvement in the sense of well being. Isolated idiopathic adult-onset GH deficiency is rare, and the utility of replacing GH in adults with idiopathic GH deficiency is debatable given the lack of robust data showing that treatment results in resolution of ill effects. Because of this uncertainty, consultation with an endocrinologist is appropriate if treatment is being considered.

KEY POINT

- Adult-onset growth hormone (GH) deficiency is the most common pituitary deficiency associated with a structural sellar or suprasellar lesion that has been treated with neurosurgical intervention and/or cranial irradiation; isolated idiopathic adult-onset GH deficiency is rare.

Gonadotropin Deficiency

In hypogonadotropic hypogonadism, the pituitary gland produces less LH and FSH, which leads to hypogonadism (reduced estrogen production and ovulatory capacity by the ovary or diminished testosterone secretion and spermatogenesis by the testis). Clinical features of hypogonadotropic hypogonadism include amenorrhea, breast atrophy, vaginal dryness, and diminished libido in women and decreased libido, erectile dysfunction, loss of skeletal muscle mass, and anemia in men. Acquired hypogonadotropic hypogonadism in women commonly results from weight loss, severe dietary restriction, anorexia nervosa, stress, heavy exercise, or severe illness, although it also may be idiopathic. MRI or CT is recommended in patients with hypogonadotropic hypogonadism to rule out structural disease. In both sexes, loss of gonadal hormones can lead to loss of bone density. Of note, hyperprolactinemia can suppress GnRH secretion and also lead to hypogonadotropic hypogonadism.

Features, diagnosis, and treatment of hypogonadism is addressed in Reproductive Disorders.

Adrenocorticotropic Hormone Deficiency

ACTH deficiency causes hypocortisolism, and low or normal ACTH levels are seen in the presence of a low measured cortisol level, in contrast to the elevated ACTH values seen in primary adrenal insufficiency. Whereas patients with primary adrenal insufficiency have increased skin pigmentation due to elevated ACTH levels, patients with ACTH deficiency do not. Symptoms of nausea, vomiting, malaise, weakness, dizziness, fatigue, fever, and hypotension can occur with ACTH deficiency, although often subacutely, with malaise and weakness being most prominent. In ACTH deficiency, adrenal production of mineralocorticoids and potassium homeostasis remain intact because the hypothalamic-pituitary-adrenal axis is controlled separately by the renin-angiotensin system. This contrasts with the frequent finding of hyperkalemia in primary adrenal insufficiency. The presentation of ACTH deficiency may be variable, and some patients may be asymptomatic, but affected patients typically exhibit symptoms of hypocortisolemia during physiologically stressful events, such as surgery or sepsis. Details regarding symptoms, diagnosis, and therapy of primary and secondary adrenal insufficiency are provided in Disorders of the Adrenal Gland.

The most common cause of ACTH deficiency is suppression of corticotropin-releasing hormone and ACTH secretion by exogenous corticosteroids for longer than 2 to 3 weeks. Similarly, megestrol acetate, which is used for appetite stimulation in cachetic patients with cancer or AIDS, has some glucocorticoid activity and can suppress ACTH secretion. Although patients who take megestrol acetate do not usually show clinical evidence of hypercortisolism (Cushing syndrome), patients should be monitored for hypocortisolism after the drug is discontinued.

When not due to medication, ACTH deficiency frequently is detected in combination with the loss of other pituitary hormones.

Thyroid-Stimulating Hormone Deficiency

In central hypothyroidism, TSH deficiency leads to reduced secretion of thyroxine (T_4), and thus a measurement of the patient's serum T_4 level is necessary to establish the diagnosis. The signs and symptoms of central hypothyroidism are similar to those of primary hypothyroidism, namely, fatigue, weight gain, cold intolerance, and constipation. In contrast to the elevated TSH level seen in primary hypothyroidism, TSH deficiency is associated with a low free T_4 level and an inappropriately normal or low TSH level. This distinction is important because a normal TSH level may be associated with significant hypothyroidism in a patient with central hypothyroidism and TSH deficiency. Acquired central hypothyroidism usually is associated with deficiencies of other pituitary hormones. Because both serum free T_4 and TSH levels can be low in central hypothyroidism, distinguishing between central hypothyroidism and the euthyroid sick syndrome may be difficult in patients with severe illness or starvation. Generally, those with euthyroid sick syndrome have elevated levels of reverse triiodothyronine (T_3), unlike those with central hypothyroidism.

Thyroid hormone dosing in patients with central hypothyroidism should be adjusted on the basis of clinical symptoms to maintain free T_4 levels within the midnormal reference range, unless doing so causes iatrogenic hyperthyroidism or hypothyroidism. TSH levels cannot be used as a measure of adequacy of replacement in these patients as they can in patients with an intact hypothalamic-pituitary axis.

Diabetes Insipidus

Diabetes insipidus is characterized by excessive urination due to a deficiency of antidiuretic hormone (also known as arginine vasopressin [AVP]) secretion, as in central diabetes insipidus, or a defect in AVP's ability to act on the kidney, as in nephrogenic diabetes insipidus. In either situation, the kidney does not concentrate urine, which results in excretion of dilute urine relative to plasma. The resultant increase in plasma osmolality leads to both polydipsia through stimulation of central osmoreceptors and polyuria because of the inability to retain free water and concentrate the urine. If patients have an adequate thirst mechanism and access to water, the serum sodium level should remain normal to high normal, although accompanied by significant polyuria and polydipsia. In partial central diabetes insipidus, the patient is largely asymptomatic because of adequate compensation through an intact thirst mechanism and ready access to water. However, with a stressor—such as water deprivation, a central nervous system event that alters the set point for stimulation of thirst, or pregnancy with degradation of AVP caused by placental vasopressinase—diabetes insipidus may become clinically apparent.

Causes of central diabetes insipidus include rare familial syndromes. In acquired cases, causes are usually mass lesions (neoplasms, such as craniopharyngioma, germinoma, and metastatic cancer), trauma (neurosurgery or traumatic brain injury), and infiltrative disorders (sarcoidosis or Langerhans cell histiocytosis) that compromise hypothalamic function. Transient central diabetes insipidus commonly occurs immediately after pituitary surgery but may resolve rapidly after the procedure.

As with polyuria, the differential diagnosis of central diabetes insipidus includes primary polydipsia due to a psychiatric disorder, medications (such as phenothiazines that cause dry mouth), or hypothalamic lesions that affect the thirst center (such as sarcoidosis); osmotic diuresis, as in uncontrolled diabetes mellitus and postobstructive diuresis; and hypercalcemia. A serum chemistry panel should be obtained to rule out osmotic causes. If the baseline serum sodium level is high normal or elevated, particularly if the urine osmolality is lower than the plasma osmolality, then diabetes insipidus is likely. If the baseline serum sodium level is less than 136 meq/L [136 mmol/L]) and urine osmolality is high, then diabetes insipidus is unlikely. (In fact, the syndrome of inappropriate antidiuretic hormone secretion is likely present.) If the baseline serum sodium level is within the normal range, a water deprivation test should be performed to differentiate diabetes insipidus from primary polydipsia.

In a water deprivation test, the serum sodium level and plasma osmolality are measured every 2 hours, and the urine volume, urine osmolality, and body weight are measured every hour. The test is finished when (1) the urine osmolality is greater than 600 mosm/kg H_2O (appropriately concentrated), (2) urine osmolality fails to concentrate for 2 consecutive hours, (3) plasma osmolality is greater than 295 mosm/kg H_2O, (4) serum sodium level is greater than 145 meq/L (145 mmol/L), or (5) the patient has lost greater than 5% body weight. The patient is then given desmopressin acetate. If any of the five parameters are met before the test begins, the water deprivation test is not recommended, and desmopressin can be administered first, followed by measurement of urine volume and osmolality every 30 minutes for 2 hours. During water deprivation and before desmopressin administration, healthy persons will increase their urine osmolality to greater than 800 mosm/kg H_2O, but those with diabetes insipidus will not increase theirs above 300 mosm/kg H_2O. In response to desmopressin, patients with central diabetes insipidus will increase their urine osmolality by at least 50%, but those with nephrogenic diabetes insipidus will not respond appreciably.

Treatment of central diabetes insipidus includes desmopressin—administered orally, by a metered nasal spray, or (if needed) by subcutaneous or intravenous injection—and the instruction to drink until no longer thirsty. Water intoxication can be avoided as long as the patient drinks only when thirsty. In the unconscious patient or someone whose thirst mechanisms are not operative, extreme care must be exerted to avoid undertreatment and overtreatment. Accurate determination of daily body weight, fixed dosages of fluid intake, and frequent monitoring of the serum sodium level are necessary.

KEY POINTS

- In the presence of polyuria, diabetes insipidus is likely if the baseline serum sodium level is high normal or clearly elevated, particularly when the urine osmolality is lower than the plasma osmolality.
- If the baseline serum sodium level is within the normal range in the setting of polyuria, a water deprivation test should be performed to differentiate diabetes insipidus from primary polydipsia.

Pituitary Tumors

Pituitary tumors (adenomas) arise from monoclonal neoplasms of the cells comprising the pituitary gland, including somatotrophs (GH), corticotrophs (ACTH), gonadotrophs (LH and FSH), lactotrophs (prolactin), and thyrotrophs (TSH). These tumors also are defined by size, with microadenomas being less than 10 mm in diameter and macroadenomas being 10 mm in diameter or greater. The most common pituitary tumor is a nonfunctioning adenoma; the most common functional pituitary tumor is a prolactinoma. Most pituitary adenomas are sporadic, although some (<5%) occur as part of the familial multiple endocrine neoplasia type 1 syndrome, which is associated with endocrine tumors of the pituitary gland, parathyroid glands, and pancreas (the three "Ps"). Although most pituitary adenomas are benign, they can be locally invasive and lead to significant compressive symptoms because of their proximity to adjacent critical structures, such as the optic chiasm. Pituitary tumors, therefore, can lead to local problems (such as visual field deficits and headaches) and also have systemic effects due to hormone hypersecretion or compression of the normal gland with resultant hypopituitarism.

Approach to a Sellar Mass

A sellar mass may be detected incidentally, for example during the evaluation of trauma, headache, sinusitis, or another disorder. If the lesion is detected on a CT scan, then MRI should be performed because an MRI provides better anatomic definition. After it is detected, the sellar mass should be characterized further by determining if hormone hypersecretion is present. Additionally, the serum prolactin level should be determined in all patients with a sellar mass to exclude a prolactinoma. If the history or physical examination is suggestive of either acromegaly or Cushing syndrome, the appropriate biochemical test should be performed. If the evaluation shows no evidence of pituitary hypersecretion, the lesion is either a clinically nonfunctioning adenoma or a nonpituitary lesion. Further evaluation for local mass effects, such as the presence of visual field compromise or hypopituitarism due to compression of the optic chiasm or normal pituitary gland, respectively, should then be performed, particularly in the setting of a macroadenoma. Therapy is warranted if the lesion is functional (such as a hormone-secreting adenoma) or if hypopituitarism or other local mass effects are found. If the lesion is nonfunctional and no accompanying mass effects are detected, serial follow-up evaluation is advised.

Mass Effects of Pituitary Tumors

Because the clinical manifestation of pituitary tumors is often insidious and slow in onset, these tumors are often large when detected. As a result, these enlarging tumors can cause mass effects on local structures. Macroadenomas with suprasellar extension compressing the optic chiasm can cause visual field defects, including bitemporal hemianopia, and invasion of the cavernous sinus area can result in cranial nerve palsies, with manifestations such as diplopia. Headaches are frequently described, and the sudden explosive onset of headache suggests possible hemorrhagic infarction of the tumor (apoplexy). Compression of the adjacent normal pituitary gland can cause hypopituitarism. Notably, diabetes insipidus is rarely caused by pituitary tumors and should instead raise the suspicion of a nonpituitary lesion, such as a cystic tumor (craniopharyngioma or Rathke cleft cyst) or a metastatic neoplasm.

Treatment of Pituitary Tumors

The goals of treating pituitary tumors are to remove or reduce the tumor mass (to decompress the local mass effects), correct pituitary hormone hypersecretion, maintain normal pituitary gland function, and prevent recurrence. Surgery is first-line therapy for macroadenomas and hypersecretory pituitary tumors, except prolactinomas. The neurosurgical approach is primarily transsphenoidal by way of an endonasal route. In experienced hands, transsphenoidal surgery is extremely safe. Permanent hypopituitarism, significant hemorrhage, and optic nerve injury occur in less than 5% of patients.

Radiation therapy is used primarily as adjuvant treatment for patients with residual disease or continued hormone hypersecretion after surgery. Irradiation is used as primary therapy only for patients who cannot undergo surgery. Because of the prolonged time needed to normalize hypersecretory states and shrink tumors, which often do not change in size after irradiation, surgery is preferred. Conventional, fractionated radiation therapy may take as long as 6 weeks. In contrast, stereotactic radiosurgery, intensity-modulated radiation therapy, and proton beam therapy may take only one or a few sessions and may be preferable from the standpoint of convenience. Complications of radiation therapy include long-term hypopituitarism in approximately 40% of treated patients and secondary neoplasms in approximately 1.5%.

Medical therapy is generally used adjuvantly after unsuccessful surgery, except with prolactinomas for which dopamine agonist therapy is first-line treatment.

KEY POINTS

- Surgery is first-line therapy for macroadenomas and hypersecretory pituitary tumors, except prolactinomas for which medical therapy with a dopamine agonist is preferred.
- Radiation therapy is used primarily as adjuvant treatment for patients with residual disease after pituitary tumor removal or continued hormone hypersecretion after surgery and as primary therapy for patients who cannot undergo surgery.

Hyperprolactinemia and Prolactinomas

Causes

Prolactin is secreted by the pituitary lactotroph cells under tonic inhibition by dopamine. This hormone is secreted in a pulsatile fashion, with the highest mean levels produced during sleep. Physiologic causes of hyperprolactinemia include pregnancy, nipple stimulation, exercise, and food intake. Therefore, in a woman with modest hyperprolactinemia, pregnancy should first be excluded, and the prolactin test should be repeated in a fasting state, with no strenuous exercise before testing. A routine breast examination usually does not raise serum prolactin levels enough to cause concern.

The most common cause of hyperprolactinemia is a prolactinoma, which is a benign adenoma. Microprolactinomas are less than 10 mm in diameter, and macroprolactinomas are 10 mm or greater in diameter. Although prolactinomas are the most common type of secretory pituitary adenoma (25%-40%), not all patients with hyperprolactinemia have prolactinomas (**Table 14**). Hyperprolactinemia is present in hypothyroidism, liver disease, and kidney failure, with a serum creatinine level typically less than 2 mg/dL (177 micromoles/L).

Many medications increase prolactin secretion by blocking dopamine release or action. This occurs most commonly with antipsychotic medications (including haloperidol, risperidone, and other antidopaminergic drugs), opiates, gastric motility drugs (metoclopramide and domperidone), and the calcium channel blocker verapamil. Estrogens increase prolactin secretion in a dose-response fashion, but the usual estrogen dose in oral contraceptives rarely causes symptomatic hyperprolactinemia.

Any hypothalamic or sellar mass that impinges on the pituitary stalk and disrupts dopamine flow can increase serum prolactin levels. Because serum prolactin levels correspond to prolactinoma size, the presence of a large sellar or suprasellar mass with only a modest increase in serum prolactin level (<150 ng/mL [150 micrograms/L]) usually indicates a cause other than a prolactinoma. Smaller prolactinomas also can result in a modest elevation of prolactin levels.

A patient with hyperprolactinemia without a clear secondary or drug-induced cause should be assessed by an imaging study (preferably, MRI of the pituitary gland) to exclude a mass lesion.

KEY POINT

- The most common cause of hyperprolactinemia is a prolactinoma.

Clinical Features and Therapy of Hyperprolactinemia and Prolactinomas

Common signs and symptoms of hyperprolactinemia include galactorrhea, oligomenorrhea, amenorrhea, and hirsutism in premenopausal women; erectile dysfunction in men; and decreased libido, infertility, headache, and osteopenia in both sexes. The presence of an underlying sellar, suprasellar, or hypothalamic mass may cause headache

TABLE 14. Causes of Hyperprolactinemia

Cause	Result
Pituitary disease	Prolactinomas
	Growth hormone–secreting tumors (cosecretion of prolactin or pituitary stalk effects)
	Nonfunctioning pituitary tumors (pituitary stalk effects)
	Lymphocytic hypophysitis (pituitary stalk effects)
	Empty sella syndrome (pituitary stalk effects)
	Cushing disease (cosecretion of prolactin or pituitary stalk effects)
Nonpituitary sellar and parasellar lesions	Craniopharyngioma
	Hypothalamic disease (sarcoidosis, Langerhans cell histiocytosis, lymphoma)
	Metastatic tumors to pituitary/hypothalamus
	Meningiomas
	Dysgerminomas
	Irradiation
Neurogenic	Chest wall or spinal cord disease
	Breast stimulation/lesions
Drugs	Psychotropic agents (butyrophenones and phenothiazines, monoamine oxidase inhibitors, tricyclic antidepressants, fluoxetine, molindone, risperidone, cocaine)
	Antihypertensive agents (verapamil, methyldopa, reserpine)
	Metoclopramide
	(Estrogen in conventionally used doses does not cause hyperprolactinemia.)
Other	Pregnancy
	Physiologic cause (coitus, nipple stimulation, strenuous exercise, stress)
	Hypothyroidism
	Chronic kidney failure
	Cirrhosis
	Macroprolactinoma
	Idiopathic
	Adrenal insufficiency
	Ectopic secretion

and mass effects, including peripheral visual field loss and ophthalmoplegia.

The indications to treat hyperprolactinemia in women include estrogen deficiency (in a premenopausal patient with amenorrhea and oligomenorrhea), infertility, bothersome galactorrhea, and hirsutism. In men, indications to treat include symptomatic testosterone deficiency, with symptoms such as erectile dysfunction, reduced libido, or gynecomastia. Headache, mass effects in patients with underlying sellar and suprasellar lesions, and osteopenia and osteoporosis due to gonadal insufficiency are indications to treat in both men and women.

When treatment is necessary, medical therapy with a dopamine agonist is the treatment of choice for most symptomatic patients (**Table 15**). A dopamine agonist can cause a rapid decrease in the serum prolactin level and shrinkage of the prolactinoma. More specifically, in as many as 90% of patients, it can normalize prolactin levels, reverse hypogonadism, and shrink tumors by at least 50%. Because of these rapid decreases in tumor size, dopamine agonists can be used as first-line therapy, even in patients with mild visual field defects, as long as visual acuity is not threatened by rapid progression of the tumor or recent tumor hemorrhage. Secondary causes of hyperprolactinemia must first be excluded because treatment of underlying conditions, such as hypothyroidism, should normalize the serum prolactin level. In patients with drug-induced hyperprolactinemia (prolactin levels rarely >200 ng/mL [200 micrograms/L]), especially those with psychiatric disorders, a change to a different medication is preferable but not always advisable, and dopamine agonists may be contraindicated because of reported worsening of psychiatric disease. When dopamine agonists are used in this setting, close consultation with the patient's psychiatrist is warranted. In women with

TABLE 15. Medical Therapies for Pituitary Adenomas

Type of Pituitary Adenoma	Medication
Prolactinoma	Cabergoline
	Bromocriptine
Adenomas causing acromegaly	Somatostatin analogues (octreotide, lanreotide)
	Cabergoline
	Pegvisomant
Adenomas causing Cushing disease	Ketoconazole
	Mifepristone
	Cabergoline
	Mitotane
	Etomidate (parenteral)
TSH-secreting adenomas	Somatostatin analogues (octreotide, lanreotide)
Nonfunctioning adenomas	Cabergoline
	Somatostatin analogues (octreotide, lanreotide)

TSH = thyroid-stimulating hormone.

prolactinomas who do not desire pregnancy, estrogen deficiency may be treated by estrogen replacement (in the form of an oral contraceptive, for example) alone to maintain normal vaginal health and bone mass. Although estrogen replacement may result in a modest increase in the serum prolactin level, the dose of estrogens used in most oral contraceptives poses little risk of prolactinoma enlargement. Nevertheless, the serum prolactin level should be monitored in these women.

Bromocriptine and cabergoline are the two oral dopamine agonists available in the United States to treat prolactin disorders: Bromocriptine is administered daily, and cabergoline is administered once or twice weekly. Although the more expensive drug, cabergoline is associated with more tumor shrinkage and normalization of prolactin levels and generally is better tolerated than bromocriptine. Adverse effects of dopamine agonists include gastrointestinal upset, nasal congestion, headache, and dizziness. Some studies have associated cabergoline with cardiac valve abnormalities, primarily in patients with Parkinson disease for which the cabergoline dosage is much higher than that used for prolactin disorders. Most subsequent studies have not shown a definitive connection between cabergoline use and cardiac valvular disease in prolactinoma management.

Permanent withdrawal of the dopamine agonist can be considered in some patients. The current recommendation is to consider withdrawal of the agonist if the prolactin level has been normal for at least 2 years and no visible tumor is seen on a pituitary MRI. Patients with these findings still require close follow-up evaluation with serial measurement of prolactin levels to assess for recurrence. Recurrence rates of up to 50% have been reported.

Neurosurgery is considered in patients with prolactinomas who are unresponsive to or poorly tolerant of dopamine agonist therapy and always should be considered in patients with a cystic prolactinoma because the cystic component will be unresponsive to medical therapy. Remission rates after transsphenoidal surgery have been reported to be as high as 80% for microprolactinomas but no more than 40% for macroprolactinomas. In patients with surgical remission, the long-term recurrence rate is approximately 20%. Radiation therapy, including stereotactic radiosurgery, is used less commonly for prolactinomas but is indicated for macroprolactinomas that do not respond to either medical or surgical treatment.

KEY POINTS

- Common signs and symptoms of hyperprolactinemia include galactorrhea, oligomenorrhea, amenorrhea, and hirsutism in premenopausal women; erectile dysfunction in men; and decreased libido, infertility, headache, and osteopenia in both sexes.
- For most symptomatic patients with hyperprolactinemia and prolactinomas, medical therapy with a dopamine agonist is usually the treatment of choice; permanent withdrawal of the drug can be considered in some patients, particularly those whose serum prolactin level has normalized (for at least 2 years) or whose tumor is no longer visible.

Pregnancy in a Patient with a Prolactinoma

Dopamine agonists have no documented risks of fetal malformations or other adverse outcomes in pregnancy; the collection of available data on the safety of bromocriptine is significantly larger than that for cabergoline. Nevertheless, in women taking a dopamine agonist, the standard management is to stop the drug after conception, except for women with a history of optic chiasmal compression with visual field compromise.

In normal women, the pituitary gland triples in size during pregnancy. Prolactinomas also may increase in size during pregnancy. Therefore, concern exists that the growing prolactinoma may cause worsening symptoms, including visual field defects and headache; pregnant women with prolactinomas are typically seen every 2 to 3 months for clinical assessment. If clinical evidence suggests symptomatic prolactinoma growth, then reinstitution of a dopamine agonist (with bromocriptine being the preferred agent in this setting), transsphenoidal surgical decompression, or delivery if the pregnancy is sufficiently advanced should be considered. Otherwise, dopamine agonist therapy is reinstituted after nursing is completed. Serial visual field testing may be useful to ensure maintenance of chiasmal function, although routine pituitary MRI is not necessary. Prolactin level measurement has no value during pregnancy.

KEY POINT

- Because prolactinomas may increase in size in pregnant women and lead to visual field loss, close clinical monitoring should be performed during pregnancy.

Other Disorders Involving Adenomas

Acromegaly

Causes and Diagnosis

Acromegaly is a disorder characterized by GH hypersecretion, most commonly by a GH-secreting pituitary adenoma. Like other pituitary tumor syndromes, acromegaly is usually sporadic, although it may occur in the setting of multiple endocrine neoplasia type 1 or familial acromegaly. When GH hypersecretion occurs before epiphyseal closure (in a child or adolescent), exaggerated linear growth of the long bones occurs, with resultant pituitary gigantism. When it occurs in adults after epiphyseal closure, acromegaly results. Clinical features include frontal bossing; prognathism, with dental malocclusion and increased spacing between the teeth; enlargement of the nose, lips, and tongue; skin tags; arthritis; carpal tunnel syndrome; sleep apnea; and excess sweating.

Patients with acromegaly have an increased incidence of type 2 diabetes mellitus, cardiovascular disease, hypertension, hypertrophic cardiomyopathy, and atherosclerotic arterial disease; they also have a two- to threefold increase in premature mortality. Because of an increased risk of premalignant polyps and colon cancer, screening with colonoscopy is recommended for all persons with GH excess.

The diagnosis of acromegaly is based on biochemical evidence of GH hypersecretion, typically with an elevated IGF-1 level. A random GH value is not useful because of the pulsatile nature of GH secretion. GH stimulates the liver to produce IGF-1, which serves as an integrated marker of GH levels. Measuring the IGF-1 level is a simple test and may be done randomly. Results correlate well with clinical symptoms. An oral glucose tolerance test also can be useful in a patient in whom the diagnosis of acromegaly is not clear. A nadir GH level of less than 1 ng/mL (1 microgram/L) excludes the disease.

A pituitary MRI can reveal the size and location of the pituitary adenoma and confirm the presence of mass effects. Approximately 80% of patients with acromegaly have macroadenomas. Patients with acromegaly should be referred to an endocrinologist for definitive diagnostic testing and therapy.

Treatment

The goals of therapy for acromegaly are to normalize the IGF-1 level, control the GH levels, reduce tumor bulk, prevent or decrease the number of comorbidities, and reduce the risk of premature death. Reduction of GH hypersecretion will lead to lessening of soft tissue abnormalities, but bony changes will persist. In addition, normalization of biochemical parameters will result in improvements in cardiac function, glucose control, hypertension, and sleep apnea and will help decrease the risk of premature mortality. The primary therapy is transsphenoidal surgery by an experienced neurosurgeon, which will normalize biochemical parameters in as many as 90% of patients with microadenomas and 40% of patients with macroadenomas.

Medical therapy is used mostly in the adjuvant setting in patients with residual disease after surgery (such as a residual tumor outside of the sella in the cavernous sinus, which is not surgically accessible). Somatostatin analogues are commonly used and normalize GH and IGF-1 levels in approximately 40% to 65% of patients. Long-acting preparations of octreotide and lanreotide are administered as monthly injections. Somatostatin analogues can shrink tumors modestly but usually not to the extent that dopamine agonists can shrink prolactinomas. Adverse effects of somatostatin analogues include diarrhea, abdominal bloating, and an increased risk of cholelithiasis. Cabergoline, a dopamine agonist, also may be considered because it is administered orally and is relatively inexpensive (compared with a somatostatin analogue). This drug normalizes biochemical parameters in 30% to 40% of patients with acromegaly, particularly those with modest disease activity.

A third type of drug used for medical therapy is a GH receptor antagonist, specifically pegvisomant, which blocks GH and thus causes a decline in IGF-1 values. Pegvisomant administered as a daily or twice weekly injection normalizes the IGF-1 level in more than 90% of patients and has associated clinical benefits. Safety monitoring of pegvisomant includes serial liver chemistry testing (elevations in serum values are uncommonly detected) and brain MRI (to monitor for tumor growth, which has been described with use of this drug). Pegvisomant is generally recommended as second-line medical therapy, either as a substitution for or in combination with a somatostatin analogue.

Radiation therapy also is used adjuvantly for management of residual disease after surgery, for disease unresponsive to medical therapy, or for patients in whom medical therapy is poorly tolerated.

KEY POINTS

- An elevated insulin-like growth factor 1 level in the setting of signs or symptoms of growth hormone excess is consistent with acromegaly.
- The primary therapy for acromegaly is transsphenoidal surgery to remove the causative growth hormone–secreting pituitary adenoma.
- Somatostatin analogues and dopamine agonists can be used adjuvantly in patients with acromegaly who have residual disease after surgery.

Cushing Disease

Cushing disease is Cushing syndrome caused by excess production of ACTH by a pituitary adenoma. Cushing syndrome is discussed in Disorders of the Adrenal Glands.

Clinically Nonfunctioning and Gonadotropin-Producing Adenomas

Clinically nonfunctioning adenomas are pituitary tumors that have no clinical manifestation of pituitary hormone hypersecretion. Because these tumors are not associated with a pituitary hormone hypersecretory syndrome, such as Cushing disease or acromegaly, they often are detected later and are macroadenomas at diagnosis. Therefore, these tumors often manifest with signs and symptoms of mass effects, such as headache, visual field loss, or hypopituitarism, but also may be detected incidentally. Occasionally, serum LH or FSH is produced at high levels, which results in high serum levels, and these tumors are referred to as LH- or FSH-producing gonadotroph adenomas.

Therapy of clinically nonfunctioning and gonadotropin-producing adenomas is largely surgical, with the goal of decompressing local structures, maintaining or improving pituitary function, and removing tumor mass. Indications for surgery include visual field loss, compression of adjacent structures, headache, hemorrhage into the tumor (apoplexy), and hypopituitarism. Visual field defects and pituitary dysfunction may improve after successful surgery, depending on the extent and duration of compromise. Radiation therapy is often used adjuvantly to control residual tumor after surgery. Medical therapy has been largely unsuccessful in tumor shrinkage in affected patients.

Incidentalomas

A pituitary incidentaloma refers to a sellar lesion that is detected during imaging for other reasons. Most incidentalomas are pituitary in origin, followed by cystic lesions, such as small craniopharyngiomas or Rathke cleft cysts (see Disorders of the Adrenal Gland, Incidentaloma). As with a sellar mass, a thorough history, physical examination, and laboratory evaluation should be performed for assessment of pituitary hormone hypersecretion (see Pituitary Tumors, Approach to a Sellar Mass). Notably, serum prolactin levels are often modestly elevated with any mass that causes pituitary stalk compression and disruption of dopamine flow. Macroincidentalomas should be evaluated with imaging studies for the presence of local mass effects and hypopituitarism. If the imaging study reveals that the lesion abuts the optic chiasm, then visual field testing should be performed.

Treatment (usually surgery) is indicated for patients with visual field compromise, oculomotor palsies, optic chiasm compression, or evidence of hormone hypersecretion. Surgery should be considered in the setting of tumor growth or loss of pituitary function. Therefore, monitoring with pituitary MRI at 6- to 12-month intervals for at least 3 years is warranted for a microadenoma to detect an enlarging tumor that may require surgery, with more frequent and protracted monitoring of any macroadenoma.

KEY POINT

- Treatment (usually surgery) is indicated for patients with pituitary incidentalomas causing visual field compromise, oculomotor palsies, optic chiasm compression, or hormone hypersecretion; surgery also should be considered in the setting of tumor growth or loss of pituitary function

Thyroid-Stimulating Hormone–Secreting Tumors

TSH- or thyrotropin-secreting pituitary adenomas are the least common type of pituitary tumor and reflect overproduction of TSH by the pituitary thyrotroph cells. The diagnosis usually is made during the evaluation of hyperthyroidism. In contrast to patients with primary hyperthyroidism, whose TSH level is suppressed, biochemical testing of patients with a TSH-secreting adenoma reveals an elevated T_4 level and an elevated or nonsuppressed TSH level. The diagnosis should be confirmed with a pituitary MRI. TSH-secreting pituitary adenomas are often macroadenomas, and the primary therapy is neurosurgical resection. For residual disease after surgery, medical therapy with a somatostatin analogue is highly effective in lowering the TSH level and controlling the hyperthyroidism in as many as 80% of patients. Adjuvant radiation therapy also may be needed for control of any residual tumor.

Disorders of the Thyroid Gland

Thyroid Physiology

The hypothalamic-pituitary axis controls thyroid hormone synthesis, production, and secretion by releasing thyrotropin-releasing hormone and thyroid-stimulating hormone (TSH) through a negative feedback loop involving thyroxine (T_4) and triiodothyronine (T_3). The thyroid gland primarily produces T_4 and a small amount of T_3. Approximately 85% of the body's circulating T_3 is produced by extrathyroidal peripheral conversion of T_4 by 5′-deiodinase enzymes, mainly in the liver and kidney. Most ambulatory patients with thyroid dysfunction have a normal hypothalamic-pituitary axis with either low serum TSH levels (indicating thyrotoxicosis) or elevated TSH levels (indicating primary hypothyroidism). Occasionally, a patient will have disease mediated by pituitary or hypothalamic dysfunction.

Only relatively small, unbound concentrations of T_4 and T_3 are biologically active (free T_4 and T_3). When bound to circulating proteins (primarily thyroxine-binding globulin [TBG] and, to a lesser extent, transthyretin and albumin), these hormones are inactive and act as large storage reservoirs. Conditions affecting protein binding of thyroid hormone can significantly affect measured levels of total thyroid hormone, which makes measurement of total T_4 and T_3 levels inaccurate and relatively uninterpretable (see later discussion).

Iodide is required for thyroid hormone synthesis, and adequate dietary iodine intake (from, for example, seafood, dairy products, iodized salt, or other iodine-rich food sources) is essential for thyroid hormone production. Although iodine deficiency is a worldwide health problem, iodine intake in the United States is generally adequate, according to the National Health and Nutrition Examination Survey (NHANES) study. The recommended iodine intake for persons older than 13 years is 150 micrograms/d but is higher for pregnant and lactating women (220 and 290 micrograms/d, respectively).

KEY POINT

- Adequate iodine intake is critical for thyroid hormone production.

Evaluation of Thyroid Function

Although various tests exist for evaluating thyroid function (**Table 16**), the serum TSH level is the most sensitive

TABLE 16. Common Tests of Thyroid Function

Measurement	Normal Range	Indication	Comment
Serum TSH	0.5-5.0 µU/mL (0.5-5.0 mU/L)	Suspected thyroid dysfunction	Misleading results in central hypothyroidism in which TSH level is inappropriately low or normal
Serum free T_4	0.9-2.4 ng/dL (12-31 pmol/L)	Suspected thyroid dysfunction with concern for pituitary dysfunction; or evidence of TSH abnormality	Variable normal ranges depending on assay
Serum free T_3	3.6-5.6 ng/L (5.6-8.6 pmol/L)	T_3 thyrotoxicosis	May substitute with total T_3 (In contrast to free thyroid hormone assays, total T_4 or T_3 measurement is affected by the serum-binding protein level.)
Serum thyroglobulin	3-40 ng/mL (3-40 µg/L)	Suspected subacute thyroiditis or suspected surreptitious ingestion of thyroid hormone or analogues; followed as a tumor marker in patients with well-differentiated thyroid cancer	Goal of an undetectable level in patients with prior thyroidectomy and radioactive iodine remnant therapy for differentiated thyroid cancer; difficult to interpret serum thyroglobulin levels in the presence of thyroglobulin antibodies
Serum TSI	0-125%	Graves disease; (euthyroid) ophthalmopathy	Not generally needed to diagnose Graves disease
Serum TBII	<10%	Similar to TSI	Not generally needed to diagnose Graves disease; detection of both blocking and stimulating antibodies against the TSH receptor
Anti–thyroid peroxidase antibodies	<2 units/mL	Suspected Hashimoto thyroiditis	Not generally needed; has predictive value for determining risk of development of overt hypothyroidism
RAIU	10%-30% of dose at 24 hours	Determination of the cause of thyrotoxicosis	Contraindicated in pregnancy and breast feeding

µg = microgram(s); µU = microunit(s); mU = milliunit(s); RAIU = radioactive iodine uptake; T_3 = triiodothyronine; T_4 = thyroxine; TBII = thyrotropin-binding inhibitory immunoglobulin; TSH = thyroid-stimulating hormone; TSI = thyroid-stimulating immunoglobulin.

indicator of thyroid function in ambulatory patients with a normal pituitary gland. Therefore, determination of the TSH level should be the first test used for patients with symptoms or signs that may be due to thyroid dysfunction. A free T_4 level may be measured concurrently with the TSH level if the clinical suspicion of thyroid or pituitary disease is high. In patients with a risk of pituitary gland dysfunction, such as those with a history of cranial irradiation, pituitary surgery, or massive head trauma, TSH and free T_4 levels should be measured to determine if central hypothyroidism is present.

Because levels of total T_4, which comprises both bound and free T_4, are affected by variations in binding protein levels, they may not accurately reflect free T_4 levels. Free T_4 is available for conversion to active T_3 but represents only a small fraction of the total T_4. Present techniques are able to estimate the free T_4 level with relatively high accuracy by determining the direct free T_4 level, by using equilibrium dialysis, or by using analogue assays.

If the TSH level is abnormal, measurement of other thyroid hormone levels is then recommended. For example, measurement of the free T_4 level is recommended to ascertain the severity of the patient's hypothyroidism if the TSH level is elevated. If the TSH level is suppressed, then measurement of free T_4 and T_3 levels is recommended to ascertain the severity of the patient's thyrotoxicosis. Most patients with thyrotoxicosis will have elevations of both levels; only rarely is the T_3 level alone elevated (T_3 thyrotoxicosis). Measurement of the T_3 level is not indicated in patients with hypothyroidism because the T_3 level is conserved and may remain within the normal range, even in patients with significant hypothyroidism.

The major thyroid antibodies are anti–thyroid peroxidase (anti-TPO) antibodies, antithyroglobulin antibodies, and anti-TSH receptor antibodies (thyroid-stimulating immunoglobulins [TSIs] and thyrotropin-binding inhibitory immunoglobulins [TBIIs]). Elevated titers of anti-TPO and antithyroglobulin antibodies are associated with autoimmune hypothyroidism (Hashimoto thyroiditis), and elevated levels of TSI or TSII antibodies are associated with autoimmune hyperthyroidism (Graves disease). In the presence of a normal TSH level, a positive thyroid antibody titer does not indicate the need for treatment but instead confers an increased risk for future thyroid dysfunction. In a person with a strong family history of autoimmune thyroid disease, measurement of anti-TPO antibody titers assesses future risk of developing hypothyroidism. Measurement of antithyroglobulin antibody titers is not as sensitive and thus is not the preferred test. Repeated or serial measurements of antithyroid antibody titers are not recommended because the degree of a titer's elevation does not indicate a need for treatment; only an abnormal TSH level does. An exception to this recommendation is in women who are or wish to become pregnant whose anti-TPO titer is positive and whose TSH level is in the normal range. This special population has a higher risk of infertility, preterm delivery, and miscarriage, and thus serial measurements are appropriate.

TSIs and TBIIs are highly associated with Graves disease. When the diagnosis of Graves disease cannot be made clinically in a patient with hyperthyroidism, measurement of the serum level of these antibodies is recommended, especially if radioactive iodine uptake studies are not available or if radioactive iodine exposure is contraindicated, as in pregnancy and breastfeeding.

Thyroglobulin is a glycoprotein that stores thyroid hormone within the thyroid gland. This glycoprotein is released into the blood stream, and serum levels can be elevated in both hyperthyroidism and destructive thyroiditis and decreased in factitious thyrotoxicosis after ingestion of exogenous thyroid hormone. Obtaining a serum thyroglobulin level is thus helpful diagnostically in patients who are euthyroid when assessing for factitious ingestion of thyroid hormone. Measurement of the serum thyroglobulin level also is recommended in patients with a history of well-differentiated thyroid cancer (papillary or follicular thyroid cancer) because the glycoprotein is an effective tumor marker used to detect thyroid cancer recurrence or persistence at the earliest possible stage. In patients who have undergone thyroidectomy and radioactive iodine ablation as initial treatment for thyroid cancer, detectable serum thyroglobulin levels likely indicate the presence of thyroid cancer cells. In most immunometric assays, thyroglobulin antibodies interfere with accurate measurement and lead to falsely low serum thyroglobulin levels. Therefore, whenever the serum thyroglobulin level is measured, thyroglobulin antibodies also are measured; if antibodies are present, the serum thyroglobulin level may not be reliable.

In clinical settings, calcitonin, which is secreted by C cells of the thyroid gland, is used primarily as a tumor marker in patients with a history of medullary thyroid cancer. Although routine measurement of the serum calcitonin level is not recommended in all patients with thyroid nodules or thyroid dysfunction, its measurement is recommended in patients with thyroid nodules who are at higher risk for medullary thyroid cancer, such as those with a positive family history of medullary thyroid cancer, with features of multiple endocrine neoplasia type 2 (MEN2), or with thyroid biopsy results suggestive of medullary thyroid cancer.

The radioactive iodine uptake (RAIU) test measures iodine uptake by the thyroid gland over a specified time period (for example, at 4 and 24 hours after iodine injection). Patients with thyrotoxicosis (hyperthyroidism) typically have an elevated (higher than 30% at 24 hours) or high-normal RAIU, which indicates endogenous production of thyroid hormones. In patients with subacute, silent, or postpartum thyroiditis or exposure to exogenous thyroid hormones, the RAIU will be very low (<5% at 24 hours), which indicates very little endogenous production. A thyroid scan will show diffuse uptake of the radioactive iodine in Graves disease or more focal uptake in toxic multinodular goiter or toxic adenoma. These radionuclide studies are contraindicated during pregnancy and in women who are breast feeding. Postpartum thyroiditis occurs in approximately 30% of women with an elevated serum thyroid peroxidase antibody level.

KEY POINT

- The serum thyroid-stimulating hormone level is the most sensitive indicator of thyroid function in ambulatory patients with intact pituitary function, and its measurement is the test of choice for detecting thyroid dysfunction.

Functional Thyroid Disorders

Thyrotoxicosis

The term thyrotoxicosis denotes thyroid hormone excess from any cause (**Figure 3**). Hyperthyroidism specifically refers to endogenous thyroid gland overactivity, most commonly caused by Graves disease, toxic multinodular goiter, or toxic adenoma. Fatigue, anxiety, insomnia, weight loss (despite increased appetite), tremulousness, tremor, heat intolerance, oligo- or amenorrhea, hyperdefecation, palpitations, shortness of breath or dyspnea on exertion, and muscle weakness are among the diverse signs and symptoms of thyrotoxicosis. The severity of symptoms may not correlate with the extent of thyroid hormone elevation. Older patients with apathetic hyperthyroidism, for example, may have minimal hyperadrenergic symptoms and instead may have atrial fibrillation or heart failure at presentation. Thyrotoxicosis may be associated with stare (due to lid retraction), dry itchy eyes, and tearing.

A thorough history and physical examination should be performed, as should appropriate laboratory and anatomic studies (**Table 17**). Typical laboratory findings of thyrotoxicosis include a suppressed TSH level and an elevated free T_4 and/or T_3 level; the TSH level is undetectable when the patient has overt hyperthyroidism. Anti-TPO and antithyroglobulin antibody levels also may be elevated with thyrotoxicosis. Thyroid ultrasonography is recommended for patients with thyrotoxicosis if a palpable nodule, a hypofunctioning area on an isotope scan, or a personal or family history of thyroid cancer is present.

Rarely, a patient may have a TSH-secreting pituitary tumor that stimulates the thyroid gland to secrete excessive T_4 and/or T_3. In contrast to more common causes of hyperthyroidism, TSH-secreting pituitary tumors may be associated with a detectable or even normal TSH level in the context of an elevated free T_4 or T_3 level. A pituitary MRI will show a pituitary tumor, and the α-subunit to serum TSH ratio will be greater than 1. Treatment is directed at the pituitary adenoma because thyroid gland–directed treatment typically is ineffective.

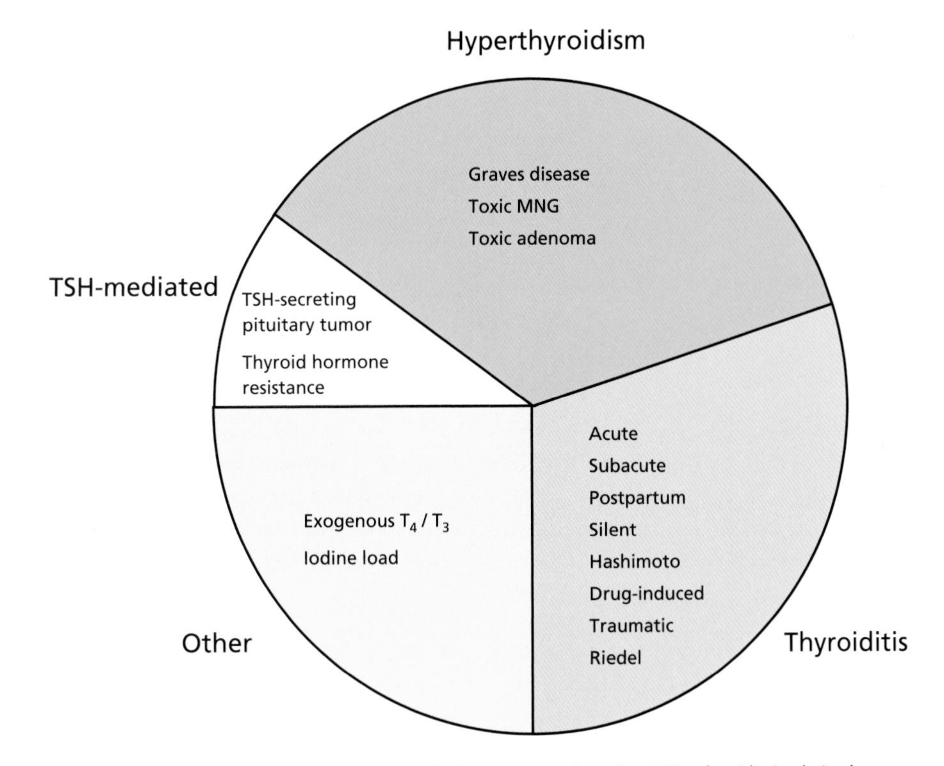

FIGURE 3. Types of thyrotoxicosis. MNG = multinodular goiter; T_3 = triiodothyronine; T_4 = thyroxine; TSH = thyroid-stimulating hormone.

TABLE 17. Classic Test Result Patterns in Thyrotoxicosis

Test	Graves Disease	Toxic Adenoma/ MNG	SAT Thyrotoxic Phase	Postpartum Thyroiditis	Exogenous T_4	Exogenous T_3	TSH-Secreting Pituitary Tumor	Reference Range
TSH	↓	↓	↓	↓	↓	↓	Normal or elevated	0.5-5.0 µU/mL (0.5-5.0 mU/L)
FT_4	↑	↑	↑	↑	↑	Normal/↓	↑	0.9-2.4 ng/dL (12-31 pmol/L)
FT_3	↑	↑	↑	↑	Normal/↑	↑	Normal/↑	3.6-5.6 ng/dL (5.6-8.6 pmol/L)
TPO Ab	+/–	+/–	+/–	+/–				<35 units/mL
TSI	+							<125%
TBII	+							<16%
RAIU	↑	↑	<5%	<5%	<5%	<5%	Normal/↑	10%-30% at 24 h

Ab = antibody; FT_3 = free triiodothyronine; FT_4 = free thyroxine; µU = microunit(s); mU = milliunits; MNG = multinodular goiter; RAIU = radioactive iodine uptake; SAT = subacute thyroiditis; TBII = thyrotropin-binding inhibitory immunoglobulin; TG = thyroglobulin; TPO = anti–thyroid peroxidase; TSH = thyroid-stimulating hormone; TSI = thyroid-stimulating immunoglobulin; ↓ = decreased; ↑ = increased; + = present; – = absent.

KEY POINTS

- Typical laboratory findings of thyrotoxicosis include a suppressed thyroid-stimulating hormone level (usually undetectable) and an elevated free thyroxine and/or triiodothyronine level.
- Radioactive iodine uptake by the thyroid gland is elevated in hyperthyroidism and decreased in destructive thyroiditis and exogenous thyroid hormone exposure.

Graves Disease

Graves disease is an autoimmune disease that can affect the thyroid gland, ocular muscles, orbital fat, and skin. Hyperthyroidism is by far its most common manifestation. In Graves disease, antibodies against the TSH receptor are produced. These antibodies stimulate autonomous thyroid gland function and secretion of excess T_4 and T_3.

Graves disease of the eye (ophthalmopathy) involves infiltration of the fibroblastic tissues of the ocular musculature, which leads to hypertrophy. Although the basic pathophysiology of Graves ophthalmopathy is not well understood, it is thought to involve stimulation of TSH receptors in orbital tissues (such as fibroblasts and adipose tissue), which results in increased cellular proliferation and local production of glycosaminoglycans. These processes result in inflammation and edema of extraocular muscles and an increase in retro-orbital tissues that causes proptosis, diplopia, chemosis, and, rarely, decreased visual acuity. Severity varies from mild to severe. Exophthalmos, orbital muscle dysfunction (as in diplopia), and conjunctival irritation may be important manifestations. Diagnosed clinically or with orbital CT or MRI, ophthalmopathy occurs in as many as 25% of patients with Graves hyperthyroidism but also may occur in patients with normal findings on thyroid function tests who have elevated TSH receptor antibodies.

Graves disease of the skin (pretibial myxedema) involves infiltration of the dermis (usually of the anterior shin). Graves disease of the skin occurs in less than 5% of patients but almost always in patients who already have Graves hyperthyroidism and eye disease.

The main risk factor for Graves disease is a family history of autoimmune thyroid disease. Physical examination of the thyroid gland may reveal the classic smooth, rubbery, firm goiter, often characterized by a bruit.

Adrenergic symptoms from thyrotoxicosis should be treated promptly with β-blocker therapy; cardioselective β-blockers, such as atenolol, are preferred. Propranolol decreases (minimally) T_4 to T_3 conversion, but the decreased amount of T_3 is thought to be relatively clinically insignificant. The benefits of the cardioselective action of β-blockers are considered more clinically relevant, and once-daily administration of atenolol leads to increased adherence to the medical regimen.

Graves hyperthyroidism can be treated with antithyroid drugs, radioactive iodine (^{131}I) ablation, or thyroid surgery. Two antithyroid drugs are available in the United States, namely, methimazole and propylthiouracil. Methimazole is the first choice because of its increased potency, once-daily dosing regimen, and lower incidence of serious adverse effects (mainly hepatic). Propylthiouracil is used in women in the first trimester of pregnancy (because of the teratogenicity of methimazole) or patients unable to tolerate methimazole.

Antithyroid drugs can be used either for short-term control of hyperthyroidism before thyroidectomy or radioactive iodine treatment or for longer periods (12-24 months) to achieve spontaneous disease remission. Whether this remission is due to the natural history of Graves hyperthyroidism or to treatment with antithyroid drugs is unknown, but 30% to 50% of treated patients will experience a remission. Patients with small goiters, mild elevations in their T_4 and T_3 levels, and lower initial drug doses are more likely to have a remission. Although most patients will have a recurrence of hyperthyroidism, prolonged remission occurs in 20% to 30% of patients with remission induced by antithyroid agents. Methimazole and propylthiouracil may start to lower free T_4 and T_3 levels within several days, but the full beneficial effect may not be seen for several weeks, depending on the severity of the hyperthyroidism and on the medication dosage. TSH suppression may persist even after a decrease in or normalization of free T_4 and/or T_3 levels. Therefore, serial TSH measurements should not be used to routinely monitor patients with hyperthyroidism.

Although generally well tolerated, antithyroid drugs have some notable adverse effects. Approximately 5% to 10% of patients taking antithyroid drugs develop drug rashes. Of more serious concern, these drugs are associated (albeit rarely) with agranulocytosis and hepatotoxicity. Propylthiouracil has been associated with elevated aminotransferase levels and a higher rate of serious hepatic injury than methimazole, and for that reason methimazole is preferred. A mild and usually reversible cholestatic pattern on liver chemistry tests can be seen with methimazole. Baseline liver chemistry studies and a complete blood count (with leukocyte differential) are thus recommended before initiation of antithyroid drugs. Patients taking antithyroid drugs who develop high fever, sore throat, prominent flulike symptoms, rash, jaundice, icterus, or other symptoms of serious illness should be immediately assessed for an adverse reaction to the medication.

A single appropriate dose of radioactive iodine can ablate an overactive thyroid in Graves disease in greater than 90% of patients. Adverse effects are uncommon, but patients may develop transient anterior neck pain or tenderness from radiation thyroiditis. An exacerbation of the thyrotoxic state for several weeks can occur because of the release of preformed hormone. The expected and desired outcome is permanent hypothyroidism, which typically occurs within 2 to 3 months of therapy, at which time thyroid hormone replacement therapy is begun.

Graves ophthalmopathy occurs more commonly in smokers and persons with a family history of the disorder. Its severity varies from mild to severe and may involve exophthalmos, inflammatory eye changes (chemosis, conjunctival injection, periorbital edema, or iritis), extraocular muscle palsies causing double vision, and optic nerve compression causing reduced visual acuity and (rarely) blindness. A primary focus in managing Graves ophthalmopathy should be to establish a euthyroid state. Because radioactive iodine treatment has been associated with (at least transient) worsening of Graves ophthalmopathy, its use is not recommended in patients with severe Graves ophthalmopathy. A thyroidectomy is preferred when definitive therapy for hyperthyroidism is required in a patient with severe Graves ophthalmopathy. Patients with advanced ophthalmopathy should be cared for by an experienced ophthalmologist, who may treat with local measures (such as artificial tears), corticosteroids, orbital irradiation, or orbital decompression, as necessary.

KEY POINT

- Radioactive iodine can effectively ablate an overactive thyroid in Graves disease in greater than 90% of patients, usually after a single dose; this treatment should be avoided in patients with significant Graves ophthalmopathy.

Toxic Multinodular Goiter and Toxic Adenoma

Toxic multinodular goiter and toxic adenoma result from an activating somatic mutation in the TSH receptor gene, which leads to autonomy of function and secretion of excess T_4 and T_3 from the nodule(s) affected. Recent iodine exposure from acute iodine loads, usually from iodinated contrast dye used in CT scans and angiographic procedures (such as cardiac catheterization), can induce thyrotoxicosis in patients with preexisting autonomy of thyroid function (Jod-Basedow phenomenon). MRI and ultrasonography should be used preferentially in patients with autonomy of thyroid function to avoid iodine exposure from iodinated contrast.

Physical examination usually reveals one or more palpable nodule(s) or overall gland enlargement. Therefore, obtaining a thyroid ultrasound is recommended to assess any detected nodule for cancer risk and the need for biopsy. Thyroid cancer is not often diagnosed in a patient with hyperthyroidism, but any nodule found should be considered for biopsy on the basis of its size and imaging characteristics (see later discussion of thyroid nodules). A multinodular goiter associated with hyperthyroidism can be treated with either radioactive iodine or surgery depending on multiple factors, including the size of the thyroid gland, evidence of obstruction (such as hoarseness with recurrent laryngeal nerve impairment), dyspnea, or local symptoms suggestive of cervical venous obstruction (such as engorgement of neck veins, especially when raising the hands above the head). Radioactive iodine therapy may effectively treat the hyperthyroidism, but surgery usually is indicated for large goiters with local compressive symptoms, except in patients who are not good surgical candidates. Radioactive iodine generally results in a modest decrease in goiter size (approximately 30% to 50%) over many months.

With toxic adenoma, a thyroid scan with radioactive iodine (^{131}I) will reveal a solitary overactive ("hot") nodule with suppression of the rest of the gland. With toxic multinodular goiter, the scan will reveal patchy uptake of radioactive iodine that is increased in autonomous regions and reduced outside those areas. In areas of decreased uptake, if a distinct "cold" nodule is present (confirmed as a nodule on a thyroid ultrasound), a biopsy is recommended before any treatment with radioactive iodine. Close monitoring with thyroid function tests is indicated approximately every 6 to 8 weeks.

Radioactive iodine ablation is the treatment of choice. Ideally, the hyperactive nodule(s) is(are) ablated over several months, and the normal thyroid tissue returns to normal function, which negates the need for lifelong thyroid hormone replacement therapy. The limitation of this treatment is the avidity of the nodule(s) for iodine. If the radioactive iodine uptake is not sufficiently high, the nodule(s) will not be ablated and the hyperthyroidism will persist. Surgical removal of the involved lobe (in patients with toxic adenoma) and total thyroidectomy (in patients with toxic multinodular goiter) is usually offered to those whose gland is not sufficiently avid for the radioactive iodine to result in ablation or who have proven thyroid cancer by biopsy. Antithyroid drugs modulate thyroid hormone production in toxic multinodular goiter and toxic adenoma and thus must be administered continuously to control hyperthyroidism.

KEY POINT

- Radioactive iodine ablation is the preferred treatment of toxic multinodular goiter and toxic adenoma.

Destructive Thyroiditis

Thyroiditis involves transient destruction of thyroid tissue, which disrupts follicles and causes the release of preformed thyroid hormone into the circulation. Forms of destructive thyroiditis include subacute (de Quervain), silent, and postpartum thyroiditis. Subacute thyroiditis most commonly occurs after a viral infection and usually involves severe thyroid and neck pain; fever, fatigue, malaise, anorexia, and myalgia are common. Silent thyroiditis is painless. Postpartum thyroiditis is a subset of painless autoimmune thyroiditis and can occur up to 12 months after parturition. It affects 5% to 8% of pregnant women in the United States and can recur with each pregnancy.

Subacute thyroiditis is associated with systemic signs of inflammation (such as an elevated erythrocyte sedimentation rate or C-reactive protein level), elevated serum free T_4 and T_3 levels, and a low serum TSH level. The disorder usually follows a classic course of approximately 6 weeks of thyrotoxicosis, a shorter period of euthyroidism, 4 to 6 weeks of hypothyroidism, and then restoration of euthyroidism. The severity and duration of an episode of destructive thyroiditis vary among patients. The clinical courses of silent and postpartum thyroiditis are more variable than that of subacute thyroiditis. Those who have had any type of thyroiditis are at increased risk for subsequent bouts. The hypothyroid phase is usually mild but can be prolonged or permanent and require thyroid hormone replacement. This more severe presentation is more likely to occur in patients with postpartum thyroiditis. When necessary, levothyroxine generally is given for approximately 6 months to allow time for thyroid gland recovery and then is tapered and stopped, with ongoing monitoring for recurrent hypothyroidism.

Figure 4 shows typical results of thyroid function and RAIU tests in patients with destructive thyroiditis. Antithyroid agents, such as methimazole or propylthiouracil, have no role in the treatment of destructive thyroiditis because endogenous production of thyroid hormone is very low. β-Adrenergic blocker therapy is recommended in specific patients during the thyrotoxic phase. NSAIDs are the first line of therapy for the neck pain of subacute thyroiditis; corticosteroid therapy is indicated in patients with severe pain unresponsive to NSAIDs and in patients with markedly elevated free T_4 or T_3 levels.

KEY POINT

- The hypothyroid phase of destructive thyroiditis can be so severe that replacement therapy with levothyroxine should be considered; this therapy is most commonly necessary in postpartum thyroiditis.

Drug-Induced Thyrotoxicosis

Multiple agents can cause thyrotoxicosis, including amiodarone (most common), interferon alfa, interleukin-2, and lithium carbonate. Iodine loads from drugs, iodinated contrast, or, in rare cases, significant povidone-iodine exposure can trigger hyperthyroidism in persons with preexisting or

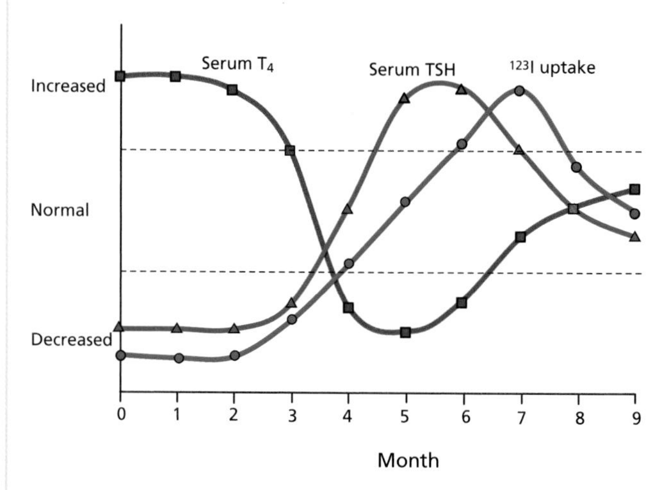

FIGURE 4. Triphasic changes in thyroid hormone levels associated with destructive thyroiditis. Measurement of serum T_4, serum TSH, and radioactive iodine (^{123}I) uptake shows thyrotoxicosis during the first 3 months, followed by hypothyroidism for 3 months, and then by euthyroidism. ^{123}I = radioactive iodine; T_4 = thyroxine; TSH = thyroid-stimulating hormone.

Adapted with permission from Pearce EN, Farwell AP, Braverman LE. Thyroiditis [erratum in N Engl J Med. 2003;349(6):620]. N Engl J Med. 2003;348(26):2650. [PMID: 12826640]

underlying thyroid autonomy. Lithium is more commonly associated with hypothyroidism than hyperthyroidism. Although the average diet in the United States contains approximately 150 to 200 micrograms/d of iodine, amiodarone contains 75 mg (75,000 micrograms) of iodine per tablet and has a half-life of months while stored in tissues. Persistent effects on thyroid function can be seen for up to 1 year after drug discontinuation.

Iodine-induced hyperthyroidism (type 1) and destructive thyroiditis (type 2) are the two forms of amiodarone-induced thyrotoxicosis. Type 1 thyrotoxicosis is more common in iodine-deficient geographic areas in patients with multinodular goiter and is treated with antithyroid agents. Type 2 thyrotoxicosis generally occurs in iodine-sufficient regions, such as the United States, and is treated with corticosteroid therapy. In practice, however, the distinction between the two types of disease is not clear, and many patients have overlapping disease, which is treated with both antithyroid agents and corticosteroids. In patients who are unresponsive to antithyroid drugs and corticosteroid therapy, a thyroidectomy may be recommended. These patients typically have multiple clinical issues and also are hyperthyroid. Therefore, the decision regarding thyroidectomy must be based on individual circumstances.

Because the management of amiodarone-induced thyrotoxicosis can be complex, involvement of an endocrinologist is appropriate. If possible, discontinuation of amiodarone should be attempted, although stopping the drug may (rarely) not be possible from a cardiac perspective. Consultation with the patient's cardiologist is thus important.

KEY POINT

- The most common cause of drug-induced thyrotoxicosis is amiodarone, which has high iodine content and can cause an iodine-induced thyrotoxicosis or destructive thyroiditis.

Subclinical Hyperthyroidism

Subclinical hyperthyroidism is characterized by a suppressed serum TSH level with concomitant T_4 and T_3 levels within the reference range. Repeat thyroid hormone levels should be obtained in 3 or 6 months to confirm that this is a continuing problem. Symptoms are mild, and most patients are asymptomatic.

Persistent mild hyperthyroidism has potential negative effects on cardiac function, the central nervous system, and bone mass. Which patients should receive treatment remains a matter of debate, but consensus supports intervention when the TSH level is less than 0.1 microunit/mL (0.1 milliunit/L), especially in patients who are 65 years and older, have tachyarrhythmias or heart disease, are postmenopausal with low bone mass, or are markedly symptomatic. The management of TSH levels less than the normal range but 0.1 microunit/mL (0.1 milliunit/L) or greater is less certain. Data suggest an increased risk of atrial fibrillation when the TSH level is less than 0.3 microunit/mL (0.3 milliunit/L). Postmenopausal patients with a TSH level less than 0.1 microunit/mL (0.1 milliunit/L) also have a higher risk of bone loss. When treatment is warranted, radioactive iodine ablation may be preferred. Often, however, the gland is not avid enough to trap sufficient iodine, and methimazole must be used to normalize the TSH level.

Hypothyroidism

A common disorder, hypothyroidism has a higher prevalence in women than men (2% versus 0.2%) and in persons with other underlying autoimmune diseases. The most frequent cause is Hashimoto thyroiditis, followed distantly by iatrogenic hypothyroidism (which can occur after radioactive iodine ablation for Graves disease, external beam radiation to the thyroid bed, or surgical removal of the thyroid gland). Amiodarone, lithium carbonate, interferon alfa, interleukin-2, and other medications can cause hypothyroidism; amiodarone causes hypothyroidism in approximately 10% of North Americans who take it chronically. Pituitary disease, pituitary tumors, and pituitary surgery can cause central hypothyroidism. Congenital forms of hypothyroidism, such as thyroid agenesis or dyshormonogenesis (a genetic defect in the synthesis of thyroid hormone), are rarer causes of hypothyroidism. Celiac disease, which occurs more frequently in patients with autoimmune thyroid disease than in the general population, is sometimes associated with inadequate levothyroxine absorption and resultant increased levothyroxine dosing requirements in patients with established hypothyroidism.

The numerous and largely nonspecific clinical manifestations of hypothyroidism include fatigue, reduced endurance, weight gain, cold intolerance, constipation, impaired concentration and short-term memory, dry skin, edema, mood changes, depression, psychomotor retardation, muscle cramps, myalgia, menorrhagia, and reduced fertility. Physical examination findings can include a reduced basal temperature, diastolic hypertension, an enlarged thyroid gland, bradycardia, pallor, dry and cold skin, brittle hair, hoarseness, and a delayed recovery phase of deep tendon reflexes. Some patients with mild hypothyroidism will exhibit few or none of these signs and symptoms. Results of laboratory studies can confirm hypothyroidism (**Table 18**). Measurement of serum TSH and total or free T_4 levels is required, but measurement of the serum T_3 level is generally not needed. Anti-TPO or thyroglobulin antibodies in the serum suggest Hashimoto thyroiditis as the cause of hypothyroidism. A thyroid scan and RAIU test are not useful. In patients with hypothyroidism in whom a goiter or nodule is palpated, imaging the gland with ultrasonography to evaluate for nodular disease requiring biopsy is appropriate.

Levothyroxine therapy is the mainstay of thyroid hormone replacement. The drug should be taken on an empty

TABLE 18. Classic Test Result Patterns in Hypothyroidism

	Hashimoto Thyroiditis	Subclinical Hypothyroidism	SAT Recovery Phase	Postpartum Thyroiditis Hypothyroid Phase	Central Hypothyroidism	Reference Range
TSH	↑	↑	↑	↑	↓/Normal	0.5-5.0 µU/mL (0.5-5.0 mU/L)
FT_4	Normal/↓	Normal	Normal/↓	Normal/↓	↓/Normal	0.9-2.4 ng/dL (12-31 pmol/L)
FT_3	Normal/↓	Normal	Normal/↓	Normal/↓	Normal/↓	3.6-5.6 ng/dL (5.6-8.6 pmol/L)
TPO Ab	+	+/–	+/–	+/–		<35 units/mL
TG Ab	+/–	+/–	+/–	+/–		<20 units/mL

Ab = antibody; FT_3 = free triiodothyronine; FT_4 = free thyroxine; µU = microunit(s); mU = milliunit(s); SAT = subacute thyroiditis; TG = thyroglobulin; TPO = anti–thyroid peroxidase; TSH = thyroid-stimulating hormone; ↓ = decreased; ↑ = increased; + = present; – = absent.

stomach 1 hour before or 2 to 3 hours after intake of food or calcium- or iron-containing supplements. Although attention recently has focused on liothyronine therapy and combination T_3-T_4 therapy that uses either thyroid hormone extract or synthetic T_3-T_4 combinations, most evidence to date shows that neither has a clinical advantage over traditional levothyroxine treatment. T_3 preparations have a short half-life and have been associated with acute spikes in serum T_3 levels, which are of particular concern in older adult patients or patients with cardiac abnormalities.

For patients receiving thyroid hormone replacement therapy, an appropriate target for the TSH level is 0.5 to 4.3 microunits/mL (0.5-4.3 milliunits/L). Discussion of the utility of aiming for a TSH level of 1.0 to 3.0 microunits/mL (1.0-3.0 milliunits/L) in most patients has occurred because of concerns that older patients and patients with positive antithyroid antibodies or a family history of thyroid disease tend to have higher TSH levels. However, no robust evidence supports this lower TSH goal. Patients age 80 years and older with subclinical or overt hypothyroidism are more likely to survive to age 89 years than their peers with normal or low serum TSH values. Increasing evidence suggests that the normal reference range for persons age 80 years and older is approximately 1 to 7 microunits/mL (1-7 milliunits/L), although further studies in this area are required. It is now recognized that patients in this age range generally should not be placed on exogenous levothyroxine solely for an elevated TSH level but that a complete consideration of the patient and the clinical context is necessary.

KEY POINT

- A target range of 0.5 to 4.3 microunits/mL (0.5-4.3 milliunits/L) for the thyroid-stimulating hormone level is appropriate for most patients with defined thyroid disease taking levothyroxine; a higher range may be appropriate for persons age 80 years and older.

Subclinical Hypothyroidism

In subclinical hypothyroidism, the serum TSH level is greater than the reference range, with concomitant serum T_4 and T_3 levels in the reference range. Patients typically have mild or no symptoms of hypothyroidism. The causes of subclinical hypothyroidism are the same as for overt hypothyroidism. Patients with subclinical hypothyroidism may have mild elevations in total cholesterol, LDL cholesterol, and even C-reactive protein levels, and some meta-analyses have shown an increased risk for atherosclerosis and cardiac events. However, evidence is insufficient to conclude that treatment with levothyroxine minimizes risks or improves outcomes when the TSH level is 10 microunits/mL (10 milliunits/L) or less. Treatment is recommended when serum TSH levels are greater than 10 microunits/mL (10 milliunits/L). Levothyroxine therapy also can be considered for patients who are markedly symptomatic, have a goiter, are pregnant or are planning to become pregnant, or have positive anti-TPO antibodies. The evidence currently is most compelling for treating pregnant patients with subclinical hypothyroidism; the normal ranges of the TSH level in patients who are pregnant are 0.1 to 2.5 microunits/mL (0.1-2.5 milliunits/L) in the first trimester, 0.2 to 3.0 microunits/mL (0.2-3.0 milliunits/L) in the second trimester, and 0.3 to 3.0 microunits/mL (0.3-3.0 milliunits/L) in the third trimester. Patients desirous of becoming pregnant should have a TSH level between 0.5 and 2.5 microunits/mL (0.5-2.5 milliunits/L).

KEY POINT

- Pregnant women or women desirous of becoming pregnant who have subclinical hypothyroidism should receive thyroid hormone replacement therapy if their thyroid-stimulating hormone level is greater than the normal range for their condition.

Structural Disorders of the Thyroid Gland

The primary structural disorders of the thyroid gland are nodules, goiters, and cancers. Rarer causes include aberrant or ectopic structural disorders, such as agenesis, hemiagenesis, substernal and lingual abnormalities, and struma ovarii.

Thyroid Nodules

Palpable thyroid nodules have a prevalence of approximately 5% in women and 1% in men in iodine-sufficient areas, such as the United States, and the prevalence increases with age. The differential diagnosis of thyroid nodules is varied (**Table 19**). Because most thyroid nodules are benign, the clinician's task is to identify malignant lesions (5%-15%) in the most accurate, efficient, and cost-effective manner (**Figure 5**). Factors associated with an increased cancer risk include age less than 20 or greater than 60 years, male gender, previous head or neck irradiation, a family history of thyroid (especially medullary) cancer, rapid nodule growth, and hoarseness. Pain is uncommon and is more often associated with benign than malignant nodules. The presence of a hard palpable nodule (or nodules), local cervical lymphadenopathy, fixation to adjacent tissue, and vocal cord paralysis increases the likelihood of cancer.

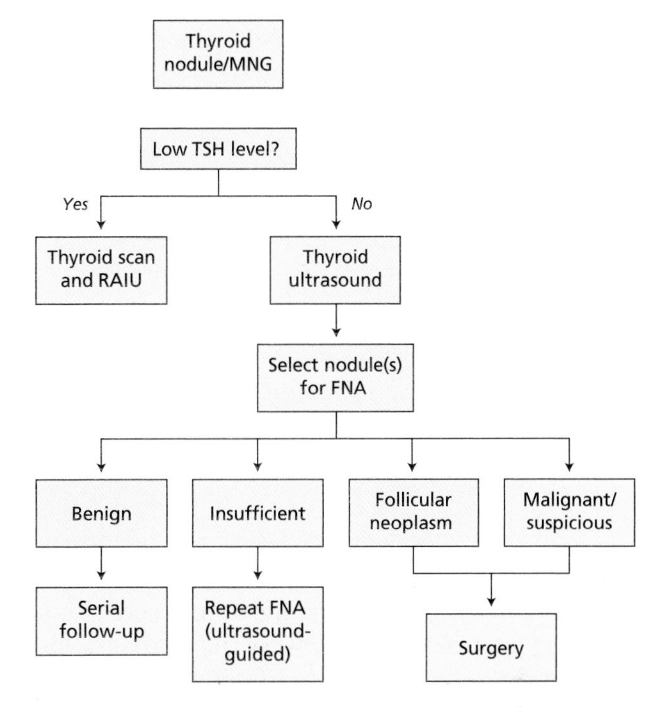

FIGURE 5. Evaluation of a thyroid nodule. Algorithm showing the suggested evaluation of a thyroid nodule. FNA = fine-needle aspiration; MNG = multinodular goiter; RAIU = radioactive iodine uptake; TSH = thyroid-stimulating hormone.

TABLE 19. Differential Diagnosis of Thyroid Nodules

Diagnosis	Notes
Benign	
Thyroid nodule	Adenomatoid hyperplasia, colloid nodule, adenomatoid nodule, follicular or Hürthle cell adenoma, and hyalinizing trabecular adenoma
Thyroglossal duct cyst	Midline cystic mass at level of hyoid bone; moves upward with protrusion of the tongue; may become infected; rarely malignant
Pyramidal lobe of thyroid	Cephalad projection of thyroid tissue from isthmus; may be palpable in autoimmune thyroid disease
Lipoma	Benign focal subcutaneous accumulation of fat
Dermoid cyst	Soft mass in the suprasternal notch
Teratoma	Type of germ cell tumor that may contain several different types of tissue (such as hair, muscle, and bone); mediastinal location at times
Branchial cyst	Soft lateral neck mass anterior to upper third of sternocleidomastoid muscle; usually seen in adults; cholesterol crystals in cyst fluid
Cervical lymphadenopathy	Possibly benign or may be associated with malignancy, including thyroid cancer
Malignant	
Thyroid cancer (primary)	Papillary (variants: follicular, diffuse sclerosing, columnar, tall cell) Follicular (variants: Hürthle cell [oncocytic]) Medullary Anaplastic
Thyroid lymphoma	Rapidly enlarging, firm neck mass; often bilateral; classically seen in older women with a history of Hashimoto thyroiditis
Metastatic cancer	Metastases of other primary cancer to thyroid (breast, melanoma, kidney)
Sarcoma	Tumors usually arising from connective tissue, with most being malignant

Measurement of the serum TSH level should be the first test performed in a patient with a thyroid nodule. If the level is suppressed, free T_4 and T_3 levels should be measured and a radionuclide scan considered. Treatment for incidentally discovered hyperthyroidism should then be undertaken. Less than 1% of hyperfunctioning nodules contain malignancy. If the TSH level is normal or elevated, thyroid ultrasonography should be performed as soon as possible to allow for timely fine-needle aspiration (FNA) biopsy, if indicated. Measurement of thyroid antibody levels is also appropriate, especially in patients with multinodular goiters or patients in whom autoimmune thyroid disease is suspected. Routine calcitonin measurement is not recommended for patients with thyroid nodules but is used to follow disease activity in patients with medullary thyroid cancer and should be considered in persons with a family history of medullary thyroid cancer. This test also should be considered in patients with MEN2 (or related disorders) or symptoms suggestive of this disease. The serum thyroglobulin level is the primary tumor marker in patients with well-differentiated thyroid cancer who have had thyroidectomy and radioactive iodine ablation.

Thyroid ultrasonography is the imaging test of choice in patients with palpable thyroid nodules and enables accurate detection and sizing of all nodules in the thyroid gland. Ultrasound characteristics are used to further delineate cancer risk in any detected nodule (**Table 20**). Additional characteristics suggestive of malignancy include size greater than 3 cm, hypoechogenicity, shape taller than wide, irregular infiltrative margins, microcalcifications within the nodule, and high intranodular vascular flow. Nodules that are purely cystic with a surrounding hypolucency (halo) or peripheral vascular flow are less likely to harbor cancer. Although ultrasound findings have reasonable specificity, they have poor sensitivity for predicting thyroid cancer and cannot by themselves be used to determine the presence or absence of cancer. CT and MRI without contrast are not routinely used but may sometimes be indicated, as in the presence of a substernal goiter, cervical lymphadenopathy, or tracheal compression. Use of intravenous dye with CT scans should be avoided, if possible, because this dye may induce hyperthyroidism in a patient with a multinodular goiter or interfere with other tests (such as an isotope radionuclide scan) or treatments.

TABLE 20. Ultrasound Characteristics of Thyroid Nodules

Cancerous Nodules	Benign Nodules
Microcalcifications	Comet tail
Increased intranodular vascularity	Increased peripheral nodule vascularity
Hypoechogenicity	Hyperechogenicity
Irregular border	Halo present
Taller than wide (sagittal view)	Pure cyst

A thyroid scan and RAIU test are appropriate in the presence of a suppressed serum TSH level because a toxic nodule (or toxic multinodular goiter) may be present.

FNA biopsy, performed either by nodule palpation or under ultrasonographic guidance, is essential in the evaluation of thyroid nodules. This procedure, when performed correctly, is a safe, simple, and relatively inexpensive method of determining the presence of cancer in a nodule. Its sensitivity is approximately 95%, with a false-negative rate of approximately 4%, depending to some extent on the nodule size. FNA biopsy is recommended for any nodule greater than 1 cm in diameter that is solid and hypoechoic on ultrasonography and for any nodule 2 cm or greater that is mixed cystic-solid without worrisome sonographic characteristics Consideration of biopsy may be appropriate for smaller nodules (at least 5 mm in diameter) in patients with risk factors, such as a history of radiation exposure, a family or personal history of thyroid cancer, cervical lymphadenopathy, or suspicious ultrasound characteristics. FNA biopsy is not routinely recommended for thyroid nodules less than 1 cm in diameter. Because large nodules (>4 cm) may be associated with sampling error, resampling of such nodules in the future is prudent, even when the nodule remains stable in size.

Patients with nodules greater than 4 cm who have associated worrisome clinical findings (such as abnormal cervical lymphadenopathy or hoarseness), radiologic features (such as a history of external radiation to the neck; see also Table 20), or laboratory findings but benign results of FNA biopsy can be considered for thyroidectomy. The Bethesda classification system has six possible cytopathologic diagnoses: (1) benign nodule, (2) malignant nodule, (3) nondiagnostic sample, (4) nodule suspicious for malignancy, (5) follicular neoplasm, and (6) follicular lesion of undetermined significance. The last three diagnoses imply an increased risk of malignancy, even though clearly malignant cells were not detected, and surgery is typically recommended to allow for histologic evaluation. Histopathologic analysis yields a diagnosis of frank malignancy in approximately 15% to 30% of these surgical samples.

Benign nodules should be monitored by periodic neck examination and ultrasonography (every 6-18 months), with repeat FNA biopsy recommended if the nodule has significant growth in the interval (50% by volume or 20% in two dimensions) or when subsequent ultrasound or clinical findings are suspicious. If the nodules are stable in both size and ultrasound characteristics after at least 18 months, the timing of clinical evaluation and ultrasonography could be extended to longer intervals (every 3-5 years).

Malignant nodules require prompt surgical removal. Surgical complications of thyroidectomy include hypoparathyroidism and recurrent laryngeal nerve paresis. The lowest complication rates are associated with thyroid surgery performed by experienced thyroid surgeons at large-volume medical centers.

The previous practice of giving patients levothyroxine to shrink thyroid nodules has been abandoned because of its inefficacy, the usefulness of FNA biopsy, and the morbidities associated with iatrogenic thyrotoxicosis.

KEY POINT

- In the evaluation of thyroid nodules that may be malignant, ultrasonography is recommended for imaging, followed by fine-needle aspiration biopsy for nodules larger than 1 cm in diameter.

Goiters

Multinodular Goiter

Multinodular goiters are more frequent with advancing age, iodine deficiency, and Hashimoto disease. Cancer risk is the same for a thyroid gland with a solitary nodule or with multiple nodules (approximately 5%-10%), and thus evaluation and management of multiple nodules also is basically the same as for a solitary nodule. In a multinodular gland, nodules with suspicious ultrasound characteristics are preferentially chosen for biopsy; in the absence of suspicious characteristics (see Table 20), the largest nodules are chosen for biopsy. Large multinodular goiters, especially those with a substernal extension, may present with local compressive symptoms, such as dysphagia, hoarseness, or even dyspnea. To confirm the presence and quantify the severity of mass effect caused by a multinodular goiter, barium swallow, direct vocal cord visualization, spirometry with flow volume loops, or neck and chest CT without contrast may be necessary. In select circumstances, radioactive iodine can be used to shrink (to a limited degree) a multinodular goiter but is not the first-line option in the United States, except in patients with thyrotoxicosis due to autonomous function. Thyroid surgery may be indicated if (1) local compressive symptoms are prominent and clinically significant, (2) malignancy is suspected, or (3) cosmetic intervention is desired by the patient.

Simple Goiter

A simple goiter is the presence of an enlarged thyroid gland without nodules. Dyshormonogenesis occasionally causes a simple goiter. On ultrasound, simple goiters can be homogeneous or heterogeneous. Patients with asymptomatic, stable simple goiters can be serially monitored clinically, but serial ultrasound in not recommended because of the lack of nodular disease. Primary thyroid lymphoma, which is rare and more likely to occur in older patients with Hashimoto thyroiditis, can present as a symptomatic rapidly enlarging goiter, usually with a very firm texture and often with systemic symptoms associated with temperature elevation. FNA biopsy of rapidly expanding firm goiters is recommended.

KEY POINT

- Barium swallow, direct vocal cord visualization, spirometry with flow volume loops, or neck and chest CT without contrast may be necessary to confirm the presence of and quantify the severity of mass effect caused by a multinodular goiter.

Thyroid Cancer

More than 95% of thyroid cancer is well differentiated and typically associated with long-term survival and low morbidity. The major forms of thyroid cancer are papillary (85%), follicular (10%), and medullary (4%); approximately 1% consists of poorly differentiated aggressive types, like anaplastic. Even less frequent are primary thyroid lymphoma and metastases to the thyroid of other cancers, such as breast cancer, kidney cancer, and melanoma. Medullary thyroid cancer can be a component of MEN2A and can be associated with hyperparathyroidism with hypercalcemia and hypertension due to a pheochromocytoma. Medullary thyroid cancer typically is characterized by plasmacytoid, spindle, round, or polygonal cells on biopsy. All patients with medullary thyroid cancer should have *RET* proto-oncogene sequencing after other appropriate evaluation, including measurement of plasma free metanephrine and normetanephrine levels to detect or exclude the presence of a pheochromocytoma.

Staging and prognosis of well-differentiated thyroid cancer (papillary and follicular) are based on American Joint Committee on Cancer criteria, which include age (<45 or ≥45 years), primary tumor size, local and distant metastases, and capsular and lymphovascular invasion. In brief, in patients younger than 45 years, stage I disease includes thyroid cancer of any size, with or without cervical lymph node involvement and without distant spread; stage II refers to patients who have distant spread of disease. In patients 45 years and older, stage I thyroid cancer denotes tumors 2 cm or less in size without local invasion or positive cervical lymph nodes, stage II denotes tumors greater than 2 cm but no more than 4 cm in size without local invasion or positive cervical lymph nodes, stage III denotes tumors larger than 4 cm in size with slight local invasion with or without cervical lymph node involvement, and stage IV denotes thyroid cancer that either has invaded nearby neck structures or superior mediastinal lymph nodes or may or may not have invaded local tissues or lymph nodes but has spread to distant sites.

Patients with stage I and II disease tend to do very well, with patients younger than 40 years having a less than 2% mortality rate at 30 years. Patients with stage III and IV disease have 10-year survival rates of approximately 82% and 38%, respectively. Treatment of well-differentiated thyroid cancer involves a combination of thyroidectomy, radioactive iodine therapy, and suppression of TSH secretion with levothyroxine therapy. Radioactive iodine therapy frequently is administered for stage III and IV disease, especially with lymph node involvement, to decrease the risk of recurrence and death.

The extent of thyroid gland removal required varies and generally depends on tumor size, with solitary tumors less than 1 cm in diameter generally effectively managed by lobectomy. Patients with larger tumors, multifocal disease, known cervical lymph node metastasis, and a history of irradiation are best treated with total or near-total thyroidectomy. Suppression of TSH secretion has been associated with long-term improvement in morbidity and mortality in patients with stage III and IV disease. The degree of TSH suppression targeted varies with risk of recurrence and is based on several factors, including stage of disease, presence of residual tumor, time since original diagnosis, and patient tolerance of TSH suppression.

The 2009, American Thyroid Association Guidelines regarding thyroid cancer recommended that patients with persistent disease should have a goal TSH level of less than 0.1 microunit/mL (0.1 milliunit/L). Patients who are currently disease free but at high risk of recurrence should have a goal TSH level of 0.1 to 0.5 microunit/mL (0.1-0.5 milliunit/L) for 5 to 10 years, and those who are disease free and at low risk of recurrence should have a goal TSH level of 0.3 to 2.0 microunits/mL (0.3-2.0 milliunits/L).

KEY POINT

- Treatment of well-differentiated thyroid cancer involves a combination of thyroidectomy, radioactive iodine therapy, and suppression of TSH secretion with levothyroxine therapy.

H Effects of Nonthyroidal Illness on Thyroid Function Tests

Nonthyroidal illness can alter the results of thyroid function tests, an effect referred to as the euthyroid sick syndrome, which is more common in critically ill patients but can occur in more stable hospitalized patients. Most commonly, T_3 levels decline sharply, and reverse T_3 (an inactive thyroid hormone metabolite) levels increase. Free T_4 levels typically decrease but remain in the reference range. A frankly low free T_4 level is usually seen in critical illness and is a poor prognostic indicator. The TSH response is less consistent, with low, normal, and elevated levels reported. However, in a patient with a nonthyroidal illness only, it is unusual for TSH levels to become undetectable or increase to greater than approximately 10 microunits/mL (10 milliunits/L) because these elevated TSH levels suggest the presence of primary hypothyroidism.

Cytokines and various other inflammatory mediators released during systemic illness also play a role in euthyroid sick syndrome. The thyroid hormone patterns seen in nonthyroidal illness appear to be an adaptive response to mitigate catabolism associated with severe physiologic stress and provide a protective effect by way of transient central hypothyroidism. Intervention with thyroid hormone therapy has not proved beneficial and is not indicated in patients with altered thyroid function test results most likely caused by nonthyroidal illness. Almost all patients have a normal TSH level after their recovery, and all thyroid hormone levels typically normalize by 8 weeks after recovery. H

KEY POINT

- Nonthyroidal illness (usually severe) can alter thyroid function test results, an effect known as euthyroid sick syndrome; results usually normalize by 8 weeks after recovery from the illness.

Thyroid Function and Disease in Pregnancy

Abnormal thyroid function during pregnancy can greatly affect the health of both mother and fetus. Elevated estrogen levels increase the TBG level, which increases the total T_4 and T_3 levels. To compensate for the increase in the TBG level and altered T_4 and T_3 kinetics and to keep the free T_4 level stable, women who take levothyroxine for hypothyroidism usually require an increased dosage (approximately 30%-50%) during pregnancy. Increasing the levothyroxine dosage at the start of pregnancy or early in pregnancy is recommended to anticipate this increased requirement, maintain normal maternal thyroid function, and provide adequate thyroid hormone to the fetus.

During the first trimester of pregnancy, increased levels of human chorionic gonadotropin (HCG) can stimulate thyroid hormone production by way of cross-reactivity with the TSH receptor because of the common α-subunit shared by HCG and TSH. Serum TSH levels may decrease to low-normal or even below-normal ranges in the first trimester, but this is rarely associated with thyrotoxicosis. The TSH level slowly increases to normal by 16 weeks' gestation.

Maternal or fetal thyroid hormone deficiency can negatively affect fetal neurocognitive development. The goal TSH level during the first trimester is approximately 0.1 to 2.5 microunits/mL (0.1-2.5 milliunits/L); in the second and third trimesters, it is approximately 0.1 to 3.0 microunits/mL (0.1-3.0 milliunits/L). The value of general prenatal maternal evaluation of thyroid function is still debated. At a minimum, thyroid function tests should be obtained in patients with strong risk factors for thyroid disease, and close monitoring is required in those with a known history of a thyroid disorder. In women planning pregnancy who have known hypothyroidism, the TSH level should be maintained at 0.5 to 2.5 microunits/mL (0.5-2.5 milliunits/L) during the preconception period.

Pregnant women receiving thyroid replacement therapy should have their thyroid hormone status monitored frequently to assess the effect of levothyroxine dose adjustments. Levothyroxine requirements increase in most patients with hypothyroidism during pregnancy. The levothyroxine dosage can be increased by giving two extra doses a week. Another reasonable approach is to attempt to maintain the TSH level at less than 2.5 microunits/mL (2.5 milliunits/L) by making frequent adjustments to the dosage, as dictated by the results of laboratory studies every 2 weeks during the first half of pregnancy and every 4 to 6 weeks during the second half. The increased levothyroxine requirements occur mainly in the first trimester of pregnancy.

Because some symptoms of thyrotoxicosis (tachycardia, heat intolerance, fatigue) overlap with symptoms of normal pregnancy, changes in thyroid function test results associated with normal pregnancy may be difficult to discern from true thyrotoxicosis. Compounding this difficulty is the contraindication during pregnancy (and in women who are breastfeeding) to some diagnostic techniques, such as thyroid scans and radioiodine uptake tests, to avoid radiation exposure of the fetus. The presence of a moderate goiter or ophthalmopathy can indicate the presence of Graves disease. Although HCG–mediated TSH receptor stimulation tends to resolve by 16 weeks' gestation, changes of primary thyroid disease persist longer, albeit with some improvement. When true hyperthyroidism is diagnosed during pregnancy, prompt referral to an endocrinologist and a high-risk obstetrician is recommended.

KEY POINT

- Thyroid scans and radioactive iodine uptake testing are contraindicated in pregnant patients and in patients who are breastfeeding or have done so recently.

H

Thyroid Emergencies

Whereas most thyroid conditions are not urgent, thyroid storm and myxedema coma are life-threatening conditions that require prompt diagnosis and intervention, typically in consultation with an endocrinologist.

Thyroid Storm

Thyroid storm is a life threatening condition that presents as severe thyrotoxicosis, coupled with secondary systemic decompensation. This disorder can be differentiated from other forms of thyrotoxicosis by the presence of temperature elevation, significant tachycardia, heart failure, gastrointestinal disorders, diarrhea, nausea, vomiting, and sometimes jaundice. Neurologically, agitation and disorientation can occur. Thyroid storm most commonly occurs in Graves disease and has a higher frequency in younger women, but it also can be due to a toxic adenoma or multinodular goiter. This disorder can occur in long-standing, untreated hyperthyroidism but usually is precipitated by an underlying condition, such as surgery, infection, trauma, parturition, acute iodine exposure, radioactive iodine (^{131}I) therapy, or ingestion of medications, including salicylates and pseudoephedrine. Signs include marked hyperthermia, marked sinus and supraventricular tachycardia, severe mental status changes (from psychosis to coma), features of heart failure (such as pulmonary edema), and gastrointestinal and hepatic abnormalities (such as nausea and vomiting, jaundice, hepatic failure).

Successful treatment of thyroid storm reduces thyroid hormone production and secretion by the thyroid gland, decreases peripheral conversion of T_4 to bioactive T_3, addresses associated adrenergic and thermoregulatory changes, treats all precipitating factors, and aggressively reverses any systemic decompensation. Definitive therapy for the causative thyroid disorder should be considered when the patient is stable. A combination of antithyroid drugs (propylthiouracil or methimazole), iodine solution, high-dose corticosteroids, β-blockers, and (rarely) lithium are used for treatment. Compared with atenolol and methimazole, propranolol and propylthiouracil have a slight added benefit of reducing T_4 to T_3 conversion, although the clinical benefits of this advantage are not clear because high-dose corticosteroid therapy is a potent inhibitor of this conversion. Intravenous corticosteroids also are routinely administered until it is clear that endogenous adrenal function is adequate to ensure that adrenal insufficiency is not present or has not been precipitated by levothyroxine therapy. Even with aggressive therapy and supportive measures, mortality rates are as high as 15% to 20%. H

KEY POINT

- Therapeutic interventions for thyroid storm are a combination of antithyroid drugs, iodine solution, corticosteroids, β-blockers, and (rarely) lithium.

Myxedema Coma

H

A severe manifestation of hypothyroidism, often to the point of systemic decompensation, myxedema coma is potentially life threatening, especially without prompt diagnosis and treatment. Myxedema coma occurs more frequently in women than men and in older adult patients. Onset is usually insidious. This disorder usually is seen in patients with a history of hypothyroidism, thyroidectomy, or radioactive iodine therapy. Primary hypothyroidism accounts for greater than 95% of all occurrences, but episodes also have been reported in patients with central hypothyroidism. Precipitating factors are numerous and varied, including chronic poor (or no) adherence to daily thyroid hormone replacement therapy, stroke, heart failure, myocardial infarction, infection, metabolic disturbances, cold exposure (more common in the winter), trauma, gastrointestinal bleeding, acidosis, and hypoglycemia.

The two most common findings of myxedema coma are mental status changes and hypothermia. Mental status changes

H CONT.

occur in greater than 90% of patients and can manifest as lethargy, stupor, coma, or sometimes psychosis ("myxedema madness"). Hypothermia (temperature less than 34.4 °C [94.0 °F]) occurs in 88% of patients; the lower the temperature, the worse the prognosis. Virtually all organ systems and biochemical pathways are slowed by myxedema coma. Hypoventilation leading to hypoxemia and hypercapnia are also common findings, as are (to a lesser degree) bradycardia, hypotension, hyponatremia, and hypoglycemia. The mortality rate of myxedema coma is high (20% or greater). Older patients generally do worse, as do patients with evidence of severe illness (high Acute Physiology and Chronic Health Evaluation [APACHE] Scale score, low Glasgow Coma Scale score).

If myxedema coma is suspected, the TSH and free T_4 levels should be checked promptly. The diagnosis is made clinically, but the TSH level is typically markedly elevated and the free T_4 level is usually low. A random cortisol level also should be obtained to assess for concomitant adrenal insufficiency.

No consensus exists about the most effective thyroid hormone replacement regimen for myxedema coma. Intravenous levothyroxine has traditionally been administered, with an initial bolus of 200 to 500 micrograms followed by daily doses between 50 and 100 micrograms until transition to oral administration is feasible. These relatively high doses of levothyroxine are recommended to replenish the depleted tissue stores of thyroid hormone. However, they may be associated with cardiac irregularities and should be used cautiously, with a more common starting dose of 100 to 200 micrograms used, especially in patients with known or suspected cardiac disorders. Supplementation with liothyronine (oral or intravenous) at doses between 5 and 10 micrograms twice daily has been proposed but is controversial, especially because a definitive benefit of this therapy has not been shown. If liothyronine is used, it should be administered cautiously in lower doses and in combination with levothyroxine. If high doses of levothyroxine are administered for myxedema coma (or any severe hypopituitarism), concurrent treatment with high-dose glucocorticoids (such as hydrocortisone) is recommended until adrenal insufficiency is excluded and appropriate adrenal function is confirmed. As with thyroid storm, all underlying precipitating conditions must be addressed. H

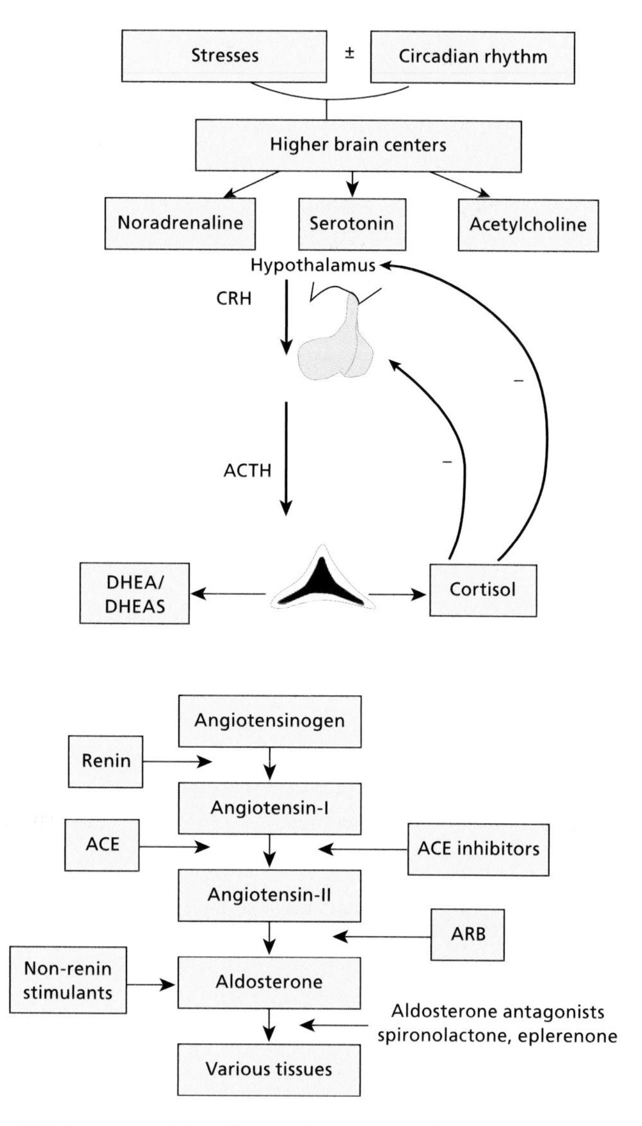

FIGURE 6. Regulation of hypothalamic-pituitary-adrenal function and the renin-angiotensin system. *Top*, hypothalamic secretion of CRH is mediated by several neurotransmitters in response to changes in stress levels and circadian rhythm. ACTH stimulates the zona fasciculata of the adrenal cortex to synthesize cortisol, which in turn feeds back centrally by negatively inhibiting CRH and ACTH secretion. ACTH also stimulates zona reticularis to synthesize the adrenal androgens DHEA and DHEAS, but these hormones do not participate in the feedback mechanism. *Bottom*, regulation of the renin-angiotensin system involves aldosterone being secreted by the outermost layer of the adrenal cortex (zona glomerulosa) as a result of angiotensin II stimulation. The site of action of commonly used drugs that interfere with the system is shown. ACTH = adrenocorticotropic hormone; ARB = angiotensin receptor blocker; CRH = corticotropin-releasing hormone; DHEA = dehydroepiandrosterone; DHEAS = DHEA sulfate.

Disorders of the Adrenal Glands

Adrenal Insufficiency

Physiologic Regulation of Adrenal Function

The three layers of the adrenal cortex secrete three distinct classes of corticosteroids under separate regulatory mechanisms (**Figure 6**). Cortisol is the primary glucocorticoid and is produced by the zona fasciculata; dehydroepiandrosterone (DHEA) and its sulfated form, DHEA sulfate (DHEAS), are the primary adrenal androgens and are produced by the zona reticularis. The production of these corticosteroids is tightly controlled by pituitary secretion of adrenocorticotropic hormone (ACTH), which, in turn, is regulated by hypothalamic secretion of corticotropin-releasing hormone (CRH).

Secreted cortisol provides negative feedback on pituitary synthesis of ACTH and hypothalamic synthesis of CRH. This integrated system keeps cortisol secretion tightly controlled. The adrenal androgens DHEA and DHEAS do not participate in negative feedback on pituitary and hypothalamic secretion. Aldosterone, the primary adrenal mineralocorticoid, is produced by the zona glomerulosa and is regulated by the renin-angiotensin system. Renin, an enzyme secreted by the kidney, regulates the conversion of angiotensinogen to angiotensin I. Angiotensin I is converted into angiotensin II, which stimulates aldosterone secretion.

Description, Causes, and Diagnosis of Adrenal Insufficiency

Adrenal insufficiency is a clinical and biochemical entity characterized by partial or complete loss of secretion of adrenocortical steroids (corticosteroids). Diseases involving the adrenal glands themselves, such as autoimmune adrenalitis, lead to primary adrenal insufficiency, in which secretion of all corticosteroids (aldosterone, cortisol, DHEA, and DHEAS) is impaired. In contrast, central adrenal insufficiency is caused either by ACTH secretion by a disease process that destroys the pituitary corticotrophs (secondary adrenal insufficiency) or by a hypothalamic disease that destroys the cells secreting CRH (tertiary adrenal insufficiency). Distinguishing between the secondary and tertiary forms of the disease can be difficult.

The most common cause of adrenal insufficiency in adults is the use of exogenous glucocorticoids administered chronically for their anti-inflammatory effect in the treatment of other medical conditions. Chronic glucocorticoid use leads to suppression of CRH and ACTH secretion centrally and, ultimately, to atrophy of the zona fasciculata and zona reticularis in the adrenal glands, with impairment of their ability to secrete physiologically regulated cortisol, particularly under stress conditions. Secretion of aldosterone from the zona glomerulosa is not affected because it is under control of the renin-angiotensin system. Common causes of primary and central adrenal insufficiency are shown in **Table 21**.

The clinical manifestations of adrenal insufficiency are often insidious, with fatigue and malaise being the dominant symptoms (**Table 22**); a high degree of clinical suspicion may be needed to pursue the diagnosis in the presence of subtle

TABLE 21. Causes of Adrenal Insufficiency

Primary Adrenal Insufficiency	Central Adrenal Insufficiency
Autoimmune adrenalitis	Exogenous glucocorticoid therapy
Infection (tuberculosis, mycosis, bacterial, HIV-associated)	Hypothalamic/pituitary diseases or surgery
Metastatic cancer	Cranial irradiation
Adrenal hemorrhage (acute disease)	Chronic administration of drugs with glucocorticoid activity (such as megestrol)
Medications (such as etomidate, ketoconazole, mitotane, and metyrapone)	

TABLE 22. Characteristics of Adrenal Insufficiency

Deficiency	Type of Adrenal Insufficiency	Symptoms	Signs	Crucial Laboratory Findings	Additional Laboratory Findings
Cortisol	Primary and central	Fatigue, nausea, anorexia, weight loss, abdominal pain, arthralgias, low-grade fever	Hyperpigmentation (in primary disease only),[a] slight decrease in blood pressure (unless cortisol deficiency is complete)	Low basal serum cortisol level (<5 µg/dL [138 nmol/L]) with suboptimal response (<18.0 µg/dL [497 nmol/L]) to cosyntropin; high plasma ACTH level (in primary disease only)	Hyponatremia; normal potassium level; azotemia; anemia; leukopenia, with high percentage of eosinophils and lymphocytes; hypoglycemia
Aldosterone	Primary	Salt craving, postural dizziness	Hypotension, dehydration	Low serum aldosterone level and high plasma renin activity	Hyponatremia; hyperkalemia
Adrenal androgen	Primary and central	Decreased libido	Decreased pubic/axillary hair (only in women)	Low serum DHEA and DHEAS levels	—

ACTH = adrenocorticotropic hormone; DHEA = dehydroepiandrosterone; DHEAS = dehydroepiandrosterone sulfate; µg = microgram(s).

[a]Results from increased secretion of ACTH and its precursor, pro-opiomelanocortin. An increase in the latter leads to increased secretion of one of its products, melanocortin-stimulating hormone, which causes the hyperpigmentation.

systemic symptoms. However, adrenal insufficiency also may present dramatically, as in addisonian crisis, in which hypotension and vascular collapse predominate. This presentation can be precipitated by severe stresses, such as concurrent illnesses or surgical procedures. Adrenal crisis is most common with primary adrenal insufficiency in which loss of both glucocorticoids and mineralocorticoids occurs and leads to vascular instability; it is less common in patients with secondary adrenal insufficiency (except under extreme circumstances) because the renin-aldosterone system is usually intact and profound hypotension and hypovolemia do not occur.

Adrenal insufficiency should be suspected in patients with suggestive signs or symptoms, especially those at increased risk for the disease (see Table 22). Adrenal insufficiency is diagnosed by demonstrating a low basal serum cortisol level that does not increase appropriately after stimulation with the ACTH analogue cosyntropin. Random serum cortisol levels vary, depending on the time of day, because of the pulsatile nature of ACTH secretion and the normal diurnal variation of cortisol levels (with the highest levels occurring in the morning and lowest in the evening). Random levels also fluctuate with the degree of physical stress present at the time of measurement. Assays for serum cortisol measurement determine the total (protein-bound and free) cortisol level. Because greater than 90% of the cortisol in the circulation is protein bound (to corticosteroid-binding globulin and albumin), an increase in binding proteins (as occurs during pregnancy or with estrogen therapy) results in increased serum cortisol levels without altering the physiologically important free hormone levels. Similarly, patients with hypoproteinemia have lower total serum cortisol levels despite having normal serum free cortisol levels. This becomes clinically relevant in critically ill patients who are hypoproteinemic (see later discussion).

When primary adrenal insufficiency is present, serum cortisol and aldosterone levels are low, but plasma renin activity and ACTH levels are increased. A minimal or no increase in the serum cortisol level from baseline in response to cosyntropin stimulation, preferably performed in the morning, confirms the diagnosis. Healthy persons increase their serum cortisol levels to greater than 18.0 micrograms/dL (497 nmol/L) after cosyntropin, 250 micrograms intravenously, is administered. Patients with central adrenal insufficiency have low plasma ACTH levels and normal aldosterone levels. Using a lower dose of cosyntropin (1 microgram instead of 250 micrograms) results in a modest increase in the plasma ACTH level that is similar to that achieved during insulin-induced hypoglycemia and, therefore, improves the diagnostic accuracy of the test in patients with central adrenal insufficiency. Serum levels of DHEA and DHEAS are characteristically low in both primary and central adrenal insufficiency.

If a diagnosis of central adrenal insufficiency is suspected on the basis of biochemical findings, imaging of the pituitary gland (preferably with MRI) should be performed to exclude other possible causes, such as a pituitary adenoma and any other sellar or perisellar mass.

Treatment of Adrenal Insufficiency

The goal of adrenal insufficiency treatment is to offer appropriate hormone replacement that closely mimics physiologic conditions, whenever possible, and to educate patients about their disease and the need to adjust their dosages with concurrent illnesses in order to avoid repeated hospital admissions and potential development of adrenal crises. Patients with primary adrenal insufficiency require glucocorticoid and mineralocorticoid replacement, but those with central disease need glucocorticoid replacement only. H

Although several agents are available for glucocorticoid replacement (**Table 23**), many endocrinologists prefer using hydrocortisone. The advantages of hydrocortisone are that it is identical to the natural product, has a shorter half-life, and

TABLE 23. Glucocorticoid Replacement Therapy in Adrenal Insufficiency

Condition	Hydrocortisone	Prednisone	Dexamethasone
Physiologic daily dosing	15-25 mg/d orally in three divided doses at 8 AM (7.5-12.5 mg), 12 PM (5-7.5 mg) and 6 PM (2.5-5 mg)	3-5 mg/d orally in two divided doses at 8 AM (2-3 mg) and 3 PM (1-2 mg)	0.375 to 0.75 mg/d orally in one dose or preferably as two divided doses
Minor stress (such as cold symptoms)	30-50 mg/d orally in three doses for 2-3 days	8-15 mg/d orally in two divided doses for 2-3 days	1-2 mg/d orally in two divided doses for 2-3 days
Moderate stress (such as a minor/moderate surgical procedure)	45-75 mg/d orally or IV in three to four divided doses for 2-3 days	15-20 mg/d orally or IV (as prednisolone) in two or three divided doses for 2-3 days; hydrocortisone can be used instead	2-3 mg/d orally in two divided doses for 2-3 days; hydrocortisone can be used instead
Severe stress (such as a major surgical procedure, sepsis)	100-150 mg/d IV in four divided doses for 1 day; taper to physiologic dose over 3-5 days	Follow hydrocortisone regimen	Follow hydrocortisone regimen
Septic shock, severe inflammatory process	150-200 mg/d IV in four divided doses; taper as clinically tolerated	Follow hydrocortisone regimen	Follow hydrocortisone regimen

IV = intravenously.

can be tightly titrated more easily to mimic normal cortisol secretion (with higher morning doses and lower afternoon and evening doses). Longer-acting medications, such as prednisone and dexamethasone, are often given once daily and are more convenient for patients, although they are susceptible to metabolism that may vary from one patient to the next, which makes optimal dosing more difficult. Whichever preparation is used, daily replacement doses should be titrated to minimize symptoms of underreplacement and adjusted to avoid overreplacement, which leads to iatrogenic Cushing syndrome. Educating patients about their illness and the need for dose adjustments (increases) with intercurrent illnesses ("sick day rules"; see Table 23) is crucial, and they should be advised to wear medical alert identification indicating their diagnosis and dependence on glucocorticoid replacement therapy.

The standard drug for mineralocorticoid replacement therapy in patients with primary adrenal insufficiency is fludrocortisone, 0.05 to 0.1 mg/d. Patients with either primary or central adrenal insufficiency are deficient in adrenal androgen, but androgen replacement therapy is not essential for survival, and the data are not clear that replacement offers a clear benefit.

H

Adrenal Function During Critical Illness

In healthy persons, glucocorticoid secretion is increased during critical illness, generally in proportion to the degree of stress associated with the illness. In patients with adrenal insufficiency, therefore, glucocorticoid replacement doses should be increased during stressful events (see Table 23).

Testing for adrenal insufficiency during critical illness occasionally can be difficult. In patients with critical illness and hypoproteinemia, measured serum cortisol levels often appear lower than they would be otherwise. Despite this limitation, adrenal function testing in these patients continues to rely on serum total cortisol measurements because determination of the free fraction is not available for clinical use in a timely manner. True adrenal insufficiency is not common in critically ill patients but should always be considered in those at increased risk. Because no agreed upon diagnostic criteria or indications for treatment of adrenal insufficiency in critical illness exist, establishing the diagnosis is difficult, as is knowing when to treat. A random serum cortisol level greater than 15 micrograms/dL (414 nmol/L) in a critically ill patient and a level greater than 12 micrograms/dL (331 nmol/L) in a critically ill patient who has hypoproteinemia (serum albumin level <2.5 g/dL [25 g/L]) make the diagnosis of adrenal insufficiency unlikely.

A stimulation test, with cosyntropin for example, is not necessary in patients during critical illness because they are already stimulated by their stressful illnesses. Some critically ill patients, such as those with septic shock, might develop severe protracted hypotension that is unresponsive to standard therapy. Most, if not all, of these patients have elevated serum total and free cortisol levels and lack other biochemical features of adrenal insufficiency. The term "relative" adrenal insufficiency continues to be mistakenly used by some to refer to a presentation such as this. High-dose hydrocortisone therapy given to patients with septic shock has not been shown to influence mortality but may result in a faster reversal of shock. This therapy, which may be associated with adverse effects, is thus directed not at treating adrenal dysfunction, but rather at controlling the associated overwhelming inflammatory response. H

KEY POINTS

- The most common cause of central adrenal insufficiency is adrenocorticotropic hormone suppression resulting from exogenous glucocorticoid replacement therapy.
- Primary adrenal insufficiency should be suspected when serum cortisol and aldosterone levels are low and plasma renin activity and adrenocorticotropic hormone levels are increased; a minimal or no increase in serum cortisol level after cosyntropin stimulation confirms the diagnosis.
- Glucocorticoid replacement therapy in primary or central adrenal insufficiency involves the use of a glucocorticoid (hydrocortisone, prednisone, or dexamethasone), whereas fludrocortisone is used for mineralocorticoid replacement therapy in primary adrenal insufficiency only.

Cushing Syndrome

Cushing syndrome comprises the constellation of signs and symptoms occurring after prolonged exposure to supraphysiologic doses of glucocorticoids. Although patients with various illnesses may have cushingoid features, some that should raise concern for true Cushing syndrome include proximal muscle weakness, multiple ecchymoses, prominent supraclavicular fat pads, violaceous striae, hypokalemia, unexplained osteoporosis, new-onset hypertension, and diabetes mellitus (**Figure 7**). Causes of Cushing syndrome are outlined in **Table 24**, with the most common being oral, intra-articular, intramuscular, inhalational, or topical administration of exogenous glucocorticoids for the treatment of various illnesses.

When the diagnosis of Cushing syndrome is suspected, it should be confirmed or satisfactorily ruled out because of its association with increased morbidity and mortality. The diagnosis is made by demonstrating unequivocal evidence of hypercortisolism, usually through the combination of initial tests and confirmatory studies, if needed (**Figure 8**). The three approaches most often used to evaluate for hypercortisolism are (1) assessment of urine free cortisol excretion in a 24-hour period, (2) documentation of loss of feedback inhibition of cortisol on the hypothalamic-pituitary axis with dexamethasone suppression testing, and (3) documentation of the loss of normal diurnal variation in cortisol secretion with late-night salivary cortisol measurement.

In evaluating patients with clinical features suggestive of Cushing syndrome, starting with any of the previously

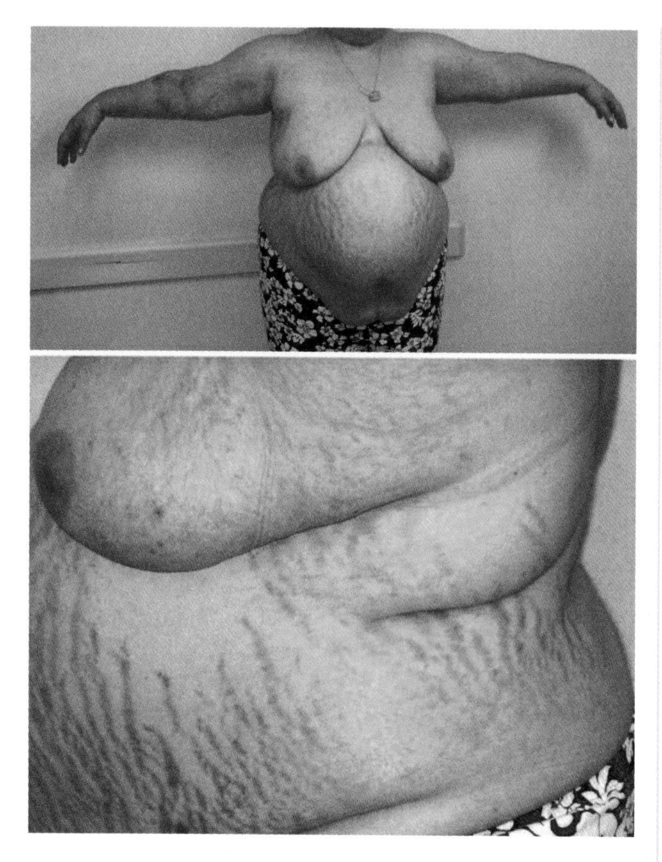

FIGURE 7. Classic features of Cushing syndrome in a patient with an adrenocorticotropic hormone–secreting pituitary adenoma. Central obesity and striae are evident (*top*). A close-up view of the striae (*bottom*) reveals their wide, violaceous nature.

mentioned approaches is appropriate. In general, however, two of the three tests are needed to confirm the diagnosis. Measurement of 24-hour urine free cortisol excretion is the gold standard test for diagnosing Cushing syndrome. A threefold to fourfold increase over normal values is diagnostic of Cushing syndrome; if this increase is present, no additional testing is required. For less dramatic increases, another diagnostic approach for hypercortisolism is required, such as the overnight dexamethasone suppression test or measurement of a late-night salivary cortisol level. The overnight dexamethasone suppression test is performed by obtaining a morning (8 or 9 AM) serum cortisol level after 1 mg of dexamethasone has been administered at 11 PM the night before; a normal response is generally considered to be a level less than 2 micrograms/dL (55 nmol/L) in healthy persons. Serum cortisol levels greater than 5 micrograms/dL (138 nmol/L) after dexamethasone administration the previous night are highly suggestive of Cushing syndrome. However, values of 2 to 5 micrograms/dL (55-138 nmol/L) require additional testing. In interpreting test results, one should consider factors that may increase corticosteroid-binding globulin levels and thus falsely increase the serum cortisol level (such as estrogen therapy or pregnancy). Caution also should be exercised in interpreting data from this test in patients taking medications that induce the cytochrome P-450 enzyme system, such as phenytoin or phenobarbital, and thereby increase the metabolism of dexamethasone.

In healthy persons, cortisol secretion exhibits a diurnal rhythm whereby serum cortisol levels reach a nadir late at night and peak in the early morning. Because loss of this diurnal rhythm is a central feature of Cushing syndrome, measurement of the nighttime cortisol level can be used as a diagnostic test. Salivary cortisol is in equilibrium with the free cortisol in the circulation. Thus, the finding of an elevated midnight salivary cortisol level on at least two separate occasions should raise concern about the possibility of Cushing syndrome, if the saliva sample was taken on a quiet, restful night.

Confirmatory testing also is needed when initial studies are suggestive of but equivocal for hypercortisolism. If not performed as an initial study, the 24-hour urine free cortisol

TABLE 24. Causes of Cushing Syndrome (Hypercortisolism)

Type of Cushing Syndrome[a]	Cause
Endogenous	
ACTH dependent (75%-80% of patients)	ACTH-secreting pituitary adenoma (60%-65% of patients)
	Ectopic ACTH secretion by tumors, such as carcinoid tumors (10%-15% of patients)
	CRH-secreting tumors (rare)
ACTH independent (20%-25% of patients)	Adrenal adenoma (10%-15% of patients)
	Adrenal carcinoma (5%-10% of patients)
Exogenous	Prolonged administration of supraphysiologic doses of glucocorticoid therapy (such as prednisone, dexamethasone, or hydrocortisone)
	Administration of drugs with glucocorticoid activity (progestational agents, such as megestrol)

ACTH = adrenocorticotropic hormone; CRH = corticotropin-releasing hormone.

[a]Patients with ACTH-dependent Cushing syndrome have hypercortisolism associated with normal or elevated plasma ACTH levels; those with ACTH-independent Cushing syndrome have hypercortisolism associated with low or undetectable plasma ACTH levels. Patients with exogenous Cushing syndrome have low or undetectable plasma ACTH levels, and their serum cortisol levels often are low unless the glucocorticoid used cross reacts in the cortisol assay.

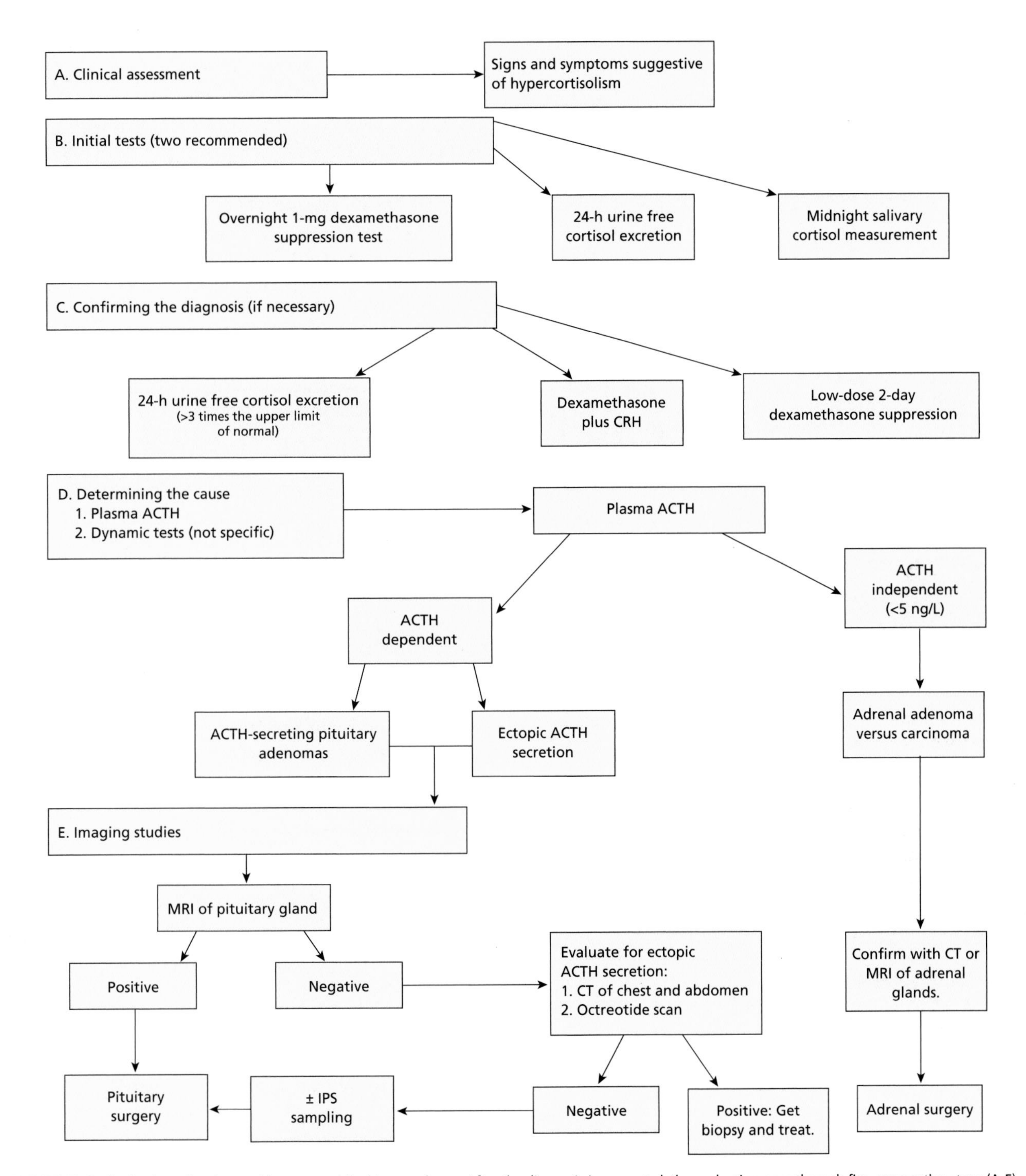

FIGURE 8. Evaluation of patients with suspected Cushing syndrome. After the diagnosis is suspected, the evaluation goes through five consecutive steps (A-E). In patients with ACTH-dependent Cushing syndrome who have normal MRIs of the pituitary gland, ectopic ACTH secretion is possible. Inferior petrosal sinus catheterization can confirm the central source of ACTH secretion in those with negative pituitary MRIs. ACTH = adrenocorticotropic hormone; CRH = corticotropin-releasing hormone; IPS = inferior petrosal sinus catheterization.

test remains the gold standard confirmatory study. The standard (as opposed to the overnight) low-dose dexamethasone suppression test also may also be used as a confirmatory study. Dexamethasone (0.5 mg) administered every 6 hours for 48 hours typically causes suppression of serum cortisol levels to less than 2 micrograms/dL (55 nmol/L) and of 24-hour urine free cortisol excretion to less than 20 micrograms/24 h (55 nmol/24 h), with higher levels consistent with Cushing syndrome. Using a CRH plus desmopressin stimulation test may be helpful in selected patients with multiple equivocal studies for hypercortisolism; however, doing so is expensive and not a routine test for diagnosing Cushing syndrome.

After hypercortisolism is firmly established, further evaluation should explore the cause, whether adrenal, pituitary, or ectopic. For example, measurement of the plasma ACTH level can differentiate ACTH-dependent hypercortisolism (ACTH level is inappropriately normal or elevated, as with a pituitary adenoma) from ACTH-independent hypercortisolism (ACTH level is low [<5 pg/mL {1.1 pmol/L}] or undetectable, as with adrenal neoplasms). The ACTH level should be measured simultaneously with the cortisol level. Other approaches used to determine the cause of hypercortisolism include dynamic testing with higher doses of dexamethasone (for example, 8 mg/d). The value of the high-dose dexamethasone suppression test is limited, however, because of significant overlap in responses observed among patients with different forms of Cushing syndrome.

Imaging studies should be obtained only after biochemical documentation of hypercortisolism is established. These studies offer no diagnostic information relevant to Cushing syndrome but instead aid in localizing any associated tumor. An MRI of the sella turcica should be obtained in patients with ACTH-dependent hypercortisolism. However, MRIs are normal in 40% to 50% of patients with documented ACTH-secreting pituitary adenomas because of the small size of these adenomas. This makes it difficult to differentiate patients with ACTH-secreting adenomas (75%) from others with ectopic ACTH secretion on the basis of an MRI. Dynamic contrast-enhanced pituitary MRI imaging can improve detection in some cases. Additionally, a significant overlap exists between these two entities in terms of their biochemical features and responsiveness to dexamethasone suppression or other dynamic testing (such as with CRH). An approach used to evaluate for a central source of ACTH secretion in patients with true-negative pituitary MRIs is bilateral inferior petrosal sinus catheterization with central and peripheral measurements of plasma ACTH levels simultaneously from both sides before and after CRH stimulation. This test is technically difficult and should only be performed at experienced centers. Instead of performing the inferior petrosal sinus catheterization, some centers with extensive experience in managing Cushing syndrome opt to proceed to surgical exploration of the pituitary gland in patients with normal MRIs who also have normal CT scans of the abdomen and chest.

In patients with hypercortisolism associated with suppressed plasma ACTH levels, a dedicated CT scan of the adrenal glands often shows a tumor (a smaller, homogeneous, more lipid-rich adenoma versus a larger, more irregular, vascular carcinoma). Although differentiating between a cortisol-secreting adrenal adenoma and a carcinoma is sometimes possible using clinical, biochemical, and imaging features, histologic confirmation of capsular invasion is necessary for larger lesions. The evaluation and management of suspected Cushing syndrome should be performed by an experienced endocrinologist.

The treatment of exogenous Cushing syndrome is to discontinue exogenous glucocorticoid replacement therapy whenever possible by using alternative therapy to treat the condition in question. Alternatively, if glucocorticoid replacement is necessary, then the smallest dose possible should be administered either once daily or every other day in the morning (9-10 AM). The treatment of endogenous Cushing syndrome depends on its cause, with ACTH-secreting pituitary adenomas (Cushing disease) best treated with pituitary adenomectomy. Immediately after this surgery, patients develop ACTH deficiency requiring daily glucocorticoid replacement therapy until endogenous ACTH production resumes, which can take as long as a year. Patients with residual disease after pituitary surgery might benefit from stereotactic radiosurgery and adjuvant medical therapy with drugs that inhibit glucocorticoid synthesis (such as ketoconazole or metyrapone) or are cytotoxic to adrenocortical cells (such as mitotane).

The preferred treatment of Cushing syndrome caused by cortisol-producing adrenal adenomas and carcinomas is surgical resection of the tumor, preferably through a laparoscopic approach. Postoperatively, most patients have resultant adrenal insufficiency lasting as long as 12 months that requires daily glucocorticoid replacement for several months. Although cortisol-secreting adenomas are generally curable with surgical resection, adrenal carcinomas might not be totally resectable and can recur. Further treatment of patients with adrenal carcinomas is discussed later. The treatment of Cushing syndrome caused by ectopic ACTH secretion should be directed at the cause, which often is difficult because many of the tumors secreting ACTH ectopically are malignant. Patients with these tumors typically have signs and symptoms of malignancy (weight loss, cachexia, and temporal wasting) and biochemical features of mineralocorticoid activity. When cortisol is secreted in large quantities, the mineralocorticoid activity becomes much more apparent and is associated with classic features, such as hypertension, hypokalemia, and excessive urine potassium loss. Most patients will require medical therapy to control their hypercortisolism and may require bilateral adrenalectomy if medical therapy is ineffective.

KEY POINTS

- The diagnosis of Cushing syndrome involves demonstration of persistent hypercortisolism associated with poor suppressibility with dexamethasone or loss of the normal diurnal variation in cortisol secretion.
- For Cushing disease caused by an adrenocorticotropic hormone–secreting pituitary adenoma, adenomectomy is the treatment of choice.
- Patients with Cushing syndrome develop transient adrenal insufficiency (lasting up to 12 months) immediately after surgical removal of any causative tumor (adrenocorticotropic hormone–secreting tumor or cortisol-producing adrenal tumor).

Adrenal Incidentaloma

The increasing use of imaging studies for various medical indications has revealed otherwise unrecognized adrenal masses in less than 1% of the population younger than 30 years and up to 7% of the population older than 70 years (**Figure 9**). Adrenal masses in younger patients are more likely to be functional and/or malignant than those found in older patients. Evaluating adrenal masses should address their potential for malignancy (whether primary or metastatic) and their functional status. Functional tumors originate from any of the three layers of the adrenal cortex or from the adrenal medulla and secrete products of the respective portion of the glands.

Initial assessment should include a thorough history and physical examination to detect any indications of malignant disease and any clinical evidence of hormone hypersecretion (**Figure 10**). Most patients with metastatic cancer of the adrenal glands have clinical evidence of disease elsewhere. Imaging characteristics and the phenotype of the mass (size, CT attenuation, and contrast washout) also provide important information relative to the risk of malignancy. The risk of malignancy (primary or metastatic) is only 2% for masses less than 4 cm in size but increases to 25% for those 6 cm or larger. Benign adrenal adenomas generally have a low CT attenuation (<10 Hounsfield units) and exhibit rapid contrast medium washout (>50% at 10 minutes). In contrast, a high CT attenuation (>20 Hounsfield units) and a delay in contrast medium washout (<50%) are typical of pheochromocytomas

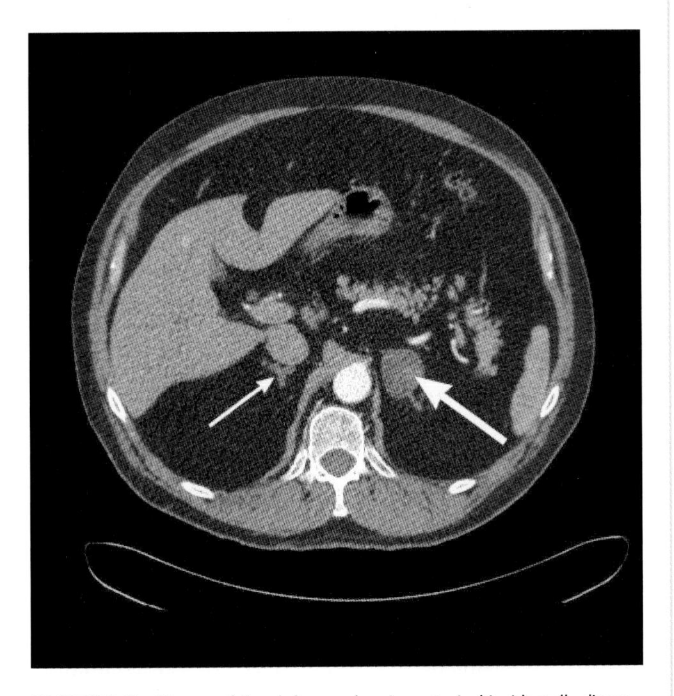

FIGURE 9. CT scan of the abdomen showing a typical incidentally discovered left adrenal mass (*thick white arrow*) in an asymptomatic man. The normal right adrenal gland is shown as an inverted Y shape (*thin white arrow*). The mass is lipid-rich and has a low attenuation factor (<10 Hounsfield units).

or malignant lesions. Primary adrenocortical carcinomas are typically large, have irregular borders, and may include areas of necrosis. Although imaging characteristics and phenotype do not predict function, they reliably predict biologic behavior. Similarly, T2-weighted MRIs are usually isointense to the liver in benign adenomas and hyperintense in adrenocortical carcinoma, pheochromocytoma, and metastatic disease. For the up to 15% of adrenal incidentalomas that are bilateral, the differential diagnosis includes bilateral adrenal hyperplasia and metastatic cancer.

Nearly 10% of adrenal incidentalomas are functional, although most have no overt clinical manifestations. Therefore, testing is usually necessary to identify functional tumors secreting catecholamines, cortisol, or aldosterone. Measurements of urine excretion or plasma levels of catecholamine metabolites (fractionated metanephrines) are good initial tests for pheochromocytoma, and further testing is reasonable when results are abnormal (see later discussion of pheochromocytoma). Notably, some patients with incidental adrenal tumors could have early-stage pheochromocytoma and thus may have negative results on biochemical testing. These patients will have imaging characteristics (high CT attenuation, delay in contrast medium washout) that raise concern for pheochromocytoma. Measurements of plasma ACTH and serum cortisol levels before and after the overnight administration of dexamethasone (1 mg) are appropriate initial tests to evaluate for possible cortisol production. Plasma ACTH levels are low in patients with cortisol-secreting adrenal tumors. Urine free cortisol measurement may also be used, either as an initial study or to confirm abnormal or equivocal results of a dexamethasone suppression test. Although the optimal upper range for the serum cortisol level after dexamethasone administration is debatable in this clinical setting, most authorities consider a value of 5 micrograms/dL (138 nmol/L) or greater to be clearly abnormal. Evaluation for aldosterone-secreting adenomas should be carried out in patients with hypertension or those with spontaneous hypokalemia by determining the plasma aldosterone level and plasma renin activity. Excess adrenal androgen production can be seen in patients with adrenal cancer and should be evaluated with determination of plasma DHEA and DHEAS levels, if suggested by the clinical presentation.

Management of an adrenal incidentaloma depends on its size, imaging characteristics (phenotype), and functional abilities (see Figure 10). Almost all adrenal tumors that are overtly functional, are larger than 6 cm in size, or have unfavorable imaging characteristics should be considered for surgical removal. The one exception is aldosterone-secreting adenomas, which may not need to be surgically removed because hyperaldosteronism often can be treated medically. Pre- and postoperative management of an adrenal incidentaloma in patients treated surgically is directed at the functionality of the tumor (see sections on Cushing Syndrome, Pheochromocytoma, and Primary Hyperaldosteronism).

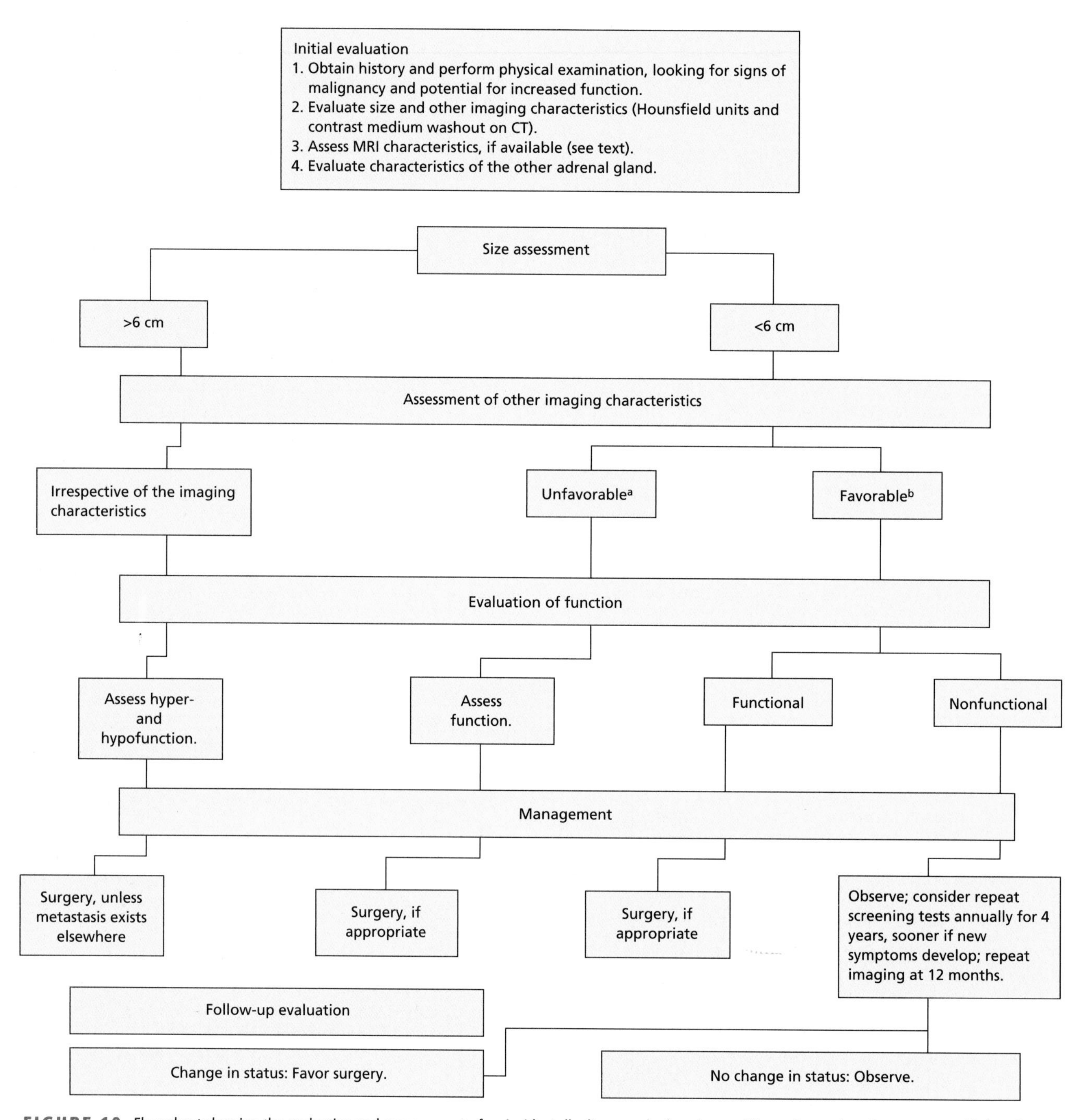

FIGURE 10. Flow sheet showing the evaluation and management of an incidentally discovered adrenal mass. Masses larger than 6 cm are more likely to be malignant.

[a]Unfavorable imaging characteristics: high CT attenuation (>20 Hounsfield units), irregular border, delayed contrast (<50%) washout.

[b]Favorable imaging characteristics: low CT attenuation (<10 Hounsfield units), smooth contour, rapid (≥50%) contrast washout.

Consensus exists that patients who have nonfunctional tumors smaller than 4 cm with favorable imaging characteristics should be followed, although agreement is lacking about how often tests (hormonal and imaging) should be repeated, if at all. CT scans of the adrenal glands (with and without contrast) provide anatomic details that are considered by many to be superior to those obtained by MRI. However, MRI's lack of radiation exposure offers some advantage. Most authorities suggest CT for follow-up studies unless concerns about exposure to radiation or contrast material exist. Although some experts recommend that hormonal evaluation be performed annually for 3 to 4 years, others advocate repeat biochemical testing only when signs or symptoms of hormonal excess are discovered. A reasonable compromise is to reevaluate patients for Cushing syndrome and pheochromocytoma at 1 year or at any time a change in clinical manifestations or imaging characteristics occurs. Regarding imaging, a repeat CT scan should be obtained at least once 6 to 12 months after the initial finding, with some advocating repeat imaging at 6, 12, and 24 months after the tumor is detected.

Testing should be repeated if significant changes in size or imaging characteristics are noted. Controversy surrounds the management of nonfunctional adrenal incidentalomas that are 4 to 6 cm in size with favorable imaging characteristics. Whereas some advocate surgical removal, others favor a management scheme similar to that for incidentalomas less than 4 cm in size.

KEY POINTS

- Assessment of incidentally discovered adrenal masses should address whether the mass is benign or malignant, primary or metastatic, and functional or nonfunctional.
- All adrenal tumors that are functional, are larger than 6 cm in size, or have unfavorable imaging characteristics should be considered for surgical removal.

Pheochromocytoma

Pheochromocytomas are rare tumors (0.1%-0.6% of persons with hypertension) composed of chromaffin cells that can secrete biogenic amines (norepinephrine, epinephrine, and dopamine) and their metabolites. Most pheochromocytomas secrete predominantly norepinephrine, which results in sustained or episodic hypertension. Less commonly, these tumors might secrete predominantly epinephrine, which can cause hypotension. Nearly 90% of pheochromocytomas arise in the adrenal medulla, and 10% are extra-adrenal, located primarily along the sympathetic chain (paragangliomas). Approximately 25% of pheochromocytomas are familial and associated with genetic disorders (such as multiple endocrine neoplasia type 2, neurofibromatosis 1, and von Hippel-Lindau disease), 10% are asymptomatic, and 10% are malignant. The familial forms of pheochromocytoma tend to occur in multiple sites, are more likely to recur after surgical resection, and are associated with other benign or malignant tumors. Genetic testing should thus be considered in patients with a family history of this tumor, in those with bilateral or extra-adrenal disease, and in younger persons with other tumors.

The clinical manifestations of pheochromocytoma vary, with hypertension (episodic or sustained) observed in greater than 90% of patients. Other signs and symptoms include episodes of diaphoresis, pallor, palpitations, headache, hyperglycemia, weight loss, arrhythmias (atrial and ventricular fibrillation), and (rarely) catecholamine-induced cardiomyopathy. The classic triad of severe headache, diaphoresis, and palpitations is highly suggestive of pheochromocytoma. Because some (10%) pheochromocytomas are diagnosed in asymptomatic patients evaluated for adrenal incidentalomas, the diagnosis should be suspected in any patient at risk (**Table 25**). Patients suspected of having a pheochromocytoma should not receive β-blockers until treated with adequate α-adrenergic blockade to avoid the potential sequela of worsened hypertension due to unopposed α stimulation.

The diagnosis of pheochromocytoma relies on the documentation of excessive secretion of catecholamines or their metabolites as measured in the plasma or in a 24-hour urine collection. Because significant catecholamine metabolism is intratumoral, measurement of catecholamine metabolites (metanephrines) is the most appropriate approach in defining catecholamine secretion. A positive test often is defined as an elevation in the plasma value or 24-hour urine excretion that is greater than twice the upper limit of normal. The upper limits of normal may vary between laboratories, with some laboratories using a hypertensive population to establish their normal value; in such assays, the distinction between patients with and without pheochromocytomas becomes easier.

In approaching the diagnosis of pheochromocytoma, one can start with measurement of either the plasma level or urine metanephrine excretion as long as the sensitivity, specificity, and limitations of the approach used are considered. There are many instances of discordance between urine and plasma measurements of catecholamine metabolites, in which case the urine levels are more specific and thus more reliable. Because the management of pheochromocytoma may involve imaging studies, it is essential first to evaluate for and then confirm the diagnosis biochemically. When clinical suspicion of pheochromocytoma is high, measurement of the plasma free metanephrine level is preferred because of the higher sensitivity of this test. When that test is positive, the 24-hour urine catecholamine metabolite excretion should be determined to confirm the diagnosis. When clinical suspicion is low, measurement of the 24-hour urine excretion of catecholamines and metanephrines is preferred because of the lower false-positive rate (higher specificity); further testing would not be necessary unless convincing clinical, familial, or genetic predisposing factors for the disease exist.

TABLE 25. Patient History Prompting Screening for Pheochromocytoma

Suggestive (hyperadrenergic) cyclic spells of hypertension, diaphoresis, palpitations, or headache
Familial predisposing syndrome (neurofibromatosis 1, MEN2, succinate dehydrogenase B mutation)
Previous vasopressor response to anesthesia or angiography
Adrenal incidentaloma
Hypertension at a young age (<20 years)
Drug-resistant hypertension
Unexplained cardiomyopathy and atrial fibrillation

MEN2 = multiple endocrine neoplasia type 2.

The preference is that patients not receive any medications during testing, but this often is not practical. Tricyclic antidepressants and other drugs with similar pharmacologic features (such as cyclobenzaprine) are among the drugs that interfere with measurement of catecholamines and metanephrines. Other interfering drugs include antihypertensive agents (such as reserpine), medications with adrenergic receptor agonist activity (such as decongestants), psychoactive drugs with dopamine or norepinephrine reuptake inhibition properties (such as buspirone), but not other selective serotonin reuptake inhibitors. In addition, acetaminophen intake can interfere with the measurement of plasma metanephrine levels in some assays. The use of medications that interfere with catecholamine and metanephrine assays should be discontinued at least 2 weeks before testing. Catecholamine and metanephrine levels that are elevated but are less than twice the upper limit of normal can occur in patients in a hyperadrenergic state, in those with anxiety disorders or high levels of psychological stress, and sometimes in those with essential hypertension. Additionally, catecholamine secretion is appropriately increased in stressful conditions, such as critical illness, and thus testing patients for pheochromocytoma in these circumstances may lead to misleading conclusions. In situations in which equivocal results are obtained, repeat testing and other biochemical studies for pheochromocytoma, such as the clonidine suppression test, may be indicated.

After the diagnosis of pheochromocytoma is biochemically confirmed, imaging studies should be performed to determine the tumor's location. Either adrenal CT with and without contrast or MRI without contrast is a reasonable option. The anatomic details are better appreciated on a CT scan, although exposure to radiation is avoided with MRI. Metaiodobenzylguanidine (MIBG), a compound with a structure similar to that of norepinephrine, is tagged with radioactive iodine (^{123}I or ^{131}I) and used for scintigraphic localization of pheochromocytomas when results of CT scans and MRIs are negative. This tagged compound also is used to localize metastasis from malignant pheochromocytoma.

Laparoscopic adrenalectomy is the most effective treatment for most pheochromocytomas. Preoperative medical therapy is instituted after the biochemical diagnosis is confirmed and before surgical resection. However, no controlled studies have shown which therapy is best. Previously, most patients were treated for 1 to 2 weeks before surgery with a competitive α-adrenergic blocking agent (phenoxybenzamine) at an initial dose of 10 mg once or twice daily, with upward titration based on blood pressure measurements every 2 to 3 days to a maximum of 80 mg/d. Because of its long-lasting effects, phenoxybenzamine contributed to the hypotension commonly observed during the first day after tumor removal. Some centers use short-acting specific α-antagonists, such as prazosin (2-5 mg, three times daily), doxazosin (2-8 mg/d), or terazosin (2-5 mg/d). In patients with tachycardia, β-blockers can be added after α-blockade is achieved, especially if blood pressure control is not achieved. The goal is to achieve a blood pressure of approximately 120/80 mm Hg. If blood pressure control is still not achieved with α- and β-blockade, other drugs, such as calcium channel blockers (amlodipine or verapamil), can be added as needed. Labetalol, a combined α- and β-blocking agent, also can be used, especially in patients with tachyarrhythmias. Patients with pheochromocytomas who are normotensive also should be treated with α-blockers because these patients often become hypertensive during surgical resection. Nitroprusside is used to control intraoperative hypertension. The anesthesiologist should be aware of the potential for changes in blood pressure during tumor manipulation and the need for volume expansion during and after tumor resection.

The long-term prognosis for patients after resection of a solitary sporadic pheochromocytoma is excellent, although some may have persistent hypertension, and as many as 17% have a recurrence. All patients should have annual follow-up evaluation for at least 10 years with repeat biochemical testing, and those with extra-adrenal lesions or familial disease should be followed clinically with blood pressure monitoring indefinitely and imaging evaluation whenever any change in status occurs. Treatment of malignant pheochromocytoma includes surgical debulking, control of catecholamine-related symptoms with α-blockers and catecholamine synthesis inhibitors, external irradiation, or targeted radiotherapy using ^{131}I-MIBG. Systemic cytotoxic chemotherapy has also been used, although response rates are usually low and short-lived.

KEY POINTS

- The diagnosis of pheochromocytoma relies on the documentation of excessive secretion of catecholamines or their metabolites.
- β-Blockers should not be given to patients suspected of having a pheochromocytoma unless these patients are already being treated with α-adrenergic blocking agents.
- Treatment of pheochromocytoma involves laparoscopic adrenalectomy after appropriate preparation with α-adrenergic blocking agents and control of blood pressure and pulse rate.

Primary Hyperaldosteronism

Primary hyperaldosteronism is a condition characterized by excessive autonomous aldosterone production by the adrenal zona glomerulosa, independent of its physiologic regulator, the renin-angiotensin system. Primary hyperaldosteronism is associated with several pathologic entities, such as solitary aldosterone-producing adrenal adenoma (40%-50%); bilateral adrenal hyperplasia, also known as idiopathic primary hyperaldosteronism (50%-60%); and, more rarely, unilateral hyperplasia or adrenal carcinoma. The main manifestations of primary hyperaldosteronism are hypertension, hypokalemia (although up to 50% of patients can be eukalemic), and metabolic alkalosis. The prevalence of primary hyperaldosteronism in patients with hypertension is variable (1%-5%). Therefore, the diagnosis should be considered in any patient with hypertension, especially hypertension resistant to treatment, associated with spontaneous (unprovoked) hypokalemia (or significant hypokalemia in response to low-dose thiazide treatment), or coexistent with an adrenal incidentaloma.

Evaluation for primary hyperaldosteronism involves the simultaneous measurements of the midmorning ambulatory plasma aldosterone level (typically increased) and plasma renin activity (typically suppressed). In most patients with hyperaldosteronism, the plasma aldosterone level exceeds 15 ng/dL (414 pmol/L), but the plasma renin activity is very low or undetectable. A ratio of plasma aldosterone (measured in ng/dL) to plasma renin activity (measured in ng/mL/h) of greater than 30 has a 90% sensitivity and specificity for the diagnosis of primary hyperaldosteronism; a ratio of 20 to 30 is suggestive of the diagnosis, especially when the plasma aldosterone level is greater than 15 ng/dL (414 pmol/L). Determining the ratio of plasma aldosterone to plasma renin activity is particularly helpful in patients receiving ACE inhibitors, angiotensin receptor blockers, or direct renin inhibitors in whom plasma renin activity is expected to be high and the aldosterone level is usually low (see Figure 6, bottom panel). Testing can be done on random blood samples, even in patients taking antihypertensive medications with the exception of spironolactone and eplerenone, both aldosterone receptor antagonists.

H The biochemical diagnosis is confirmed by demonstrating persistent elevation (poor suppressibility) of the plasma aldosterone level in response to a high-sodium load. Sodium chloride can be given orally (2 g three times daily for 3 days) or intravenously (normal saline, 500 mL per hour for 4 hours). During salt loading, plasma aldosterone levels are suppressed to less than 5 ng/dL (138 pmol/L) in healthy persons but remain elevated (often >10 ng/dL [276 pmol/L]) in patients with primary hyperaldosteronism. The decision to pursue salt loading should be made only after at least two plasma aldosterone to plasma renin activity ratios are elevated in the presence of an elevated aldosterone level. It is necessary to ensure that patients are potassium replete before beginning a salt-loading test because increased sodium intake will exacerbate hypokalemia.

Measurement of 24-hour urine aldosterone excretion (typically, <12 micrograms/24 h [33.2 nmol/24h]) during the third day of the salt loading also can confirm the diagnosis, provided adequate salt loading is achieved (as demonstrated by a high urine sodium excretion (greater than 200 meq/24 h [200 mmol/24 h]). After adequate salt loading, a plasma aldosterone level greater than 10 ng/dL (276 pmol/L) is diagnostic of hyperaldosteronism.

After the biochemical diagnosis is confirmed, further studies, such as CT of the adrenal glands, are performed to define the pathologic cause of primary hyperaldosteronism. A solitary adrenal adenoma, which is often 2 cm or less in diameter, is easy to recognize on a CT scan. Bilateral adrenal hyperplasia is characterized by diffuse or focal enlargement of both adrenal glands and is associated with unilateral or bilateral nodules; making this distinction is crucial because of its impact on therapy. However, imaging studies are not always accurate in defining the pathologic entity causing hyperaldosteronism, especially given the high prevalence of adrenal incidentalomas in persons older than 40 years. One definitive approach is to catheterize both adrenal veins and measure plasma aldosterone levels from both sides to determine if aldosterone production is unilateral or bilateral. Because this procedure is technically difficult and can be associated with adverse effects, such as adrenal vein dissection and hemorrhage, it should be used selectively in patients in whom surgery is being considered and performed only at centers with expertise in the procedure. H

Referral to an endocrinologist is recommended whenever the biochemical data are not typical because some rare conditions may also present with hypertension, hypokalemia, and metabolic alkalosis but may not be associated with an elevated aldosterone level.

The goals of therapy for hyperaldosteronism are normalization (or at least improvement) of blood pressure, resolution of hypokalemia, and attainment of normal aldosterone levels and effects. The last goal is especially important because aldosterone can have adverse effects over and above its influence on blood pressure or the potassium level. Although laparoscopic surgical resection of a solitary aldosterone-secreting adrenal adenoma is usually recommended, especially in young patients, medical therapy also can be an effective alternative approach when it includes an aldosterone receptor blocker (either spironolactone or eplerenone). After removal of the aldosterone-producing adrenal adenoma, potassium levels become normal in greater than 90% of patients; blood pressure normalizes in two thirds of patients, and its control improves in the remaining third.

The treatment of choice for primary hyperaldosteronism caused by bilateral adrenal hyperplasia is medical therapy with either spironolactone or eplerenone. Spironolactone (50-300 mg/d) is often effective in controlling hypertension and hypokalemia. Besides being an aldosterone antagonist that blocks the aldosterone receptor, spironolactone also blocks the androgen receptor and can cause gynecomastia, mastodynia, impotence, and diminished libido in men and menstrual irregularities in women. Eplerenone (25-100 mg/d) is a more selective aldosterone receptor blocker and has fewer of these adverse events. Some medically treated patients with adrenal adenomas and bilateral adrenal hyperplasia require treatment with amiloride to attain eukalemia; a low-dose thiazide diuretic (12.5-25 mg/d) also can be added to reverse hypervolemia. Patients should be followed indefinitely with monitoring of blood pressure, kidney function, and potassium levels. In premenopausal women, aldosterone antagonists are known to be teratogenic in the male fetus and thus must be avoided unless prevention of pregnancy is secured.

KEY POINTS

- Testing for primary hyperaldosteronism includes measuring simultaneous midmorning ambulatory plasma aldosterone levels and plasma renin activity; a ratio of the former over the latter greater than 20 is suggestive of the diagnosis.
- The biochemical diagnosis of primary hyperaldosteronism is confirmed by demonstrating persistent elevation (poor suppressibility) of the plasma aldosterone level in response to a high salt load.
- Primary hyperaldosteronism caused by a solitary aldosterone-secreting adenoma is best treated by adrenalectomy, whereas disease caused by bilateral adrenal hyperplasia is managed medically by using a nonselective (spironolactone) or a more selective (eplerenone) aldosterone blocking agent.

Adrenocortical Cancer

Adrenocortical cancer is a rare malignancy. As many as 60% of patients with this cancer have symptoms of hormone (cortisol) excess, whereas others have mechanical symptoms related to rapid tumor growth (abdominal fullness, nausea, and back pain) and a few have an incidentally discovered adrenal mass. Given the variable clinical presentation of this entity, diagnosis often requires integration of the clinical, biochemical, and imaging data discussed in previous sections. Most adrenocortical cancers produce multiple corticosteroids, including biologically inactive precursors. The imaging characteristics of adrenocortical cancer include a large mass with irregular borders or shape, occasional calcification, high attenuation (high Hounsfield units) on CT, and delay in contrast medium washout.

The treatment of adrenocortical cancer depends on the extent of disease at presentation. Surgical removal after appropriate biochemical assessment remains the best option, especially in patients with early disease. Even after apparent complete resection, adjuvant therapy with mitotane, a known adrenal cytotoxic drug, may be beneficial. Treatment with mitotane is recommended for patients with persistent disease and others with known metastases and is associated with objective remissions in approximately 25% of patients. The main limiting factors of mitotane use are the associated adverse events, including nausea, vomiting, lethargy, and other neurologic symptoms. Experience with other cytotoxic chemotherapy is limited, but this treatment usually has been ineffective. A poorer prognosis is associated with advanced stages of the disease, the presence of metastasis at diagnosis, an older age, and cortisol hypersecretion by the tumor. In patients without clinically evident disease after initial surgery, the median survival rate is 60% at 5 years. This rate is 20% to 25% for those with metastatic disease. Newer studies suggest that mitotane use may improve future survival, even after apparent complete tumor resection.

KEY POINTS

- The manifestations of adrenocortical cancer include hormone (cortisol) excess and mechanical symptoms due to a rapidly growing mass.
- Surgical resection is the best therapeutic option for adrenocortical cancer followed by use of the cytotoxic drug mitotane.

Reproductive Disorders

Basic Concepts and Common Features

The hypothalamic-pituitary-gonadal axes of men and women share many features. Gonadotropin-releasing hormone (GnRH) is released in a pulsatile manner from the hypothalamus. When released, GnRH stimulates the gonadotropic cells in the anterior pituitary gland to secrete follicle-stimulating hormone (FSH) and luteinizing hormone (LH). FSH and LH stimulate spermatogenesis and testosterone production in the testes and follicular development and estrogen production in the ovaries. Testosterone and estrogen decrease the release of GnRH, FSH, and LH through negative feedback inhibition on the hypothalamus and pituitary gland. Feedback inhibition of FSH is also controlled by inhibin B, a protein product of ovarian granulosa cells and testicular Sertoli cells.

Physiology of Male Reproduction

The testes are composed of seminiferous tubules, Leydig cells, and Sertoli cells. Leydig cells are responsible for testosterone production by LH stimulation, and Sertoli cells are responsible for spermatogenesis by FSH stimulation and testosterone. Testosterone is secreted in a diurnal pattern, with the highest levels achieved in the morning, and can be metabolized to dihydrotestosterone in some tissues, such as the prostate, and to estrogen in other tissues, such as fat. The male reproductive axis is shown in **Figure 11**.

Only 2% of testosterone is free testosterone, 44% is bound to sex hormone–binding globulin (SHBG), and the remaining 54% is bound to albumin. Testosterone's binding affinity for SHBG is much greater than for albumin. As a result, testosterone freely disassociates from albumin. Bioavailable testosterone is approximately the amount of free testosterone plus albumin-bound testosterone. A morning total testosterone level has long been considered the most

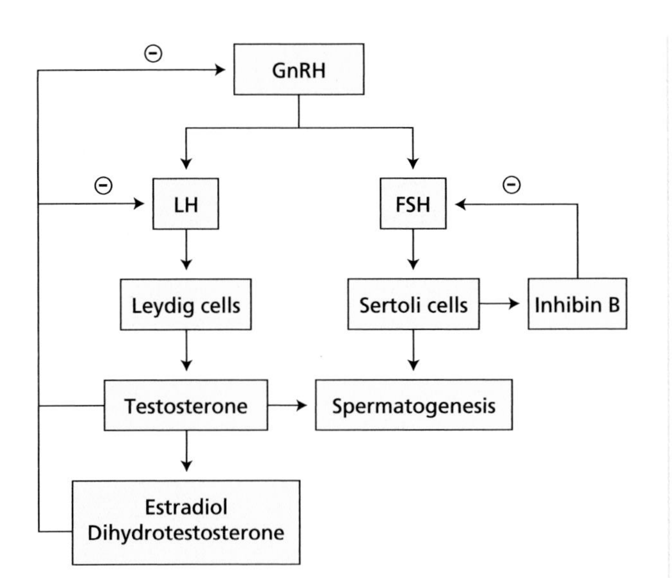

FIGURE 11. Male reproductive axis. Pulses of GnRH elicit pulses of LH and FSH. FSH acts on Sertoli cells, which assist sperm maturation and make inhibin B, the major negative regulator of basal FSH production. The Leydig cells make testosterone, which feeds back to inhibit GnRH and LH release. Some testosterone is irreversibly converted to dihydrotestosterone or estradiol, which are both more potent than testosterone in suppressing GnRH, LH, and FSH. FSH = follicle-stimulating hormone; GnRH = gonadotropin-releasing hormone; LH = luteinizing hormone; – (circled) = negative feedback.

accurate measure of a patient's androgen status except when SHBG is increased (as in the aging man) or decreased (as in obesity). In these circumstances, a serum free testosterone measurement by equilibrium dialysis or a calculated serum free testosterone level is a better measure of a patient's androgen status. Similarly, because of alterations in binding proteins in acutely ill patients, a testosterone measurement should not be obtained because it can lead to an erroneous diagnosis of testosterone deficiency.

Primary Hypogonadism

Primary hypogonadism is due to testicular failure and is defined as a low testosterone level with elevated LH and FSH levels. Primary hypogonadism can have congenital or acquired causes. The most common congenital cause is Klinefelter syndrome (XXY karyotype). Acquired causes include exposure to certain chemotherapy agents, pelvic irradiation, mumps orchitis, trauma, and testicular torsion.

Secondary Hypogonadism

Caused by a hypothalamic or pituitary defect, secondary hypogonadism is defined as a low testosterone level with simultaneously low or inappropriately normal LH and FSH levels. Secondary hypogonadism also can be due to congenital or acquired causes. Idiopathic hypogonadotropic hypogonadism, with anosmia (Kallmann syndrome) or without anosmia, is an example of congenital secondary hypogonadism. Acquired causes include hyperprolactinemia, functioning or nonfunctioning pituitary adenomas or other sellar masses, chronic opiate use, corticosteroids (exogenous use or excessive endogenous), and infiltrative diseases (such as hemochromatosis).

Androgen Deficiency in the Aging Male

Testosterone levels gradually decrease with age. The degree of decline in the testosterone level is highly variable, and many men will never become hypogonadal. The cause of this decline appears to be multifactorial, with changes in the hypothalamic-pituitary axis and Leydig cell function being the major causes.

Diagnosis and Evaluation of Male Hypogonadism

Symptoms of hypogonadism include low libido, erectile dysfunction, fatigue, and decreased muscle strength. However, these symptoms are common in the general male population and are nonspecific for hypogonadism. More specific signs and symptoms include gynecomastia, decrease in testicular size, and absence of morning erections. Laboratory testing is necessary to make a diagnosis. The best initial test is a morning (8 AM) measurement of the serum total testosterone level. If this level is normal (>350 ng/dL [12 nmol/L]), then hypogonadism is excluded. If abnormal (<200 ng/dL [6.9 nmol/L]), a second confirmatory morning measurement of the total testosterone level should be obtained, according to Endocrine Society guidelines. If the total testosterone level is more equivocal (200-350 ng/dL [6.9-12 nmol/L]) or if an SHBG abnormality is likely in the patient being evaluated, then a serum free testosterone level by equilibrium dialysis or a calculated serum free testosterone level can determine whether hypogonadism is truly present.

When hypogonadism is confirmed, the next step is to determine whether the patient has primary or secondary hypogonadism by measuring LH and FSH levels. Primary hypogonadism is indicated by supranormal LH and FSH levels. In patients with confirmed primary hypogonadism, no clear history of a testicular insult (such as chemotherapy or radiation therapy), and a consistent clinical picture, then a karyotype should be performed to exclude Klinefelter syndrome. If secondary hypogonadism is confirmed by inappropriately normal or low LH and FSH levels, measurement of the serum prolactin level to evaluate for hyperprolactinemia and iron saturation level (transferrin saturation and ferritin levels) to exclude hemochromatosis should be performed to assess for the possible cause. In addition, the presence of any additional pituitary hormone deficiencies should be assessed. An MRI of the pituitary gland should be ordered to exclude hypothalamic or pituitary masses as the cause of decreased gonadotropin production and secretion if any symptoms consistent with mass effect are present, including headaches, visual field changes, a serum total testosterone level less than 150 ng/dL (5.2 nmol/L), an increased prolactin level, or any additional pituitary hormonal deficiencies. **Figure 12** shows an algorithm for evaluating hypogonadism.

KEY POINTS

- Hypogonadism is best diagnosed after two early morning (8 AM) measurements show a decreased total testosterone level.
- After hypogonadism is diagnosed, luteinizing hormone (LH) and follicle-stimulating hormone (FSH) levels should be measured to determine whether the cause is primary (elevated LH and FSH levels) or secondary (low or inappropriately normal LH and FSH levels).
- If primary hypogonadism is confirmed in a patient with no history of a testicular insult and a consistent clinical picture, a karyotype is recommended to exclude Klinefelter syndrome; if secondary hypogonadism is confirmed, the cause should be determined by measurement of prolactin and iron saturation (transferrin saturation and ferritin) levels, evaluation of anterior pituitary function, and (possibly) a pituitary MRI.

Testosterone Replacement Therapy

Various testosterone preparations are available for treatment of male hypogonadism. Transdermal and intramuscular routes of administration are the most widely used.

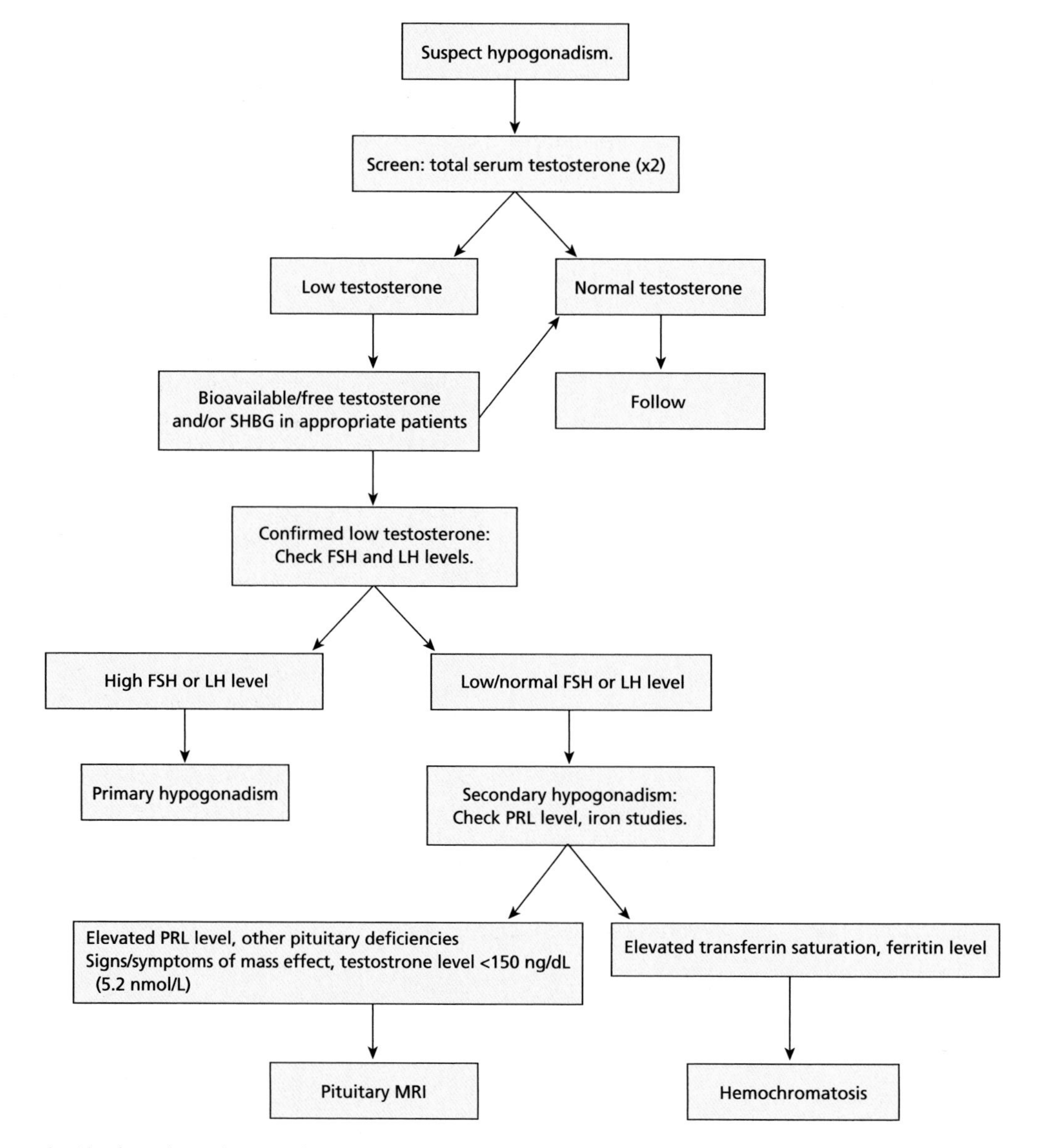

FIGURE 12. Algorithm for evaluating hypogonadism. FSH = follicle-stimulating hormone; LH = luteinizing hormone; PRL = prolactin; SHBG = sex hormone–binding globulin; ×2 = two separate measurements.

In the 1950s, intramuscular testosterone preparations became available. Current preparations include testosterone enanthate and testosterone cypionate, which are administered every 2 to 4 weeks. Advantages to these preparations include their low cost and dosing flexibility. The disadvantage is the large fluctuation in testosterone level after each injection, which can cause fluctuations in mood, energy, libido, and erectile function.

In the 1980s, transdermal preparations that were applied to the scrotum became available. Current transdermal preparations include nongenital patches. Those with an alcohol base often cause skin irritability, and those without an alcohol base can have poor skin adherence, especially in patients who are physically active.

Another testosterone preparation is a buccal tablet applied twice daily. Adverse effects include gum irritation and a bitter taste.

The most popular testosterone preparations currently are hydroalcoholic gels. Advantages to these preparations are the steady level of testosterone provided within 30 minutes of administration and the invisibility of the gel. Disadvantages include the need for daily use, cost, and possible exposure to and absorption by others who come in contact with the patient or his replacement therapy.

Patients receiving testosterone replacement therapy require monitoring of testosterone levels at 3 to 6 months after initiation and annually thereafter, with a goal testosterone level in the midnormal range. For patients receiving intramuscular testosterone preparations, the testosterone level should be checked at the midpoint between scheduled injections. For patients using transdermal preparations, testosterone levels can be checked at any time.

Some of the adverse effects of testosterone replacement—increased hematocrit, worsened sleep apnea, benign prostatic hyperplasia, dyslipidemia, and possibly increased risk of prostate cancer—also need careful monitoring. The Endocrine Society has released clinical guidelines for monitoring these adverse effects (**Table 26**). Recently, long-term adverse cardiovascular effects have been described with testosterone use, which further emphasize the danger of overdiagnosing hypogonadism or overprescribing testosterone replacement therapy.

KEY POINTS

- Advantages of using a hydroalcoholic gel for testosterone replacement therapy are the steady level of testosterone provided within 30 minutes of administration and the invisibility of the gel; disadvantages include the need for daily use, the cost, and the risk of exposure to and absorption by others who come in contact with the patient.
- After a patient begins testosterone replacement therapy, careful monitoring of testosterone levels and other parameters should occur to assess for adverse effects of treatment, such as increased hematocrit, worsened sleep apnea, benign prostatic hyperplasia, and dyslipidemia.

Anabolic Steroid Abuse in Men

Androgen abuse is common among elite and professional athletes and in young men. The exogenous androgens used for this purpose can suppress endogenous gonadotropins and, therefore, testicular testosterone production. Commonly abused androgens include injectable testosterone esters, oral alkylated testosterone preparations, human chorionic gonadotropin (HCG) injections, aromatase inhibitors, dehydroepiandrosterone (DHEA), and androstenedione supplements.

Physical examination findings may include excessive muscular bulk, acne, gynecomastia, and decreased testicular volume. Low sperm counts also may be present with exogenous androgen use. Androgen abuse can result in hypogonadism and infertility, which occasionally are irreversible. Additional adverse side effects include a low HDL cholesterol level, hepatotoxicity, erythrocytosis, and psychiatric disorders.

Male Infertility

The single best test to assess male fertility is semen analysis. The patient should abstain from sexual activity for 48 to 72 hours to ensure an adequate sample. If semen analysis

TABLE 26. Endocrine Society Clinical Guidelines for Monitoring Adverse Effects of Testosterone Replacement Therapy

Parameter	Recommended Screening Schedule	Alerts
Hematocrit	Value obtained at baseline and then at 3 months and 6 months after therapy initiation, followed by yearly measurements	Value >54%
PSA level	For patients >40 years of age with a baseline value >0.6 ng/mL (0.6 µg/L), DRE and PSA level (determined at 3 and 6 months after therapy initiation followed by regular screening)	Increase >1.4 ng/mL (1.4 µg/L) in 1 y or >0.4 ng/mL (0.4 µg/L) after 6 months of use; abnormal results on DRE; AUA prostate symptoms score/IPSS >19

AUA = American Urological Association; DRE = digital rectal examination; IPSS = International Prostate Symptom Score; µg = microgram(s); PSA = prostate-specific antigen.

Data from Bhasin S, Cunningham GR, Hayes FJ, et al. Testosterone therapy in men with androgen deficiency syndromes: an Endocrine Society Clinical Practice Guideline. J Clin Endocrinol Metab. 2010;95(6):2550. [PMID: 20525905]

results are abnormal, the test should be repeated. If confirmed as abnormal, then a referral to a reproductive endocrinologist or urologist is warranted to determine the best treatment plan.

KEY POINT

- The single best test to assess male fertility is semen analysis, which should be repeated if initial results are abnormal.

Gynecomastia

Gynecomastia is a benign but abnormal growth of breast tissue in male patients resulting from an imbalance of testosterone and estrogen, which leads to an increased estrogen-to-testosterone ratio. Causes of this imbalance include medications (such as spironolactone, cimetidine, calcium channel blockers, and ACE inhibitors), liver disease, kidney disease, male hypogonadism, testicular cancer, hyperthyroidism, adrenal tumors, HCG-secreting tumors, and androgen insensitivity syndrome. When this imbalance occurs in the neonatal period and adolescence, gynecomastia is often physiologic, resolving spontaneously most of the time.

Gynecomastia is confirmed on physical examination by the detection of subareolar glandular tissue and should be differentiated from lipomastia, or accumulation of fat in the breast. If gynecomastia is present, a careful evaluation to detect secondary causes, such as chronic illnesses, hyperthyroidism, medications, and drug abuse, is required. The initial laboratory evaluation includes obtaining serum levels of total testosterone, estradiol, HCG, LH, and thyroid-stimulating hormone (TSH). If either primary or secondary hypogonadism is diagnosed, then an evaluation to determine the cause is indicated. If the HCG level is elevated, testicular ultrasonography should be performed first. If the ultrasound is negative for any neoplasm, then chest and abdominal imaging is appropriate to detect malignancy. If the estradiol level is elevated, testicular ultrasonography is performed first; if no mass is detected, adrenal CT or MRI is performed to evaluate for an adrenal mass. If this imaging is negative, the cause is likely to be idiopathic or due to elevated peripheral aromatase activity. If both LH and testosterone levels are elevated and if the rest of the hormonal evaluation is unremarkable, androgen insensitivity syndrome is the likely diagnosis.

KEY POINT

- In a male patient with gynecomastia, a careful evaluation to detect secondary causes, such as chronic illness, hyperthyroidism, medications, and drug abuse, is required; appropriate initial laboratory evaluation includes measurement of serum levels of total testosterone, estradiol, human chorionic gonadotropin, luteinizing hormone, and thyroid-stimulating hormone.

Physiology of Female Reproduction

Normal function of the menstrual cycle requires careful coordination of inhibition and stimulation between the hormones of the hypothalamic (GnRH)–pituitary (FSH, LH)–ovarian (estradiol and progesterone) axis. The GnRH pulse frequency varies across the menstrual cycle to promote follicular development and ovulation (**Figure 13**). The FSH level increases slightly in the early follicular phase of the menstrual cycle, which begins with the onset of menstrual bleeding (day 1). This increase leads to recruitment of ovarian follicles, an increase in estradiol (which stimulates endometrial proliferation), and induction of LH receptors in the ovaries. Estradiol exerts acute positive feedback on the pituitary gland, eliciting an LH surge. This LH surge results in ovulation and initiates the luteal phase of the menstrual cycle. Additionally, LH stimulates theca cell androgen production. Androgens are aromatized to estrogen in the granulosa cells by FSH. After the LH surge, the corpus luteum secretes estradiol and progesterone. The declining progesterone levels lead to menstrual bleeding unless conception has occurred.

An average normal menstrual cycle is 28 to 35 days in length. The luteal phase length is constant and usually is 14 days. The follicular phase varies in length from 14 to 21 days, but relatively little variation characterizes follicular phase length in healthy adult women age 20 to 40 years. More cycle length variation occurs in the first 5 years of menstruation, and a decrease in follicular phase length occurs during perimenopause. Menstrual cycles less than 25 days or greater than 35 days are likely anovulatory.

Primary Amenorrhea

Primary amenorrhea is defined as the lack of menses by age 16 years accompanied by a normal body hair pattern and

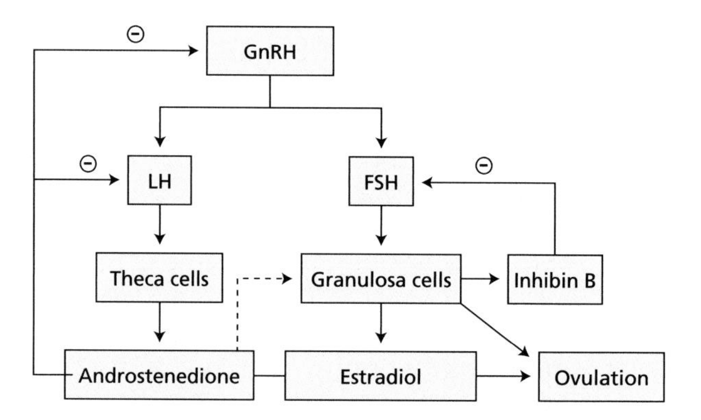

FIGURE 13. Female reproductive axis. As in the male reproductive axis, pulses of GnRH drive LH and FSH production. LH acts on theca cells to stimulate androgen (principally androstenedione) production. Androstenedione is metabolized to estradiol in granulosa cells. FSH acts on granulosa cells to enhance follicle maturation. Granulosa cells produce inhibin B as a feedback regulator of FSH production. FSH = follicle-stimulating hormone; GnRH = gonadotropin-releasing hormone; LH = luteinizing hormone; – (circled) = negative feedback.

normal breast development. Pregnancy must be ruled out in all patients with primary amenorrhea. Approximately 50% of patients with primary amenorrhea have a chromosomal abnormality, such as gonadal dysgenesis, and approximately 15% have an anatomic abnormality of the uterus, vagina, or cervix. Primary ovarian insufficiency due to Turner syndrome, a syndrome characterized by short stature and the loss of a portion or all of one X chromosome, is one of the most common causes of primary amenorrhea. The diagnosis of Turner syndrome can be made on the basis of a karyotype. Diagnosing Turner syndrome is critical because affected patients have a higher incidence of cardiovascular disease, metabolic syndrome, and thyroid dysfunction and should be evaluated annually as adults for these entities.

KEY POINT

- One of the most common causes of primary amenorrhea is primary ovarian insufficiency due to Turner syndrome, which is diagnosed by a karyotype.

Secondary Amenorrhea

Secondary amenorrhea is defined as the absence of a menstrual cycle for three cycles or 6 months in previously menstruating women. Pregnancy is the most common cause of secondary amenorrhea.

Uterine or outflow tract disorders (especially Asherman syndrome), although rare, also must always be considered as a possible cause. Asherman syndrome is due to endometrial scarring after a uterine procedure (usually, repeated dilation and curettage) and should be considered in any woman with amenorrhea and past exposure to uterine instrumentation. The classic presentation is amenorrhea with ovulatory or premenstrual symptoms. After pregnancy is excluded, approximately 40% of secondary amenorrhea will be due to ovarian causes, most commonly polycystic ovary syndrome (PCOS). Additional causes of secondary amenorrhea include hypothalamic amenorrhea, hyperprolactinemia, thyroid disease, and primary ovarian insufficiency.

Functional hypothalamic amenorrhea affects 3% of women between age 18 and 40 years and is a diagnosis of exclusion. Risk factors for this condition include a low body weight and fat percentage, rapid and substantial weight loss, eating disorders, excessive exercise, severe emotional stress, severe nutritional deficiencies, and chronic or acute illness. FSH and LH levels are inappropriately low or normal in this low-estrogen disorder, but FSH is frequently higher than LH. Recovery of menses occurs in 30% to 100% of patients, depending on the cause, with stress and weight loss exhibiting the best prognoses.

Hyperprolactinemia causes secondary amenorrhea through direct inhibition of GnRH secretion. Both hypothyroidism and hyperthyroidism also cause secondary amenorrhea. Hypothyroidism results in increased levels of thyrotropin-releasing hormone through negative feedback, and this hormone, in turn, stimulates prolactin secretion. Hyperthyroidism can cause rapid weight loss, which is known to cause functional hypothalamic amenorrhea.

Primary ovarian insufficiency is defined as amenorrhea before age 40 years in the setting of two elevated FSH levels. Possible secondary causes include Turner syndrome, a fragile X premutation carrier status, autoimmune oophoritis, and the effects of chemotherapy or radiation therapy.

Diagnosis and Evaluation of Amenorrhea

The initial evaluation of amenorrhea includes a thorough history and physical examination and measurement of serum HCG, prolactin, FSH, and TSH levels to assess for pregnancy, hyperprolactinemia, primary ovarian insufficiency, and thyroid disease, respectively. A pelvic ultrasound is required in all patients with primary amenorrhea. A pituitary MRI also is required in these patients if primary ovarian insufficiency is excluded as a cause and in patients with secondary amenorrhea that is hypothalamic in nature but has no clear cause to exclude a pituitary or hypothalamic tumor.

If the prolactin level is elevated, then an evaluation for causes of hyperprolactinemia is necessary, including a review of the patient's medications, thyroid status, and kidney function and, possibly, imaging of the pituitary gland to evaluate for pituitary adenoma. If the FSH level is elevated on two separate measurements, then the diagnosis of primary ovarian insufficiency is made. Patients with these findings also should have a karyotype to evaluate for Turner syndrome and should be tested for the fragile X mutation; a careful review of systems is necessary to assess for autoimmune disease. If the patient has thyroid dysfunction, then treatment of the underlying disorder should result in resumption of menses.

If results of the laboratory tests are normal, the next step is to assess estrogen sufficiency with a progesterone challenge test. Estradiol levels can be variable in amenorrhea of differing causes, but results of a progesterone challenge test will clearly delineate between an estrogen-deficient state (no bleeding) and an estrogen-sufficient state (withdrawal bleeding). If the patient is producing estrogen, she will have withdrawal bleeding within 1 week of completing a course of progesterone. In this case, the patient is not estrogen deficient, and PCOS (or a similar diagnosis) should be considered. If no withdrawal bleeding occurs after the progesterone challenge, then the patient has a low-estrogen state, and hypothalamic amenorrhea is the diagnosis. If no clear cause of the hypothalamic amenorrhea is present, then a pituitary MRI should be ordered to rule out a pituitary adenoma.

KEY POINT

- In a patient with amenorrhea and normal results on initial laboratory studies, the next step in evaluation is a progesterone challenge test.

Hirsutism and Polycystic Ovary Syndrome

Hirsutism is defined as an excess in terminal hair growth in women in androgen-dependent areas of the body. A patient's familial hair pattern and ethnic background should be taken into account when assessing for hirsutism. When hirsutism is present, then the patient must be assessed for virilization, which is commonly due to an ovarian or adrenal tumor. Signs and symptoms of virilization include a deepening of voice, severe acne, clitoromegaly, a decrease in breast size, and male-pattern balding. Other concerning features are rapid onset and progressive hirsutism over a short period of time (such as 1 year) or hirsutism that develops after age 30 years.

Recommended laboratory tests for moderate to severe hirsutism or virilization include measurement of the plasma DHEA sulfate level and serum levels of TSH, prolactin, total testosterone, and follicular phase 17-hydroxyprogesterone to exclude thyroid disease, hyperprolactinemia, ovarian and adrenal tumors, and late-onset congenital adrenal hyperplasia. If the serum total testosterone level is greater than 200 ng/dL (6.9 nmol/L), then a pelvic ultrasound and adrenal CT are necessary to exclude an ovarian or adrenal neoplasm; if the plasma DHEA sulfate level is greater than 700 micrograms/mL (1890 micromoles/L), then an adrenal CT is necessary to exclude an adrenal cortisol-secreting and/or androgen-secreting neoplasm. Most cases of hirsutism have benign causes, with PCOS being the most common.

PCOS is one of the most common endocrine disorders in young women, with a prevalence of approximately 7%. In 1990, the National Institutes of Health defined PCOS as occurring in women who have oligomenorrhea and clinical or biochemical evidence of hyperandrogenism when other endocrine disorders are excluded. In 2003, the American Society for Reproductive Medicine and the European Society of Human Reproduction established new, still debated diagnostic criteria (Rotterdam criteria) stating that two of the following three findings must be present to establish a diagnosis of PCOS: (1) oligo-ovulation or anovulation, (2) clinical or biochemical evidence of hyperandrogenism, and (3) polycystic ovarian morphology on an ultrasound when other endocrine disorders are excluded.

The primary clinical manifestations of PCOS are menstrual irregularity (oligomenorrhea or amenorrhea), ovulatory dysfunction with resultant infertility, insulin resistance, and hyperandrogenism. Oligo-ovulation or anovulation can result in endometrial hyperplasia and/or infertility. Hyperandrogenism presents as hirsutism, acne, or androgenic alopecia. Most patients with PCOS also have insulin resistance, and studies have shown an increased incidence of metabolic syndrome, obesity, impaired glucose tolerance, and frank type 2 diabetes mellitus. Both obese and lean women with PCOS have evidence of insulin resistance, which suggests that this finding is intrinsic to the disorder. Improvement in insulin resistance with weight loss or the use of metformin is associated with a decrease in serum androgen levels. In fact, patients treated with metformin have not only improved insulin sensitivity and androgen levels, but also improved ovulatory rates with increased pregnancy rates. These data strongly suggest that the insulin resistance of PCOS plays a role in the oligomenorrhea and hyperandrogenism seen in this disorder. More recent studies also have shown frequent associations between the insulin resistance of PCOS and both fatty liver disease and sleep apnea.

Treatment of the clinical manifestations of PCOS depends on which symptom(s) is(are) most problematic to the patient. Weight loss and exercise are mainstays of therapy for all patients with PCOS and have been shown to lessen the severity of clinical manifestations of the disorder. If a patient's major concern is hyperandrogenism, then oral contraceptive therapy is the best choice. Spironolactone may be added after 6 months if acne and hirsutism are still cosmetically bothersome to the patient. Additional treatments for hirsutism include waxing, electrolysis, laser therapy, and topical eflornithine. For the menstrual irregularities associated with PCOS, oral estrogen-progesterone contraceptives are effective and provide endometrial protection. If a patient has a contraindication to oral contraceptives or does not wish to take them, cyclical progesterone can be given to induce withdrawal bleeding. The insulin resistance of PCOS is treated with diet and exercise. Metformin also can be used, especially if acanthosis nigricans or impaired glucose tolerance is present. Infertility in PCOS is usually treated with diet, exercise, clomiphene, or metformin, depending on the patient's age, degree of insulin resistance, and personal preference.

KEY POINTS

- A woman with acute onset of rapidly progressive hirsutism should be assessed for signs of virilization (deepening of the voice, acne, clitoromegaly, decrease in breast size, and male-pattern balding) because of the risk of an androgen-secreting ovarian or adrenal tumor.
- Polycystic ovary syndrome, which is characterized by menstrual irregularities and hyperandrogenism, is associated with insulin resistance and an increased risk of metabolic syndrome, impaired glucose tolerance, and type 2 diabetes mellitus.
- Oral contraceptives are effective in treating the oligomenorrhea of polycystic ovary syndrome (PCOS) and provide endometrial protection; the insulin resistance and obesity of PCOS are best treated with weight loss and exercise, but use of metformin also should be considered.

Anabolic Steroid Abuse in Women

Some women abuse anabolic steroids to enhance their athletic performance or physique. Adverse effects include hirsutism, acne, deepening of the voice, decreased breast size, and clitoromegaly. Withdrawal of androgens does not result in severe hypogonadism, as it does in men. Symptoms of hyperandrogenism with a normal or low testosterone level may be a clue of androgen abuse.

Female Infertility

Infertility is defined as the inability to conceive in 1 year with regular unprotected sexual intercourse. If the female partner is older than 35 years, then infertility is defined as the inability to conceive within 6 months. Infertility evaluation for women includes a careful menstrual history and proper evaluation of oligomenorrhea, if present. Measuring serum TSH and prolactin levels is appropriate to exclude thyroid disease and hyperprolactinemia because even mild abnormalities in thyroid function or prolactin levels can result in infertility. If results of initial testing are normal, then referral to a reproductive endocrinologist is indicated. Further evaluation will typically include a semen analysis of the male partner, confirmation of ovulatory function with measurement of a midluteal progesterone level, ovarian reserve testing by measuring a serum FSH level on day 3 of the menstrual cycle, and hysterosalpingography performed sometime between days 6 and 10 of the menstrual cycle to evaluate for any uterine or tubal abnormalities. If no abnormalities are found, closely monitored therapy with clomiphene or gonadotropins may be initiated.

KEY POINT

- Measuring the serum thyroid-stimulating hormone and prolactin levels is appropriate to exclude thyroid disease and hyperprolactinemia in a woman with infertility; if results of initial testing are normal, then referral to a reproductive endocrinologist for further evaluation and treatment is appropriate.

Calcium and Bone Disorders

Calcium Homeostasis

Precise regulation of calcium homeostasis in the body is critical. Calcium is the main mineral component of the skeleton and plays major roles in neuronal transmission, muscle contraction, and blood clotting; it also is an important intracellular messenger regulating numerous processes throughout the body. The normal range for the total serum calcium level is 9.0 to 10.5 mg/dL (2.2-2.6 mmol/L); 50% to 60% of this calcium is bound to plasma proteins or complexed with anions, and the remaining ionized calcium controls physiologic actions. The normal level of ionized calcium is maintained in a very narrow range (4.4-5.2 mg/dL [1.1-1.3 mmol/L]).

The body regulates serum calcium by controlling its entry through the intestine, its exit through the kidney, and its storage in bone (**Figure 14**). These processes are regulated by parathyroid hormone (PTH) and 1,25-dihydroxyvitamin D. 1,25-Dihydroxyvitamin D is made when exposure of the skin to ultraviolet light triggers conversion of 7-dehydrocholesterol to vitamin D_3 or cholecalciferol. Cholecalciferol also is supplied by dietary sources or nutritional supplements, such as vitamin D_2 (ergocalciferol), a plant steroid. In the liver, vitamins D_2 and D_3 are hydroxylated to 25-hydroxyvitamin D, the storage form of vitamin D, which in turn is hydroxylated in the kidney to the active form, 1,25-dihydroxyvitamin D. PTH and 1,25-dihydroxyvitamin D maintain tight control of the plasma ionized calcium level.

The plasma ionized calcium level is monitored by a parathyroid cell membrane calcium-sensing receptor (CSR).

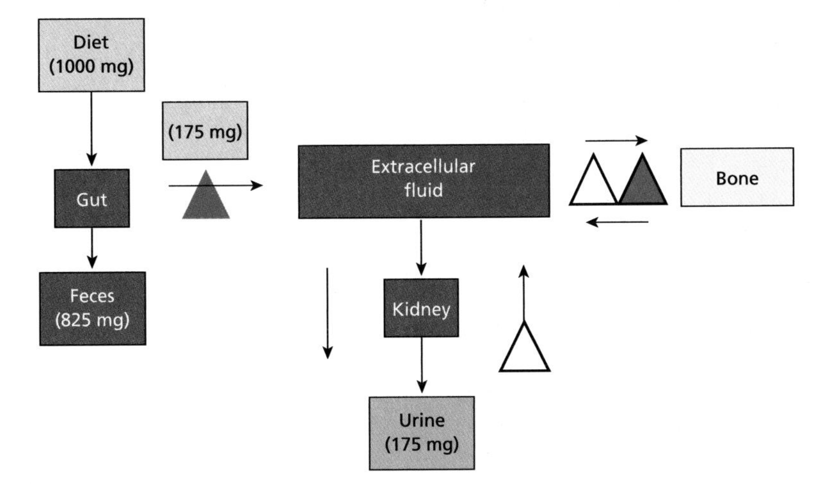

FIGURE 14. Regulation of calcium homeostasis. The flow of calcium through the body (net daily calcium flux) in a hypothetical healthy person with a typical dietary calcium intake of 1000 mg/d is shown. In this example, 175 mg is absorbed by the gut and enters the extracellular fluid compartment (plasma and interstitial fluid). The remaining 825 mg is lost in feces. After filtration of plasma by the kidney, most of the calcium is reclaimed from the filtrate, and in this example, 175 mg is released in urine to maintain net zero change in total body calcium. Processes regulated by parathyroid hormone are indicated by white triangles, and those regulated by 1,25-dihydroxyvitamin D are indicated by teal triangles.

As circulating levels of plasma ionized calcium increase, CSR signaling is activated and causes PTH secretion to decrease; when plasma ionized calcium levels are low, PTH secretion increases. PTH activates bone resorption and distal nephron calcium resorption. PTH also stimulates kidney production of 1,25-dihydroxyvitamin D, thereby increasing calcium absorption by the small intestine. If plasma ionized calcium levels increase above the normal range, PTH secretion declines, which leads to greater calcium losses by the kidneys, reduced 1,25-dihydroxyvitamin D production, and decreased calcium absorption by the intestines. Both PTH and 1,25-dihydroxyvitamin D act on bone to facilitate calcium release. Accordingly, the plasma ionized calcium level is maintained in a narrow range, even at the expense of skeletal calcium when necessary.

Hypercalcemia

Clinical Manifestations of Hypercalcemia

Clinical manifestations of hypercalcemia are the same, regardless of its underlying cause. Most persons with mild hypercalcemia (levels > the normal serum calcium level but <12 mg/dL [3.0 mmol/L]) are asymptomatic, although some report mild fatigue, depression, constipation, mild polyuria, mild increase in thirst, or vague changes in cognition. Typical manifestations of hypercalcemia are more common with serum calcium levels of 12 to 14 mg/dL (3.0-3.5 mmol/L) and include anorexia, nausea, abdominal pain, muscle weakness, and depressed mental status. Dehydration caused by polyuria also is common because hypercalciuria decreases the kidneys' ability to concentrate urine. At calcium levels greater than 14 mg/dL (3.5 mmol/L), lethargy, disorientation, and coma may develop. The severity of the symptoms is determined by the severity of the serum calcium elevation, the rate of increase, and the overall health of the affected person.

Patients with primary hyperparathyroidism (and thus, by definition, hypercalcemia) in the setting of multiple endocrine neoplasia (MEN) types 1 and 2 also may have specific manifestations of the other tumors associated with these syndromes. Patients with hypercalcemia due to sarcoidosis may have inflammatory or pulmonary symptoms. Because hypercalcemia of malignancy typically develops only when a substantial tumor burden is present, most patients with this type of hypercalcemia already have symptoms related to an established cancer diagnosis.

KEY POINT

- Typical manifestations of hypercalcemia include anorexia, nausea, abdominal pain, muscle weakness, dehydration, and depressed mental status; symptom severity is determined by the extent of the serum calcium elevation, the rate of increase, and the overall health of the affected person.

Causes and Diagnosis of Hypercalcemia

Identifying the cause of hypercalcemia (**Table 27**) requires a comprehensive history, physical examination, laboratory tests, and, occasionally, imaging studies. Medications, foods, and nutritional supplements should be reviewed. Family history suggesting inherited disorders of calcium metabolism or related conditions should be elicited. In addition to evaluating patients with suspected hypercalcemia for signs of dehydration and depressed mental status, the clinician should identify signs of common causes of hypercalcemia, such as malignancy and granulomatous diseases. Benign parathyroid conditions do not produce a neck mass. Physical evidence of osteoporosis or kidney stones should also be sought. Other findings depend on the type of hypercalcemia involved (see Table 27).

When an elevated serum calcium level is found, factitious hypercalcemia—caused by increased levels of the plasma proteins that bind calcium—must first be excluded in patients at risk for this condition, including those with HIV infection, chronic hepatitis, and multiple myeloma. The ionized calcium level in these patients remains normal.

After hypercalcemia is confirmed, the next step is the simultaneous measurement of serum PTH and serum or plasma ionized calcium levels. In the absence of plasma protein abnormalities, obtaining a total serum calcium level is usually adequate; ionized calcium samples must be drawn under anaerobic conditions and kept on ice for accurate results. With normal parathyroid glands, hypercalcemia will suppress PTH. If the serum calcium level is elevated and the PTH level is high or inappropriately normal, the diagnosis of PTH-mediated hypercalcemia or primary hyperparathyroidism is made (see later discussion) (**Figure 15**). If PTH levels are low, causes of non–PTH-mediated hypercalcemia should be considered (see later discussion). The serum creatinine level also may be acutely elevated in persons with hypercalcemia who are dehydrated or chronically elevated in those with nephrocalcinosis. The serum phosphorus level may be low in hypercalcemia associated with primary hyperparathyroidism, whereas hyperphosphatemia may occur if the cause is vitamin D intoxication. By changing the set point for the CSR, lithium therapy can lead to mild hypercalcemia and mildly elevated PTH levels that mimic primary hyperparathyroidism but do not require intervention.

Parathyroid Hormone–Mediated Hypercalcemia

Description, Evaluation, and Treatment

Primary hyperparathyroidism is the most common cause of hypercalcemia diagnosed in the outpatient setting. The annual incidence of primary hyperparathyroidism in the United States is approximately four per 100,000 persons. The incidence peaks in the fifth to sixth decade of life, with a female-to-male ratio of 3:2. The clinical manifestations of hyperparathyroidism depend on its severity and chronicity. The hypercalcemia of primary hyperparathyroidism often is

TABLE 27. Differential Diagnosis of Hypercalcemia

Parathyroid Hormone Mediated
Primary hyperparathyroidism
Parathyroid adenoma(s)
Parathyroid hyperplasia
Parathyroid carcinoma
Tertiary hyperparathyroidism
Familial hypocalciuric hypercalcemia
Lithium therapy–associated hypercalcemia
Nonparathyroid Hormone Mediated
Malignancy-associated hypercalcemia
Humoral hypercalcemia of malignancy
PTH-related protein (squamous cell carcinoma, adenocarcinoma of the breast or ovary, renal cell carcinoma, transitional cell carcinoma, T-cell lymphoma, islet cell neoplasms, myeloma)
1,25-Dihydroxyvitamin D (B-cell lymphoma)
Local osteolytic hypercalcemia (myeloma, breast cancer, lymphoma)
Granulomatous diseases (sarcoidosis, tuberculosis)
Endocrinopathies (hyperthyroidism, adrenal insufficiency)
Certain drugs (thiazide diuretics, excessive calcium supplements, vitamin D or A)
Immobilization
Other (increased plasma protein levels from factitious hypercalcemia, acute kidney failure, total parenteral nutrition, or milk alkali syndrome)

PTH = parathyroid hormone.

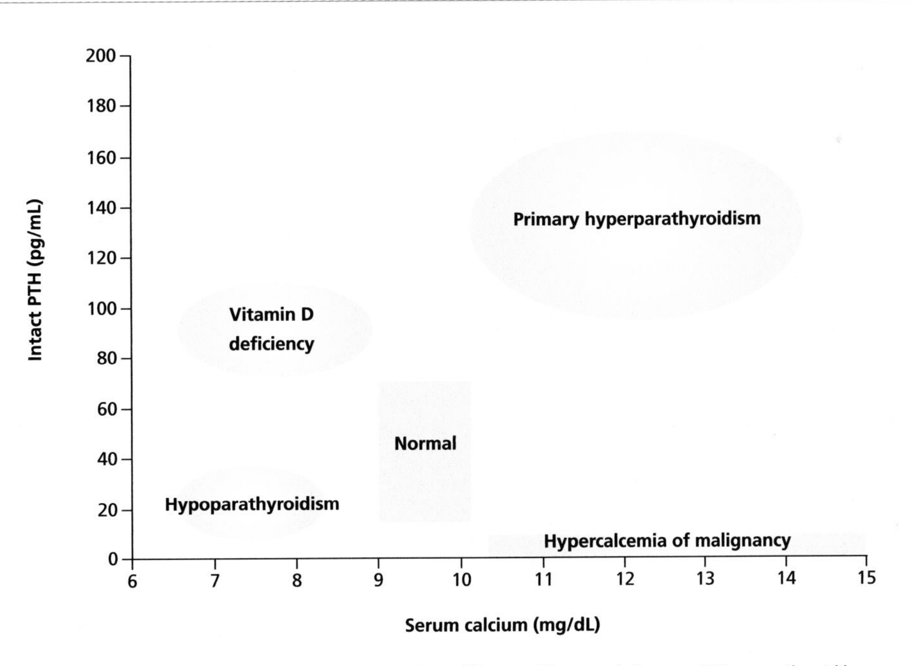

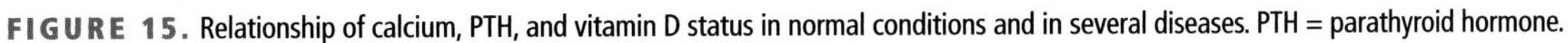

FIGURE 15. Relationship of calcium, PTH, and vitamin D status in normal conditions and in several diseases. PTH = parathyroid hormone.

diagnosed incidentally by routine blood testing before the development of symptoms. This disorder also may be found during the evaluation of osteoporosis or nephrolithiasis. In 75% to 80% of patients with primary hyperparathyroidism, a solitary parathyroid adenoma is present; hyperplasia involving multiple parathyroid glands is found in 15% to 20%, and parathyroid carcinoma is present in less than 1%. Symptoms associated with more severe or prolonged disease include nephrolithiasis, kidney disease due to nephrocalcinosis, fragility fractures, and bone pain.

After the diagnosis of primary hyperparathyroidism is established, additional testing may be necessary to determine whether parathyroidectomy is warranted. Guidelines for surgical intervention in patients with asymptomatic primary hyperparathyroidism were updated at a National Institutes of Health workshop in 2008 (**Table 28**). A parathyroid sestamibi scan or ultrasound may locate the causative adenoma but is not required to diagnose primary hyperparathyroidism.

No current medical therapy is as effective as surgery for primary hyperparathyroidism. A 15-year long-term follow-up study of patients who did not undergo parathyroidectomy showed that one third developed disease progression and most experienced additional bone loss by the study's end. Patients who do not have surgery can be monitored and, in some cases, may benefit from medication. Dietary calcium should not be restricted in these patients, and vitamin D deficiency should be corrected to prevent further elevation of PTH and bone loss. In those with low bone mass, a bisphosphonate will help slow bone loss but will not control hypercalcemia. In patients with symptomatic hypercalcemia who are not surgical candidates or whose causative parathyroid adenoma cannot be localized, the calcimimetic agent cinacalcet can control hypercalcemia. However, this agent has multiple drug interactions and is very expensive, and its long-term safety has not been established, limiting its use to specific clinical situations.

A schedule recommending follow-up testing of persons with primary hyperparathyroidism who do not undergo parathyroidectomy also was developed at the 2008 National Institutes of Health workshop (**Table 29**). Patients who develop criteria for parathyroidectomy should be referred for surgery.

Familial Forms of Hyperparathyroidism

Familial hypocalciuric hypercalcemia (FHH) is a rare autosomal dominant condition caused by inactivating mutations of the *CASR* gene. These mutations result in high serum calcium levels and inappropriately normal to mildly elevated serum PTH levels. Patients with FHH have low urine calcium excretion, although this finding may occur in those taking thiazide diuretics, proton pump inhibitors, or lithium. FHH is suspected in patients with a family history of asymptomatic, stable, mild hypercalcemia and in patients whose urine calcium to creatinine clearance ratio is very low (<0.01). The diagnosis of FHH can be made on clinical grounds in a patient with chronic mild hypercalcemia and hypocalciuria, lack of symptoms or sequelae, and a family history of similar findings. FHH can be confirmed with genetic testing for *CASR* gene mutations, although not all mutations have been characterized. FHH is usually a benign condition that requires no intervention but should be recognized to prevent unnecessary parathyroidectomy.

Familial hyperparathyroidism can occur as an isolated entity or as part of the MEN syndromes (types 1 and 2). These syndromes should be considered in all patients with primary hyperparathyroidism, particularly those who are young or have a personal or family history of a related endocrinopathy. Knowing before surgery whether the hyperparathyroidism is familial or not is essential because patients with inherited primary hyperparathyroidism often have multigland parathyroid hyperplasia, and evaluation of all parathyroid glands should occur during surgery. If MEN2 is suspected, pheochromocytoma must be excluded before the patient can safely undergo surgery, and the patient should be evaluated for medullary thyroid cancer.

TABLE 28. Indications for Surgical Intervention in Patients with Primary Hyperparathyroidism

Increase in serum calcium level ≥1 mg/dL (0.25 mmol/L) above upper limit of normal[a]
Creatinine clearance <60 mL/min (0.06 L/min)[a]
T-score (on DEXA scan) of −2.5 or worse at the lumbar spine, total hip, femoral neck, or distal radius[a]
Age <50 y[a]
Surgery also indicated in patients in whom medical surveillance is neither desired nor possible, including those with significant bone, kidney, gastrointestinal, or neuromuscular symptoms typical of primary hyperparathyroidism

DEXA = dual-energy x-ray absorptiometry.

[a]In otherwise asymptomatic patients.

Adapted from Bilezikian JP, Khan AA, Potts JT Jr; Third International Workshop on the Management of Asymptomatic Primary Hyperthyroidism. Guidelines for the management of asymptomatic primary hyperparathyroidism: summary statement from the Third International Workshop. J Clin Endocrinol Metab. 2009;94(2):336. [PMID: 19193908] Copyright 2009, The Endocrine Society.

TABLE 29. Long-Term Monitoring of Patients with Primary Hyperparathyroidism Who Do Not Undergo Parathyroidectomy

Test	Interval
Serum calcium	Annually
Serum creatinine	Annually
Bone densitometry	Every 1-2 years at three sites (such as the lumbar spine, hip, and distal radius)

Adapted from Bilezikian JP, Khan AA, Potts JT Jr; Third International Workshop on the Management of Asymptomatic Primary Hyperthyroidism. Guidelines for the management of asymptomatic primary hyperparathyroidism: summary statement from the Third International Workshop. J Clin Endocrinol Metab. 2009;94(2):336. [PMID: 19193908] Copyright 2009, The Endocrine Society.

Nonparathyroid Hormone–Mediated Hypercalcemia

Causes and Diagnosis

If a patient's serum calcium level is elevated and the PTH level is appropriately suppressed to less than normal, then PTH-independent hypercalcemia is likely. A non-PTH disorder is most often responsible for acute hypercalcemia. Cancer is the most common cause of PTH-independent hypercalcemia and the most frequent cause of acute hypercalcemia in a hospitalized patient. When the PTH level is low and the patient does not have a malignancy, diagnostic considerations should

CONT.

include nonmalignant causes, such as vitamin D intoxication or production of 1,25-dihydroxyvitamin D by granulomatous disease (such as sarcoidosis or tuberculosis) (see Table 27).

Malignancy-Associated Hypercalcemia
In malignancy-associated hypercalcemia, the serum calcium elevation is usually moderate or severe, and the PTH level is low (see Figure 15). Evidence of significant dehydration and generalized debility is evident, as are other cancer-related symptoms. In most instances, a cancer diagnosis has already been established.

Humoral hypercalcemia of malignancy (HHM) results from tumor production of a circulating factor that acts on skeletal calcium release, renal calcium handling, or intestinal calcium absorption. Rarely, this disorder can be caused by unregulated production of 1,25-dihydroxyvitamin D (as in B-cell lymphomas) or other mediators that interfere with calcium homeostasis. The most common cause of HHM is PTH-related protein (PTHrP). PTHrP is homologous to PTH, and they share a common receptor. PTHrP and PTH both activate osteoclasts to resorb bone, thereby decreasing calcium excretion and increasing phosphate clearance by the kidneys.

Tumors that cause HHM by secreting PTHrP are typically squamous cell carcinomas (often of the lung), although other tumors (such as breast and renal cell carcinoma) also can be responsible. Tumors produce PTHrP in small amounts. Therefore, HHM typically develops in patients with a large tumor burden and is seldom the presenting feature of a cancer.

Another form of malignancy-associated hypercalcemia is local osteolytic hypercalcemia, which occurs when bony metastases produce factors that activate bone resorption by osteoclasts. The classic tumor associated with this syndrome is multiple myeloma, although other neoplasms (breast cancer, lymphoma) may also be implicated.

KEY POINTS

- If the serum calcium level is elevated and the parathyroid hormone (PTH) level is high or inappropriately normal in a patient with hypercalcemia, the diagnosis is PTH-mediated primary hyperparathyroidism, most often caused by a solitary parathyroid adenoma.
- Tumors that secrete parathyroid hormone–related protein, typically squamous cell carcinomas, are the most common cause of hypercalcemia of malignancy.

Treatment of Acute Hypercalcemia

When the serum calcium level is severely elevated, treatment should include rehydration and increasing urine calcium excretion while simultaneously reducing bone resorption or intestinal calcium absorption, depending on which is the main source of the excess calcium.

Most patients with acute hypercalcemia have volume contraction, which further exacerbates their inability to excrete calcium. Therefore, the first intervention should be intravenous infusion of normal saline. Delivery of sodium and water to the distal nephron will enhance urine calcium excretion. After intravascular volume is replenished, a loop diuretic, such as furosemide, allows additional aggressive saline hydration and may further enhance calcium excretion. However, evidence for the efficacy of furosemide in this setting is lacking.

Nearly all causes of severe hypercalcemia involve increased osteoclast activity, and thus drugs that inhibit bone resorption are useful. The treatment of choice is an intravenous bisphosphonate, such as pamidronate or zoledronate. Zoledronate has greater potency and a longer duration of action than pamidronate. Caution should be exercised with these agents in the setting of kidney dysfunction.

For more rapid resolution of hypercalcemia, subcutaneous injection of calcitonin can be used, either alone or simultaneously with a bisphosphonate. Tachyphylaxis limits the effectiveness of calcitonin to a few days. In severe or refractory hypercalcemia, low-calcium bath hemodialysis may be required. Patients whose kidney function precludes the use of bisphosphonates may respond to off-label use of denosumab, which also reduces osteoclast-mediated bone resorption.

When hypercalcemia results from increased intestinal calcium absorption, as occurs in vitamin D intoxication or granulomatous diseases, glucocorticoid treatment is indicated (for example, prednisone, 10-40 mg/d). Glucocorticoids directly impair intestinal calcium transport and also inhibit kidney or granulomatous 1α-hydroxylase activity, thereby resulting in decreased production of 1,25-dihydroxyvitamin D.

Long-term management should focus on addressing the cause of hypercalcemia. Treatment of the underlying cause may not lead to immediate lowering of the serum calcium level and thus should be coupled with short-term management interventions that should be continued until stabilization is achieved.

KEY POINT

- Treatment of acute hypercalcemia involves administering intravenous fluids, increasing urine calcium excretion, and reducing either bone resorption or intestinal calcium absorption, depending on which is the main source of excess calcium.

Hypocalcemia

Diagnosis and Causes of Hypocalcemia

Hypocalcemia is present when the serum calcium level is less than normal. This diagnosis should be confirmed with repeat measurements and a serum albumin measurement, given that a low plasma calcium-binding protein level can cause a factitious low serum calcium level. The measured serum calcium level should be corrected for a low albumin level by adding 0.8 mg/dL (0.2 mmol/L) of calcium for each 1 g/dL (10 g/L) of albumin that a patient's serum albumin level is less than 4 g/dL (40 g/L). An accurate ionized calcium measurement will circumvent these pitfalls.

Chronic mild to moderate hypocalcemia is usually asymptomatic. However, when the serum calcium level is less than 7.5 to 8.0 mg/dL (1.9-2.0 mmol/L) and the serum albumin level is normal, a patient may develop symptoms of neuromuscular irritability, including tremor, muscle spasms or cramps, or paresthesias. On physical examination, Chvostek sign (contraction of the ipsilateral facial muscles with tapping of the facial nerve) and Trousseau sign (carpopedal spasm induced by prolonged application of greater-than-systolic pressure by a blood pressure cuff) may be noted. Tetany or seizures may be seen if the serum calcium level becomes severely low. Prolongation of the corrected QT interval and bradycardia may be evident on an electrocardiogram, indicating that the patient is at risk for cardiac arrhythmias.

The cause of hypocalcemia usually is identified by obtaining a careful history (**Table 30**). Dietary calcium and vitamin D intake, inadequate sun exposure, gastrointestinal malabsorption, and alcohol intake should be discussed. Information

TABLE 30. Differential Diagnosis of Hypocalcemia

Condition	Laboratory Findings	Comments
Disorders of vitamin D metabolism (vitamin D deficiency) Lack of sunlight Dermatologic disorders Dietary deficiency Malabsorption Liver disease Kidney disease Vitamin D-dependent rickets, type I (1α-hydroxylase deficiency)	Mild hypocalcemia, hypophosphatemia, elevated PTH level, and decreased 25-hydroxyvitamin D level; decreased 1,25-dihydroxyvitamin D level if kidney disease is present	Vitamin D deficiency widespread among housebound and institutionalized older persons and general medical patients with disorders that predispose to altered vitamin D metabolism
Vitamin D resistance (vitamin D–dependent rickets, type II)	Hypocalcemia, hypophosphatemia, and elevated PTH level; elevated 1,25-dihydroxyvitamin D level when treated with vitamin D	Vitamin D–receptor defect leading to resistance to 1,25-dihydroxyvitamin D
Hypoparathyroidism Postsurgical (most common cause; seen after thyroid, parathyroid, or neck surgery) After external radiation therapy to neck Autoimmune (autoimmune polyglandular syndrome) Congenital (DiGeorge syndrome) Infiltrative (hemochromatosis, sarcoidosis)	Hypocalcemia, hyperphosphatemia, and a low or inappropriately normal PTH level	—
PTH resistance (pseudohypoparathyroidism)	Hypocalcemia, hyperphosphatemia, and elevated PTH level with normal 25-hydroxyvitamin D level	Pseudohypoparathyroidism, type 1a, an autosomal dominant disorder marked by resistance to multiple hormones and Albright hereditary osteodystrophy (short stature, obesity, round facies, brachymetacarpia, and mental deficiency)
Hypomagnesemia Chronic diuretic use Alcoholism Diarrhea Malabsorption Certain drugs (amphotericin B, aminoglycosides, cisplatin)	Hypomagnesemia and hypocalcemia; PTH level potentially low, normal, or high	Hypomagnesemia potentially leading to impaired PTH secretion and PTH resistance, with impaired tissue responsiveness to PTH

(*continued on next page*)

TABLE 30. Differential Diagnosis of Hypocalcemia (*continued*)

Condition	Laboratory Findings	Comments
Medications Causing altered vitamin D metabolism (phenytoin, phenobarbital, isoniazid, theophylline, rifampin, 5-fluorouracil plus leucovorin) Causing intravascular binding (phosphate, foscarnet, EDTA, citrated blood products) Intravenous bisphosphonates (especially in vitamin D deficiency; contraindicated in hypocalcemia)	Hypocalcemia and low 25-hydroxyvitamin D or 1,25-dihydroxyvitamin D level (with agents that alter vitamin D metabolism)	Hypocalcemia potentially developing rapidly with use of some medications, especially if administered intravenously
Extravascular deposition Pancreatitis Hungry-bone syndrome Rhabdomyolysis Tumor lysis syndrome Osteoblastic metastases	Hypocalcemia and hyper- or hypophosphatemia	In pancreatitis, hypocalcemia from the deposition of calcium in the form of calcium soaps; hyperphosphatemia suggestive of rhabdomyolysis or tumor lysis syndrome with release of phosphate from the bone; hypophosphatemia seen in hungry-bone syndrome or with osteoblastic metastases (of prostate or breast cancer)
Sepsis	Hypocalcemia and low PTH and 1,25-dihydroxyvitamin D levels	Sepsis most likely mediated by the action of inflammatory cytokines on the parathyroid glands, kidneys, and bone
Acute respiratory alkalosis	Normal serum calcium but low ionized calcium levels	Alkalosis leading to increased binding of calcium ions to albumin
Artifactual hypoglycemia with hypoalbuminemia	Low serum calcium and normal ionized calcium levels	Reduced protein binding leading to lower total serum calcium level, with normal ionized fraction

EDTA = ethylenediaminetetraacetic acid; PTH = parathyroid hormone.

about previous head and neck surgery and irradiation should be elicited because these are the most common causes of acquired hypoparathyroidism. The risk for rarer conditions, such as autoimmune disease and iron overload states, also should be determined. Any history of pancreatitis, rhabdomyolysis, tumor lysis syndrome, or ongoing transfusion therapy should be investigated because all are potential causes of hypocalcemia. If the patient's history and physical examination findings do not reveal an obvious reason for the hypocalcemia, simultaneous measurement of PTH and serum calcium levels will determine whether the process is PTH mediated. A low or inappropriately normal PTH level in the setting of a low calcium level indicates hypoparathyroidism. An elevated PTH level is seen in secondary hyperparathyroidism and is an appropriate physiologic response of the parathyroid glands to a low calcium level of any cause. These measurements should be followed by kidney function testing and measurement of magnesium, phosphorus, and 25-hydroxyvitamin D levels (see Figure 15).

Unintentional removal or injury of parathyroid glands during thyroidectomy can result in hypoparathyroidism with hypocalcemia postoperatively. Patients who had severe primary hyperparathyroidism with high bone turnover may experience hungry bone syndrome after parathyroidectomy, which is protracted hypocalcemia with deposition of large quantities of calcium into the unmineralized bone matrix.

Autoimmune destruction or infiltrative diseases, such as hemochromatosis, also may impair parathyroid function. Additionally, congenital absence of the parathyroid glands occurs in DiGeorge syndrome. Functional hypoparathyroidism may result from hypomagnesemia because magnesium is necessary for PTH release and action. Patients with alcoholism can experience this type of hypoparathyroidism and hypocalcemia related to their other nutritional deficiencies. Pseudohypoparathyroidism is caused by inherited PTH resistance, which results in hypocalcemia accompanied by marked elevations of the serum PTH level.

Hypocalcemia may occur in acute pancreatitis, in which fatty acids released through the action of pancreatic enzymes complex with calcium. Hypocalcemia due to the formation of calcium phosphate complexes occurs in severe hyperphosphatemic states, such as kidney failure, rhabdomyolysis, and tumor lysis syndrome. Hypocalcemia may also be seen in patients given multiple erythrocyte transfusions using cells to which calcium chelators have been added. Hypocalcemia due to vitamin D deficiency is typically mild and asymptomatic.

KEY POINTS

- Hypocalcemia is diagnosed after the serum calcium level is less than normal on repeated measurements, even after correction for hypoalbuminemia, if present.
- If a patient's history and physical examination findings do not clearly indicate a cause of hypocalcemia, then kidney function and parathyroid hormone, magnesium, phosphorus, and vitamin D levels should be checked.

Treatment of Hypocalcemia

In patients with symptoms of marked hypocalcemia, calcium should be delivered by slow continuous intravenous infusion (for example, calcium gluconate as 0.5-1.5 mg elemental calcium/kg/h) to raise the serum calcium level until symptoms are relieved. Concurrently, any deficiency in magnesium or vitamin D should be corrected. Oral calcium should be administered as the intravenous infusion is tapered.

In patients with less severe hypocalcemia, oral administration of calcium should be sufficient. Older persons and those taking proton pump inhibitors may not absorb calcium well, and thus higher dosages may be needed. Vitamin D also should be provided. Recommended daily intake of dietary calcium and vitamin D is provided in **Table 31**. Patients who are vitamin D deficient may require replenishment of their stores before starting a standard daily dose (see later discussion).

In chronic hypoparathyroidism, long-term administration of 1,25-dihydroxyvitamin D is necessary because 1α-hydroxylase will not be active in the kidney in the absence of PTH. A starting dose of 0.25 microgram/d is typical, with titration upward as needed. In patients with hypoparathyroidism, the serum calcium level should be kept at or slightly lower than the lower limit of the normal range (sufficient to relieve symptoms and reverse tetanic signs). Higher serum calcium levels may exacerbate hypercalciuria, which increases the risk of nephrocalcinosis or kidney stones. Periodic measurement of 24-hour urine calcium excretion is recommended to exclude hypercalciuria.

KEY POINT

- In patients with hypoparathyroidism, the serum calcium level should be kept at or slightly less than the lower limit of normal, at a level sufficient to relieve symptoms and reverse tetanic signs; full normalization of this level often results in hypercalciuria, which increases the risk of nephrocalcinosis or kidney stones

Metabolic Bone Disease

Osteoporosis

Epidemiology and Physiology

Osteoporosis is defined as low bone mass involving trabecular bone microarchitecture and connectivity and a thinning of cortical bone, which lead to decreased bone strength and an increased risk of fracture (**Figure 16**). Osteoporosis results from genetic factors and diseases and medications that affect peak bone mass and contribute to the rate of bone loss with aging. Osteoporosis can be diagnosed by measuring bone mineral density (BMD), which reflects the bone calcium content and is a surrogate for bone mass. The World Health Organization (WHO) states that in postmenopausal women and men older than 50 years, osteoporosis is present when the BMD T-score is 2.5 or more standard deviations (SD) less than that of a healthy young adult reference population in whom bone density is at its peak (see later discussion). The presence of a vertebral or hip fracture sustained with low trauma is also diagnostic of osteoporosis. Osteopenia is present in this population when the T-score is 1.1 to 2.4 SDs less than peak bone density.

TABLE 31. U.S. Institute of Medicine 2010 Daily Recommended Intake of Calcium and Vitamin D[a,b]

Group	Calcium Intake (mg)	Upper Limit of Calcium Intake (mg)	Vitamin D Intake (units)	Upper Limit of Vitamin D Intake (units)
Men and Women (19-50 y, including women who are pregnant and lactating)	1000	2500	600	4000
Men (51-70 y)	1000	2000	600	4000
Women (51-70 y)	1200	2000	600	4000
Men and Women (>70 y)	1200	2000	800	4000

[a]Released November 30, 2010, before U.S. Preventive Services Task Force recent draft statement on vitamin D and calcium supplementation for prevention of cancer and osteoporotic fractures in adults.

[b]For adults age 19 years and older.

Adapted with permission from The National Academies Press, Copyright 2011, National Academy of Sciences. Institute of Medicine of the National Academies. DRIs for Calcium and Vitamin D. 11/30/2011. Available at www.iom.edu/Reports/2010/Dietary-Reference-Intakes-for-Calcium-and-Vitamin-D.aspx. Accessed June 13, 2012.

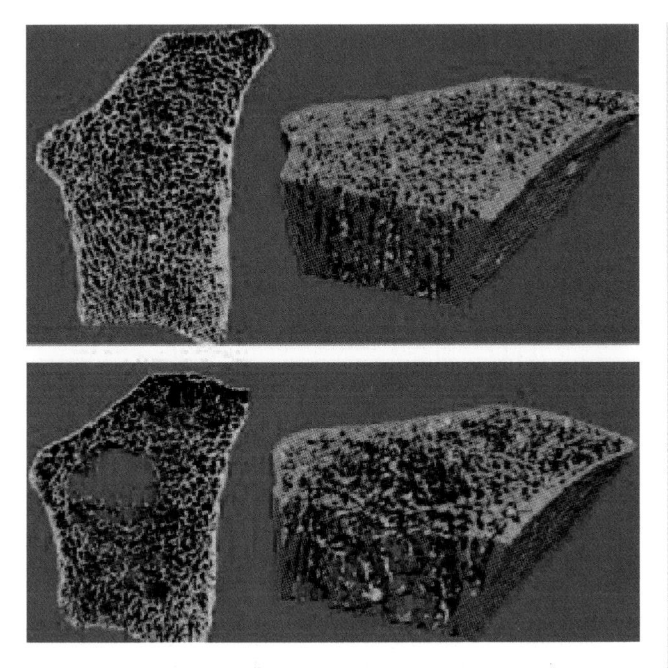

FIGURE 16. Osteoporotic bone. These images are three-dimensional micro-CT images of trabecular bone in the distal radius of a woman with normal bone density (*top*) and a woman with osteoporosis (*bottom*). Note the thinning and loss of trabeculae, which lead to loss of resistance to fracture.

Peak bone mass is achieved in the late 20s or early 30s; after this age, bone density decreases slowly. Because peak bone mass is lower in women than men, women experience higher rates of fracture. The most common sites of fragility fractures are the hips, distal forearms, and vertebrae. The lifetime risk of experiencing any fragility fracture for white women is close to 50%, and for white men is close to 20%. The incidence of hip fracture in women and men at age 65 years is approximately 300 and 150, respectively, per 100,000 person-years. These rates increase to approximately 3000 and 2000, respectively, per 100,000 by age 85 years. Black persons generally have a higher BMD and lower risk for fracture than their white, Hispanic, or Asian counterparts. Hip fracture carries the highest morbidity and mortality of all fractures. Deaths typically occur from associated complications, such as pulmonary embolism and pneumonia. At least one third of patients with hip fracture return to their previous level of functioning, but 20% will require long-term nursing care. Because of the high cost to patients and insurers, preventing hip fracture is a major focus of osteoporosis management.

Bone remodeling occurs continuously in adults. A cycle of bone remodeling begins with the recruitment of bone-resorbing osteoclasts. Osteoblasts are then recruited and fill the resorption pit with new bone matrix. The matrix is then mineralized with hydroxyapatite. Through the process of bone remodeling, the skeleton is constantly rejuvenated and mineral stores of the skeleton are made available to the body as needed. With advancing age, slightly less bone is formed than was resorbed during each remodeling cycle, which results in the gradual decline in bone mass with aging (see Figure 16). With this decrease in bone mass comes a concomitant increase in fracture risk. The age-related decline in bone mass occurs at a rate of approximately 0.1% to 0.5% per year in both sexes. In women, however, the rate of bone loss accelerates in the perimenopausal period and early menopause because of estrogen deficiency. After this period, a woman may have lost one quarter to one third of her total skeletal mass.

Risk factors for low bone mass and the resultant increased risk of fracture are shown in **Table 32**.

Evaluation

Measurement of bone density is an essential tool to assess fracture risk. Of the available modalities, dual-energy x-ray absorptiometry (DEXA) has the highest accuracy and precision and is most widely used in large clinical trials of osteoporosis medications. In a typical DEXA report, the BMD measurements are converted to T-scores and Z-scores (**Figure 17**). The T-score is the number of SDs the patient's BMD is higher or lower than the mean reference value for young, healthy, sex-matched persons at peak bone density. The Z-score represents the number of SDs the patient's BMD is higher or lower than the mean value for persons of the patient's age and sex. The T-score is used to diagnose osteoporosis and predict fracture risk. The most common sites measured by DEXA are the proximal femur and lumbar spine. In women, each SD less than the peak bone mass represents a loss of 10% to 12% of bone mineral content and corresponds to an approximately 2- to 2.5-fold increase in fracture risk at that site.

The 2010 National Osteoporosis Foundation (NOF) guidelines for osteoporosis screening appear in **Table 33**. DEXA is also appropriate to use in patients with conditions affecting bone mass (such as hyperparathyroidism) and for monitoring patients receiving osteoporosis therapy. When patients begin prescription osteoporosis therapy, their T-scores will improve slightly, but their fracture risk may decline by as much as 30% to 50%. Therefore, in patients receiving therapy for osteoporosis, BMD changes over time, rather than T-scores, should be monitored every 1 to 2 years using the same densitometer.

After the diagnosis of osteoporosis is made, the clinician should consider a selective evaluation for secondary causes of low bone mass if the patient's age and comorbid conditions do not provide an explanation (**Table 34**). A comprehensive history and physical examination can reveal underlying conditions associated with bone loss. The evaluation also should assess the patient for risk factors of low bone mass (see Table 32). Routine blood chemistry studies are reasonable, including a complete blood count and

TABLE 32. Risk Factors for Low Bone Mass and Fractures

Nonmodifiable Risk Factors
Advanced age
Female sex
First-degree relative with history of hip fracture
Personal history of fragility fracture
Postmenopausal status
White or Asian ancestry
Modifiable Risk Factors
Alcohol abuse
Low body weight
Sedentary lifestyle
Smoking
Conditions
Anorexia nervosa
Chronic kidney disease
Chronic liver disease
COPD
Cushing syndrome
Growth hormone deficiency
Hyperparathyroidism
Hypogonadism
Intestinal malabsorption
Monoclonal gammopathy
Organ transplantation
Rheumatoid arthritis
Thyrotoxicosis
Medications
Carbamazepine
Corticosteroids
Depot medroxyprogesterone acetate
Leuprolide
Phenytoin
Proton pump inhibitors
Causes of Falls
Cognitive decline
Decreased mobility
Impaired neuromuscular function
Low visual acuity
Sedative drug use

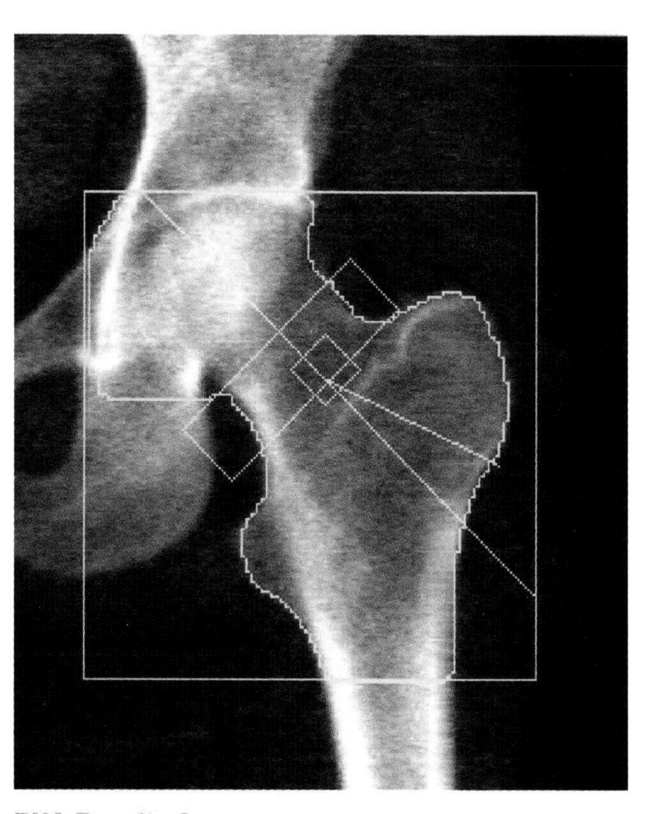

DXA Results Summary:

Region	Area (cm^2)	BMC (g)	BMD (g/cm^2)	T - Score	Z - Score
Neck	4.75	2.76	0.580	-2.4	-1.7
Troch	7.95	3.58	0.450	-2.5	-2.1
Inter	20.10	14.78	0.735	-2.4	-2.1
Total	**32.80**	**21.11**	**0.644**	**-2.4**	**-2.0**

FIGURE 17. Sample hip dual-energy x-ray absorptiometry report. The scan image of the left hip region shows positioning of the hip, with regions analyzed outlined in yellow. Of particular interest are the total hip (contents of large rectangle) and the femoral neck (contents of small rectangle). The analysis provides the bone mineral density and the patient's results expressed as Z-scores (standard deviations from same-age reference group) and T-scores (standard deviations from young adult reference group at peak bone mass). This patient has osteopenia (T-score of −2.4) in both the femoral neck and total hip. The Z-scores indicate that the bone density is considerably below the age-matched reference range, which raises concern that a condition besides aging has contributed to bone loss. BMC = bone mineral content; BMD = bone mineral density; DXA = dual-energy x-ray absorptiometry; Inter = intertrochanteric space; Troch = greater trochanter.

measurement of serum levels of calcium, phosphorus, electrolytes, creatinine, 25-hydroxyvitamin D, and alkaline phosphatase. Measurement of the serum PTH level is recommended if the serum calcium level is elevated. An elevated PTH level in the setting of a low calcium level and/or low 25-hydroxyvitamin D level indicates secondary hyperparathyroidism, which also can cause bone loss. Subclinical hyperthyroidism should be ruled out by determining the serum thyroid-stimulating hormone level. A 24-hour urine calcium level may reveal calcium malabsorption or excessive

TABLE 33. Guidelines for Osteoporosis Screening

Women age ≥65 y
Men and women age >50 y with fragility or low-trauma fracture
Postmenopausal women age <65 y with one or more of the following risk factors for future fragility fracture: personal history of fracture, secondary cause of low bone mass, low body weight, current smoker, alcohol abuse, or a first-degree family member with a hip fracture
Men and premenopausal women with secondary cause of low bone mass or personal history of low trauma or fragility fracture

Data from National Osteoporosis Foundation. Clinician's Guide to Prevention and Treatment of Osteoporosis. Available at: www.nof.org/sites/default/files/pdfs/NOF_ClinicianGuide2009_v7.pdf, p 13-14. Accessed May 11, 2012.

TABLE 34. Secondary Causes of Low Bone Mass

Endocrine disorders: hyperparathyroidism, osteomalacia, Cushing syndrome, hypogonadism, hyperthyroidism, acromegaly, and diabetes mellitus
Hematopoietic disorders: myeloma, sickle cell disease, thalassemia minor, leukemia, lymphoma, and polycythemia vera
Connective tissue disorders: systemic lupus erythematosus and rheumatoid arthritis
Kidney disease: chronic kidney disease, renal tubular acidosis, and hypercalciuria
Gastrointestinal conditions: malabsorption (gastrectomy, primary biliary cirrhosis, celiac disease, gastric bypass surgery, pancreatic insufficiency, and inflammatory bowel disease)
Exogenous: corticosteroids, proton pump inhibitors, anticonvulsants, heparin, gonadotropin-releasing hormone agonists, depot medroxyprogesterone, chemotherapeutic agents, and excessive alcohol
Genetic: osteogenesis imperfecta, homocystinuria, Marfan syndrome, cystic fibrosis, and hemochromatosis

kidney calcium losses. Testosterone levels should be checked in men who have risk factors or symptoms of hypogonadism, with replacement therapy initiated if indicated. Testing for monoclonal gammopathy in older adults may be appropriate because asymptomatic monoclonal gammopathy may cause bone loss. If no cause is found for the osteoporosis, it is considered idiopathic. Idiopathic osteoporosis is rare in premenopausal women but accounts for approximately 50% of osteoporosis in men of all ages.

Prediction of Fracture Risk

The DEXA T-score allows the prediction of a patient's relative fracture risk. The Fracture Risk Assessment Tool (FRAX) developed by the WHO was designed to predict the absolute fracture risk. Based on data from cohorts around the globe, the FRAX is a Web-based tool (http:www.shef.ac.uk/FRAX/index.jsp) that incorporates major risk factors and a patient's femoral neck T-score (if available) to calculate an absolute fracture risk over the next 10 years.

FRAX does not include all components of a patient's fracture risk, such as tendency to fall. The effect of osteoporosis drugs on fracture risk as calculated with FRAX is unknown. Nevertheless, the NOF now recommends that FRAX be used as a component of decision-making when deciding which patients with osteopenia may benefit from treatment with antiosteoporotic medications.

Prevention of Osteoporosis and Fracture

First Steps

Lifestyle modifications and adjustment of modifiable risk factors (see Table 32) are the first steps in preventing or treating osteoporosis. Physical therapy evaluation may be appropriate for patients considered at high risk for falls. For frail older patients, medications that may predispose to dizziness should be avoided.

Persons of all ages must consume adequate amounts of both calcium and vitamin D to maintain bone health. Additionally, calcium and vitamin D supplementation has a beneficial effect on postmenopausal bone loss, although not as dramatic as is seen with antiresorptive or anabolic therapies. Recently, the recommended daily allowances of calcium and vitamin D were revised by the U.S. Institute of Medicine (IOM) (see Table 31), and a new vitamin D guideline was provided by the Endocrine Society in 2011. However, controversy exists about the need for higher dosages of calcium and vitamin D supplementation in some populations. In June 2012, the U.S. Preventive Services Task Force (USPSTF) released a draft recommendation statement recommending against supplementation with greater than 1000 mg/d of calcium or with 400 units/d or more of vitamin D for primary prevention of fractures in healthy community-dwelling women who are postmenopausal because of lack of evidence showing safety or efficacy. The USPSTF does, however, recommend vitamin D supplementation for preventing falls in noninstitutionalized older persons.

Antiosteoporosis Pharmacologic Therapy

Osteoporosis is most often prevented or treated with antiresorptive agents (**Table 35**). FDA-approved antiresorptive agents for the treatment of low bone mass include bisphosphonates, selective estrogen receptor modulators, and calcitonin. All of these agents reduce vertebral and nonvertebral (multiple sites, including the hip) fracture rates by 30% to 60% over 2 to 3 years. Only some of the bisphosphonates (and estrogen) have been shown specifically to reduce hip fracture risk. For the prevention of osteoporosis in women, the antiresorptive agents approved by the FDA are alendronate, ibandronate, risedronate, zoledronate, raloxifene, and estrogen.

TABLE 35. FDA-Approved Medications for Osteoporosis and Approved Indications

Medication	Postmenopausal Osteoporosis		Osteoporosis in Men	Corticosteroid-Induced Osteoporosis	
	Prevention	Treatment	Treatment	Prevention	Treatment
Estrogens[a]	Yes	No	No	No	No
Calcitonin[a]	No	Yes[b]	No	No	No
Raloxifene	Yes	Yes	No	No	No
Alendronate[a,c]	Yes	Yes	Yes	No	Yes
Ibandronate[d]	Yes	Yes	No	No	No
Risedronate[a,e]	Yes	Yes	Yes	Yes	Yes
Zoledronate[f]	Yes	Yes	Yes	Yes	Yes
Denosumab[g]	No	Yes	No	No	No
Teriparatide	No	Yes	Yes	No	No

[a]Generic preparation available in the United States.

[b]More than 5 years after menopause.

[c]Oral daily or weekly dosing.

[d]Oral monthly dosing; intravenous dosing every 3 months.

[e]Oral daily, weekly, or monthly dosing.

[f]Intravenous dosing once yearly.

[g]Subcutaneous injection every 6 months.

Bisphosphonates bind to the bone matrix and decrease osteoclast activity, thereby slowing bone resorption while new bone formation and mineralization continue. Alendronate and risedronate have been studied most extensively; over a period of 2 to 3 years, these drugs produce a 6% increase in bone density and a 30% to 50% reduction in fracture risk at both vertebral and nonvertebral sites. Ibandronate reduces the risk of vertebral fracture by as much as 50% after 3 years of therapy but has not been shown in clinical trials to prevent hip fracture. No clear benefit of newer bisphosphonate drugs versus older agents has been demonstrated; the older drugs are available in generic form and may be more cost-effective for long-term therapy (see Table 35). Esophagitis is a risk of oral bisphosphonate therapy, and thus these agents are contraindicated in patients with active esophageal disease or swallowing disorders. Intravenous bisphosphonates are preferred for women with postmenopausal osteoporosis who are unable to take oral bisphosphonates or who desire the convenience of less frequent dosing. However, the costs of these drugs and their administration are significantly greater than those of available oral agents. Intravenous ibandronate is given every 3 months, whereas zoledronate is administered annually. Zoledronate reduces the risk of fracture of the hip and other skeletal sites. An acute-phase reaction (flulike symptoms for several days) is a common adverse effect of zoledronate. Bisphosphonate therapy is not recommended for patients with impaired kidney function (creatinine clearance less than 30-35 mL/min [0.030-0.035 L/min] [normal, 90-140 mL/min {0.09-0.14 L/min}]).

Osteonecrosis of the jaw has been described in patients taking bisphosphonates and is more likely to occur in patients undergoing treatment for cancer who receive frequent doses of intravenous bisphosphonates. The risk of this complication with the dosages used for osteoporosis treatment is estimated at 1 in 10,000. Special care is necessary when patients require dental procedures because extractions may increase the risk of osteonecrosis. Persons with any defect in jaw architecture or with upcoming jaw surgery should not take bisphosphonates. Stopping ongoing therapy for dental procedures is of limited utility because the agents remain in the bone matrix long after discontinuation. Bisphosphonates should be avoided in women of childbearing age. Because of the long biologic half-life of bisphosphonates, a theoretical risk of passage to the fetus exists, even in patients no longer taking them.

Given the persistence of bisphosphonates in the bone matrix, concern exists about adverse effects of prolonged therapy, including an association with atypical femoral fractures. To date, bisphosphonates have not been conclusively proved to be causative. Nevertheless, the FDA issued a Drug Safety Communication in 2010 recommending that patients receiving bisphosphonate therapy be reassessed periodically, particularly after 5 years of use, to determine if treatment remains appropriate. Many experts recommend that after 5 years of therapy, patients be considered for a "drug holiday" lasting 2 years or more. For patients with severe osteoporosis or ongoing fractures, treatment with teriparatide during the bisphosphonate drug holiday should be considered. Persons on drug holiday should be monitored for fracture and evidence of reactivation of bone loss (by BMD testing every 1-2 years); therapy should be restarted if reactivation of bone loss is evident.

Raloxifene, a selective estrogen receptor modulator, is an estrogen agonist in bone but an estrogen antagonist in the breast and uterus. Vertebral fracture risk reduction with raloxifene is comparable to that of estrogen or bisphosphonate therapy. Raloxifene has not been shown, however, to prevent hip fractures. Also, patients treated with raloxifene have a 1.4- to 1.5-fold increased risk of fatal stroke and thromboembolism. Raloxifene is a good choice for women whose bone loss is primarily in the spine, who have a relatively low risk of hip fracture, and who are unable to tolerate oral bisphosphonates. Although generally well tolerated, this drug may exacerbate menopausal hot flushes. Raloxifene is not approved for use in men or premenopausal women.

The beneficial effects of calcitonin are much less pronounced than those of other antiresorptive agents. Calcitonin injections and nasal spray are approved for the treatment of established osteoporosis but not for its prevention. Calcitonin has been shown to prevent primarily vertebral fractures and is generally safe and well tolerated. Because of the availability of other safe and more potent drugs, calcitonin is rarely used for osteoporosis treatment except when other options are lacking.

The use of estrogen to maintain bone health has fallen out of favor because of data from the Women's Health Initiative indicating that estrogen increases the risk of cardiovascular disease and breast cancer. Therefore, estrogen use for osteoporosis prevention should be limited to women who also require its beneficial effects for hot flushes or vaginal dryness.

Denosumab is the newest available antiresorptive agent. This drug is a humanized monoclonal antibody directed against the receptor activator of nuclear factor κB (RANK) ligand, a key signal in activating bone resorption. This leads to decreased osteoclastogenesis. Approved only for women with postmenopausal osteoporosis and a high risk of fracture, denosumab is administered by injection every 6 months. Fracture prevention by denosumab is comparable to that seen with bisphosphonate therapy. Common adverse effects include musculoskeletal pain, hyperlipidemia, and cystitis. An increased risk of infections, particularly skin infections, and osteonecrosis of the jaw also have been reported in association with denosumab use. Denosumab is not appropriate for use in persons who are immunosuppressed or who have hypocalcemia. Given its similar efficacy for fracture prevention as bisphosphonates and its significant risk factor profile and expense, denosumab is not generally used for routine treatment of postmenopausal osteoporosis.

Teriparatide (recombinant human PTH [1-34]) is currently the only available anabolic agent for osteoporosis therapy in the United States and is generally used in patients with severe osteoporosis (T-score ≤−3.5), recurrent fractures, or continuing bone loss while taking other medications. Although chronic elevation of the serum PTH level results in bone loss, transient spikes have anabolic effects on bone. A daily subcutaneous injection of teriparatide provides a brief increase in the serum PTH level and results in increased BMD. The effects are particularly dramatic in the spine; one study comparing 14 months of teriparatide therapy with alendronate treatment showed that alendronate-treated patients had a 5.6% increase in lumbar spine BMD, whereas teriparatide-treated patients had a 12.2% increase. Teriparatide has a "black box" warning from the FDA concerning a risk of osteosarcoma, which is based on the increased incidence seen in rats. For this reason, the drug is administered for no longer than 2 years, and its use is contraindicated in patients with hyperparathyroidism, Paget disease, unexplained elevation of the alkaline phosphatase level, malignancy involving bone, or a history of radiation therapy. Selection of patients for this costly and potent drug requires care, and consultation with an endocrinologist should be considered.

Simultaneous administration of teriparatide and oral bisphosphonates impairs the anabolic effects of teriparatide and thus is not recommended. When bisphosphonates are used after completion of a course of teriparatide, the increase in BMD due to teriparatide therapy is preserved and followed by additional gain during subsequent bisphosphonate treatment. In clinical practice, many patients being considered for teriparatide therapy have already received long-term bisphosphonate therapy. Whether these patients benefit as much from teriparatide as bisphosphonate-naïve patients do is unclear.

The most comprehensive set of guidelines for identifying patients who will benefit from treatment of low bone mass were updated by the NOF in 2010 (**Table 36**). Follow-up DEXA (using the same machine, if possible) is recommended every 1 to 2 years initially to monitor response to therapy. Stable or improved bone density indicates appropriate response to therapy. Bone loss while receiving

TABLE 36. NOF 2010 Guidelines for Pharmacologic Treatment of Patients with Osteoporosis

Men age >50 y or postmenopausal women with osteoporosis *OR* prior vertebral or hip fracture
Men age >50 y or postmenopausal women with osteopenia *AND* a prior fragility fracture or other medical issues that increase fracture risk
Men and women with osteopenia *AND* a 3% or greater probability of hip fracture or a 20% or greater probability of other major osteoporotic fracture over the next 10 years[a]

NOF = National Osteoporosis Foundation.

[a]Percentages determined by using the U.S.-adapted WHO Fracture Risk Assessment Tool (FRAX) algorithm.

Data from National Osteoporosis Foundation. Clinician's Guide to Prevention and Treatment of Osteoporosis. Available at: www.nof.org/sites/default/files/pdfs/NOF_ClinicianGuide2009_v7.pdf. Accessed July 5, 2012.

therapy should prompt evaluation of medication adherence and unrecognized secondary causes of bone loss (as discussed previously).

KEY POINTS

- Dual-energy x-ray absorptiometry has the highest accuracy and precision of the modalities available for measuring bone mineral density and assessing fracture risk and is most widely used in large clinical trials of osteoporosis medications.
- Osteoporosis is most often treated with antiresorptive agents, such as bisphosphonates, selective estrogen receptor modulators, and calcitonin; teriparatide is currently the only available anabolic agent for osteoporosis treatment in the United States.

Osteomalacia

In osteomalacia, the bone matrix is normal in quantity but weakened by insufficient mineral content. Osteomalacia in the growing skeleton is termed rickets and is associated with bony deformities, including bowing of the legs. Causes of osteomalacia include deficiencies of calcium, phosphate, or vitamin D, but inhibition of mineralization from any cause may be responsible. These deficiencies may result from nutritional insufficiency, intestinal malabsorption, or abnormalities in vitamin D metabolism due to liver disease, kidney disease (renal tubular acidosis, chronic kidney disease), or antiepileptic drugs. Rarely, osteomalacia occurs because of genetic vitamin D resistance, inherited kidney disorders of phosphate wasting, or oncogenic osteomalacia (a humoral syndrome of increased urine phosphate loss associated with rare tumors of mesenchymal origin). Osteomalacia presents in adults as proximal muscle weakness and diffuse or focal skeletal pain. Osteomalacia also can be asymptomatic, with diagnosis based on clinical evaluation and laboratory and imaging results. Decreased or low-normal levels of calcium and phosphorus are noted, as is an elevated alkaline phosphatase level. Depending on the cause, decreased levels of either 25-hydroxyvitamin D or 1,25-dihydroxyvitamin D may be seen. Plain films may show osteopenia or pseudofractures. When necessary, the diagnosis can be confirmed with a bone biopsy analyzed by an experienced bone pathologist.

The treatment of osteomalacia depends on the pathogenesis of the condition. For patients with dietary insufficiency or malabsorption of vitamin D, high doses of cholecalciferol and calcium (see Table 31) will rapidly correct deficits and heal the bone. An assessment for underlying disorders (such as celiac disease, which may be asymptomatic) should be performed, with other evaluations if indicated. Phosphate-wasting conditions require a different approach, such as phosphate supplementation or localization and removal of any causative tumor.

KEY POINT

- For most patients with osteomalacia caused by dietary insufficiency or malabsorption of vitamin D, administration of high doses of cholecalciferol and calcium will rapidly correct deficits and heal the bone.

Vitamin D Deficiency

Guidelines for screening for vitamin D deficiency are lacking, but risk factors include advanced age, dark skin, low sun exposure, and fat malabsorption. Vitamin D deficiency is diagnosed in patients with a low serum 25-hydroxyvitamin D level. The optimal level is currently a matter of debate, with the IOM recommending a level of 20 ng/mL (50 nmol/L) and the Endocrine Society endorsing a level of 30 ng/mL (75 nmol/L). Vitamin D levels are adequate for skeletal health at 20 ng/mL (50 nmol/L), but nonskeletal benefits may require a level of 30 ng/mL (75 nmol/L). The evidence supporting skeletal benefits at a vitamin D level of 20 ng/mL (50 nmol/L) is more robust than is the evidence for the nonskeletal benefits achieved at a level of 30 ng/mL (75 nmol/L). The IOM (see Table 31) and the Endocrine Society recommend the same daily vitamin D dose for each demographic group, but the Endocrine Society cautions that adults may need doses as high as 1500 to 2000 units/d to achieve their recommended serum target level of 30 ng/mL (75 nmol/L) (but see previous discussion of the draft recommendation statement from the USPSTF). For those found to be vitamin D deficient (defined as a 25-hydroxyvitamin D level less than 20 ng/mL [50 nmol/L]), the Endocrine Society recommends a course of ergocalciferol, 50,000 units weekly for 8 weeks, followed by confirmation of a normal serum 25-hydroxyvitamin D level.

Paget Disease of Bone

Clinical Features and Evaluation

Paget disease of bone is a condition in which abnormal osteoclast function leads to accelerated and disordered bone remodeling, which produces highly disorganized and brittle bone microarchitecture in affected areas. This process sometimes leads to deformity of affected bones, increased bone vascularity, nerve impingement syndromes, and a propensity to fracture. Paget disease of bone is commonly seen in older persons and may be familial. The precise cause is unknown, although an inherited or viral origin (or a combination of the two) is suspected. Most persons with Paget disease are asymptomatic, with increased serum alkaline phosphatase levels detected incidentally on blood testing or pathognomonic changes discovered on radiographs. If the disease is severe or extensive, bony deformity and pain result, either from the bony lesions themselves or from complications of the abnormal bone, such as nerve compression, degenerative arthritis or osteosarcoma. The skull may be enlarged, and significant bowing of the long bones of the legs may occur. Skull involvement may cause a sensorineural hearing loss, and bony overgrowth may lead to local impingement on spinal nerve roots with pain or neurologic deficits. Rare complications include high-output heart failure from multiple vascular shunts in bone and transformation to osteosarcoma.

The diagnosis of Paget disease typically is made after finding isolated elevation of the serum alkaline phosphatase level without other evidence of liver disease. A nuclear bone scan is then performed to locate the involved areas (**Figure 18**). Plain radiographs of these areas should be evaluated to exclude metastatic disease and confirm the pagetic findings.

Treatment

Treatment of Paget disease is indicated for patients with bone pain and for patients with involvement of the skull, weight-bearing bones, or joints. The goal of treatment is to decrease pain and reduce risk of pathologic fracture. High-dose antiresorptive agents are given, such as a 2-month course of risedronate, 30 mg/d orally, or a single dose of an injectable bisphosphonate (see previous discussion). Injectable calcitonin is less effective but can be used in patients with impaired kidney function. Disease activity and response to therapy are assessed by serial measurement of alkaline phosphatase levels. The goal of treatment is normalization of the alkaline phosphatase level. Retreatment is indicated if the alkaline phosphatase level (checked every 3 to 6 months) is greater than normal. Patients with skull involvement should also have periodic audiometry to exclude hearing loss.

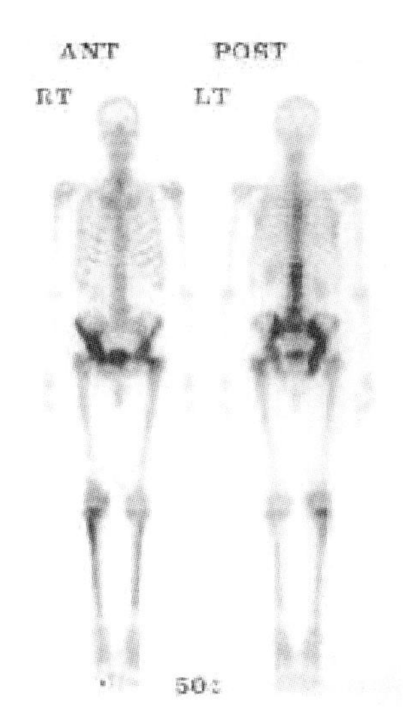

FIGURE 18. Whole-body bone scan images from a patient with Paget disease showing intense tracer uptake in the right proximal tibia, pelvis, left proximal femur and lumbar spine. ANT = anterior; LT = left; POST = posterior; RT = right.

KEY POINT

- In Paget disease of bone, disease activity and response to therapy are assessed by serial measurement of the alkaline phosphatase level.

Bibliography

Diabetes Mellitus

ACCORD Study Group, Cushman WC, Evans GW, Byington RP, et al. Effects of intensive blood-pressure control in type 2 diabetes mellitus. N Engl J Med. 2010;362(17):1575-1585. [PMID: 20228401]

Athyros VG, Tziomalos K, Gossios TD, et al; GREACE Study Collaborative Group. Safety and efficacy of long-term statin treatment for cardiovascular events in patients with coronary heart disease and abnormal liver tests in the Greek Atorvastatin and Coronary Heart Disease Evaluation (GREACE) Study: a post-hoc analysis. Lancet. 2010;376(9756):1916-1922. [PMID: 21109302]

Calles-Escandón J, Lovato LC, Simons-Morton DG, et al. Effect of intensive compared with standard glycemia treatment strategies on mortality by baseline subgroup characteristics: the Action to Control Cardiovascular Risk in Diabetes (ACCORD) trial. Diabetes Care. 2010;33(4):721-727. [PMID: 20103550]

Cengiz E, Tamborlane WV, Martin-Fredericksen M, Dziura J, Weinzimer SA. Early pharmacokinetic and pharmacodynamic effects of mixing lispro with glargine insulin: results of glucose clamp studies in youth with type 1 diabetes. Diabetes Care. 2010;33(5):1009-1012. [PMID: 20150302]

International Association of Diabetes and Pregnancy Study Groups Consensus Panel, Metzger BE, Gabbe SJ, Persson B, et al. International Association of Diabetes and Pregnancy Study Groups recommendations on the diagnosis and classification of hyperglycemia in pregnancy. Diabetes Care. 2010;33(3):676-682. [PMID: 20190296]

Juvenile Diabetes Research Foundation Continuous Glucose Monitoring Study Group, Tamborlane WV, Beck RW, Bode BW, et al. Continuous glucose monitoring and intensive treatment of type 1 diabetes. N Engl J Med. 2008;359(14):1464-1476. [PMID: 18779236]

Moghissi ES, Korytkowski MT, DiNardo M, et al; American Association of Clinical Endocrinologists; American Diabetes Association. American Association of Clinical Endocrinologists and American Diabetes Association consensus statement on inpatient glycemic control. Diabetes Care. 2009;32(6):1119-1131. [PMID: 19429873]

O'Kane MJ, Bunting B, Copeland M, Coates VE; ESMON Study Group. Efficacy of self monitoring of blood glucose in patients with newly diagnosed type 2 diabetes (ESMON study): randomised controlled trial. BMJ. 2008;336(7654):1174-1177. [PMID: 18420662]

Poolsup N, Suksomboon N, Rattanasookchit S. Meta-analysis of the benefits of self-monitoring of blood glucose on glycemic control in type 2 diabetes patients: an update. Diabetes Technol Ther. 2009;11(12):775-784. [PMID: 20001678]

Umpierrez GE, Hellman R, Korytkowski MT, et al; Endocrine Society. Management of hyperglycemia in hospitalized patients in non-critical care setting: an Endocrine Society clinical practice guideline. J Clin Endocrinol Metab. 2012;97(1):16-38. [PMID: 22223765]

Zeller M, Danchin N, Simon D, et al; French Registry of Acute ST-Elevation and Non–ST-Elevation Myocardial Infarction Investigators. Impact of type of preadmission sulfonylureas on mortality and cardiovascular outcomes in diabetic patients with acute myocardial infarction. J Clin Endocrinol Metab. 2010;95(11):4993-5002. [PMID: 20702526]

Disorders of the Pituitary Gland

Cook DM, Yuen KC, Biller BM, Kemp SF, Vance ML; American Association of Clinical Endocrinologists. American Association of Clinical Endocrinologists medical guidelines for clinical practice for growth hormone use in growth hormone–deficient adults and transition patients—2009 update. Endocr Pract. 2009;15(Supppl 2):1-29. [PMID: 20228036]

Freda PU, Beckers AM, Katznelson L, et al; Endocrine Society. Pituitary incidentaloma: an Endocrine Society clinical practice guideline. J Clin Endocrinol Metab. 2011;96(4):894-904. [PMID: 21474686]

Laws ER, Jane JA Jr. Neurosurgical approach to treating pituitary adenomas. Growth Horm IGF Res. 2005;15(Suppl A):S36-S41. [PMID: 16039890]

Loh JA, Verbalis JG. Disorders of water and salt metabolism associated with pituitary disease. Endocrinol Metab Clin North Am. 2008;37(1):213-234. [PMID: 18226738]

Melmed S, Casanueva FF, Hoffman AR, et al; Endocrine Society. Diagnosis and treatment of hyperprolactinemia: an Endocrine Society clinical practice guideline. J Clin Endocrinol Metab. 2011;96(2):273-288. [PMID: 21296991]

Melmed S, Colao A, Barkan A, et al; Acromegaly Consensus Group. Guidelines for acromegaly management: an update. J Clin Endocrinol Metab. 2009;94(5):1509-1517. [PMID: 19208732]

Molitch ME. Prolactinomas and pregnancy. Clin Endocrinol (Oxf). 2010;73(2):147-148. [PMID: 20550542]

Sheehan JP, Pouratian N, Steiner L, Laws ER, Vance ML. Gamma Knife surgery for pituitary adenomas: factors related to radiological and endocrine outcomes. J Neurosurg. 2011;114(2):303-309. [PMID: 20540596]

Toogood AA, Stewart PM. Hypopituitarism: clinical features, diagnosis, and management. Endocrinol Metab Clin North Am. 2008;37(1):235-261. [PMID: 18226739]

Disorders of the Thyroid Gland

American Thyroid Association (ATA) Guidelines Taskforce on Thyroid Nodules and Differentiated Thyroid Cancer, Cooper DS, Doherty GM, Haugen BR, et al. Revised American Thyroid Association management guidelines for patients with thyroid nodules and differentiated thyroid cancer [errata in Thyroid. 2010;20(6):674-675 and Thyroid. 2010;20(8):942]. Thyroid. 2009;19(11):1167-1214. [PMID: 19860577] Also available at: www.thyroidguidelines.org/revised/taskforce. Accessed June 8, 2012.

American Thyroid Association Guidelines Taskforce, Kloos RT, Eng C, Evans DB, et al. Medullary thyroid cancer: management guidelines of the American Thyroid Association [erratum in Thyroid. 2009;19(11):1295]. Thyroid. 2009;19(6):565-612. [PMID: 19469690] Also available at: http://thyroidguidelines.net/medullary/taskforce. Accessed June 8, 2012.

Bahn RS, Burch HB, Cooper DS, et al; American Thyroid Association; American Association of Clinical Endocrinologists. Hyperthyroidism and other causes of thyrotoxicosis: management guidelines of the American Thyroid Association and American Association of Clinical Endocrinologists. Endocr Pract. 2011;17(3):456-520. [PMID: 21700562] Also available at: http://thyroidguidelines.net/hyperthyroidism. Accessed June 8, 2012.

Cooper DS. Approach to the patient with subclinical hyperthyroidism. J Clin Endocrinol Metab. 2007;92(1):3-9. [PMID: 17209221]

Devdhar M, Ousman YH, Burman KD. Hypothyroidism. Endocrinol Metab Clin North Am. 2007;36(3):595-615. [PMID: 17673121]

Franklyn JA. Subclinical thyroid disorders—consequences and implications for treatment. Ann Endocrinol (Paris). 2007;68(4):229-230. [PMID: 17651685]

Kwaku MP, Burman KD. Myxedema coma. J Intensive Care Med. 2007;22(4):224-231. [PMID: 17712058]

Nayak B, Burman K. Thyrotoxicosis and thyroid storm. Endocrinol Metab Clin North Am. 2006;35(4):663-686. [PMID: 17127140]

Poppe K, Velkeniers B, Glinoer D. Thyroid disease and female reproduction. Clin Endocrinol (Oxf). 2007;66(3):309-321. [PMID: 17302862]

Stagnaro-Green A, Abalovich M, Alexander E, et al; American Thyroid Association Taskforce on Thyroid Disease During Pregnancy and Postpartum. Thyroid. 2011;21(10):1081-1125. [PMID: 21787128]

Surks MI, Boucai L. Age- and race-based serum thyrotropin reference limits. J Clin Endocrinol Metab. 2010;95(2):496-502. [PMID: 19965925]

Surks MI, Ortiz E, Daniels GH, et al. Subclinical thyroid disease: scientific review and guidelines for diagnosis and management. JAMA. 2004;291(2):228-238. [PMID: 14722150]

Wartofsky L. Myxedema coma. Endocrinol Metab Clin North Am. 2006;35(4):687-698. [PMID: 17127141]

Yassa L, Marqusee E, Fawcett R, Alexander EK. Thyroid hormone early adjustment in pregnancy (the THERAPY) trial. J Clin Endocrinol Metab. 2010;95(7):3234-3241. [PMID: 20463094]

Disorders of the Adrenal Glands

Al-Aridi R, Abdelmannan D, Arafah BM. Biochemical diagnosis of adrenal insufficiency: the added value of dehydroepiandrosterone sulfate measurements. Endocr Pract. 2011;17(2):261-270. [PMID: 21134877]

Allolio B, Fassnacht M. Clinical review: adrenocortical carcinoma: clinical update. J Clin Endocrinol Metab. 2006;91(6):2027-2037. [PMID: 16551738]

Arafah BM. Hypothalamic pituitary adrenal function during critical illness: limitations of current assessment methods. J Clin Endocrinol Metab. 2006;91(10):3725-3745. [PMID: 16882746]

Bornstein SR. Predisposing factors for adrenal insufficiency. N Engl J Med. 2009;360(22):2328-2339. [PMID: 19474430]

Funder JW, Carey RM, Fardella C, et al; Endocrine Society. Case detection, diagnosis, and treatment of patients with primary hyperaldosteronism: an Endocrine Society clinical practice guideline. J Clin Endocrinol Metab. 2008;93(9):3266-3281. [PMID: 18552288]

Lenders JW, Eisenhofer G, Mannelli M, Pacak K. Phaeochromocytoma. Lancet. 2005;366(9486):665-675. [PMID: 16112304]

Nieman LK. Approach to the patient with an adrenal incidentaloma. J Clin Endocrinol Metab. 2010;95(9):4106-4113. [PMID: 20823463]

Nieman LK, Biller BM, Findling JW, et al. The diagnosis of Cushing's syndrome: an Endocrine Society clinical practice guideline. J Clin Endocrinol Metab. 2008;93(5):1526-1540. [PMID: 18334580]

Sprung CL, Annane D, Keh D, et al; CORTICUS Study Group. Hydrocortisone therapy for patients with septic shock. N Engl J Med. 2008;358(2):111-124. [PMID: 18184957]

Young WF Jr. Clinical practice. The incidentally discovered adrenal mass. N Engl J Med. 2007;356(6):601-610. [PMID: 17287480]

Reproductive Disorders

Basaria S, Coviello AD, Travison TG, et al. Adverse events associated with testosterone administration. N Engl J Med. 2010;363(2):109-122. [PMID: 20592293]

Bhasin S, Cunningham GR, Hayes FJ, et al; Task Force, Endocrine Society. Testosterone therapy in men with androgen deficiency syndromes: an Endocrine Society clinical practice guideline. J Clin Endocrinol Metab. 2010;95(6):2536-2559. [PMID: 20525905]

Gordon CM. Clinical practice. Functional hypothalamic amenorrhea. N Engl J Med. 2010;363(4):365-371. [PMID: 20660404]

Hoffman LK, Ehrmann DA. Cardiometabolic features of polycystic ovary syndrome. Nat Clin Pract Endocrinol Metab. 2008;4(4):215-222. [PMID: 18250636]

Martin KA, Chang RJ, Ehrmann DA, et al. Evaluation and treatment of hirsutism in premenopausal women: an Endocrine Society clinical practice guideline. J Clin Endocrinol Metab. 2008;93(4):1105-1120. [PMID: 18252793]

Nelson LM. Clinical practice. Primary ovarian insufficiency. N Engl J Med. 2009;360(6):606-614. [PMID: 19196677]

Nestler JE. Metformin for the treatment of the polycystic ovary syndrome. N Engl J Med. 2008;358(1):47-54. [PMID: 18172174]

Qaseem A, Snow V, Denberg TD, et al; Clinical Efficacy Assessment Subcommittee of the American College of Physicians. Hormonal testing and pharmacologic treatment of erectile dysfunction: a clinical practice guideline from the American College of Physicians. Ann Intern Med. 2009;151(9):639-649. [PMID: 19884625]

Rosner W, Vesper H; Endocrine Society; American Association for Clinical Chemistry; American Association of Clinical Endocrinologists; Androgen Excess/PCOS Society; American Society for Bone and Mineral Research; American Society for Reproductive Medicine; American Urological Association; Association of Public Health Laboratories; Laboratory Corporation of America; North American Menopause Society; Pediatric Endocrine Society. Toward excellence in testosterone testing: a consensus statement. J Clin Endocrinol Metab. 2010;95(10):4542-4548. [PMID: 20926540]

Yeap BB. Testosterone and ill-health in aging men. Nat Clin Pract Endocrinol Metab. 2009;5(2):113-121. [PMID: 19165223]

Calcium and Bone Disorders

Bilezikian JP, Khan AA, Potts JT Jr; Third International Workshop on the Management of Asymptomatic Primary Hyperthyroidism. Guidelines for the management of asymptomatic primary hyperparathyroidism: summary statement from the third international workshop. J Clin Endocrinol Metab. 2009;94(2):335-339. [PMID: 19193908]

Body JJ, Gaich GA, Scheele WH, et al. A randomized double-blind trial to compare the efficacy of teriparatide [recombinant human parathyroid hormone (1-34)] with alendronate in postmenopausal women with osteoporosis. J Clin Endocrinol Metab. 2002;87(10):4528-4535. [PMID: 12364430]

Holick, MF. Vitamin D deficiency. New Engl J Med. 2007;357(3):266-281. [PMID: 17634462]

Inzucchi SE. Management of hypercalcemia. Diagnostic workup, therapeutic options for hyperparathyroidism and other common causes. Postgrad Med. 2004;115(5):27-36. [PMID: 15171076]

Khan AA, Bilezikian JP, Kung AW, et al. Alendronate in primary hyperparathyroidism: a double-blind, randomized, placebo-controlled trial. J Clin Endocrinol Metab. 2004;89(7):3319-3325. [PMID: 15240609]

Rittmaster RS, Bolognese M, Ettinger MP, et al. Enhancement of bone mass in osteoporotic women with parathyroid hormone followed by alendronate. J Clin Endocrinol Metab. 2000;85(6):2129-2134. [PMID: 10852440]

Rubin MR, Bilezikian JP, McMahon DJ, et al. The natural history of primary hyperparathyroidism with or without parathyroid surgery after 15 years. J Clin Endocrinol Metab. 2008;93(9):3462-3470. [PMID: 18544625]

Silverberg SJ, Shane E, Jacobs TP, Siris E, Bilezikian JP. A 10-year prospective study of primary hyperparathyroidism with or without parathyroid surgery [erratum in N Engl J Med. 2000;342(2):144]. N Engl J Med. 1999;341(17):1249-1255. [PMID: 10528034]

U.S. Preventive Services Task Force. Vitamin D and Calcium Supplementation to Prevent Cancer and Osteoporotic Fractures in Adults: Draft Recommendation Statement. AHRQ Publication No. 12-05163-EF-2. Available at: www.uspreventiveservicestaskforce.org/draftrec3.htm. Accessed June 13, 2012.

Endocrinology and Metabolism Self-Assessment Test

This self-assessment test contains one-best-answer multiple-choice questions. Please read these directions carefully before answering the questions. Answers, critiques, and bibliographies immediately follow these multiple-choice questions. The American College of Physicians is accredited by the Accreditation Council for Continuing Medical Education (ACCME) to provide continuing medical education for physicians.

The American College of Physicians designates MKSAP 16 Endocrinology and Metabolism for a maximum of 12 *AMA PRA Category 1 Credits*™. Physicians should claim only the credit commensurate with the extent of their participation in the activity.

Earn "Same-Day" CME Credits Online

For the first time, print subscribers can enter their answers online to earn CME credits in 24 hours or less. You can submit your answers using online answer sheets that are provided at mksap.acponline.org, where a record of your MKSAP 16 credits will be available. To earn CME credits, you need to answer all of the questions in a test and earn a score of at least 50% correct (number of correct answers divided by the total number of questions). Take any of the following approaches:

- Use the printed answer sheet at the back of this book to record your answers. Go to mksap.acponline.org, access the appropriate online answer sheet, transcribe your answers, and submit your test for same-day CME credits. There is no additional fee for this service.
- Go to mksap.acponline.org, access the appropriate online answer sheet, directly enter your answers, and submit your test for same-day CME credits. There is no additional fee for this service.
- Pay a $10 processing fee per answer sheet and submit the printed answer sheet at the back of this book by mail or fax, as instructed on the answer sheet. Make sure you calculate your score and fax the answer sheet to 215-351-2799 or mail the answer sheet to Member and Customer Service, American College of Physicians, 190 N. Independence Mall West, Philadelphia, PA 19106-1572, using the courtesy envelope provided in your MKSAP 16 slipcase. You will need your 10-digit order number and 8-digit ACP ID number, which are printed on your packing slip. Please allow 4 to 6 weeks for your score report to be emailed back to you. Be sure to include your email address for a response.

If you do not have a 10-digit order number and 8-digit ACP ID number or if you need help creating a username and password to access the MKSAP 16 online answer sheets, go to mksap.acponline.org or email custserv@acponline.org.

CME credit is available from the publication date of December 31, 2012, until December 31, 2015. You may submit your answer sheets at any time during this period.

Directions

*Each of the numbered items is followed by lettered answers. Select the **ONE** lettered answer that is **BEST** in each case.*

Item 1

A 62-year-old man is evaluated before having panretinal laser photocoagulation therapy in both eyes. He has an 18-year history of type 2 diabetes mellitus. He also has diabetic neuropathy and hypertension. At his annual retinal eye examination last week, his vision had deteriorated to 20/30 in his right eye and 20/40 in his left eye; new blood vessels are seen growing on the optic discs of both eyes. Medications are metformin, insulin glargine, simvastatin, ramipril, enteric-coated aspirin, and hydrochlorothiazide.

On physical examination, temperature is 36.9 °C (98.4 °F), blood pressure is 147/86 mm Hg, pulse rate is 88/min, and respiration rate is14/min; BMI is 34. Other than the presence of proliferative diabetic retinopathy, physical examination findings are unremarkable.

Which of the following is the most likely outcome of the planned procedure?

(A) Diminished central vision with retention of peripheral vision
(B) Diminished peripheral and night vision with retention of central vision
(C) Improvement of vision (to 20/20) in both eyes
(D) Loss of binocular vision and depth perception

Item 2

A 61-year-old man is evaluated after a CT scan obtained because of right epigastric pain showed a 7-cm right adrenal mass. The patient reports no change in weight or appetite and no history of hypertension, palpitations, headaches, or excess sweating. He takes no medication.

Physical examination shows a man with normal features. Temperature is 36.7 °C (98.1 °F), blood pressure is 122/76 mm Hg, pulse rate is 74/min and regular, and respiration rate is 16/min; BMI is 29. No plethora, muscle wasting, weakness, or ecchymosis is noted.

Results of laboratory studies, including measurement of serum electrolyte, cortisol, and adrenocorticotropic hormone levels and of the 24-hour urine metanephrine level, are normal, as are results of a dexamethasone suppression test.

The previously obtained CT scan shows a 7-cm right adrenal mass with an attenuation factor of 77 Hounsfield units and a normally sized left adrenal gland. No lymphadenopathy or other masses were detected.

Which of the following is the most appropriate management?

(A) Biopsy of the adrenal mass
(B) Right adrenalectomy
(C) Serum aldosterone to plasma renin activity ratio determination
(D) 24-Hour measurement of urine cortisol excretion

Item 3

An 18-year-old woman is evaluated for a 6-month history of amenorrhea. The patient underwent menarche at age 13 years and had normal menstrual cycles until 6 months ago. She reports no hot flushes, night sweats, weight changes, or cold or heat intolerance. She has had no uterine procedures and has no family history of thyroid disease or primary ovarian insufficiency.

On physical examination, vital signs are normal; BMI is 22. No evidence of hirsutism, acne, alopecia, clitoromegaly, or galactorrhea is found.

Results of laboratory studies are normal, including serum follicle-stimulating hormone, human chorionic gonadotropin, prolactin, free thyroxine (T_4), and thyroid-stimulating hormone levels.

Which of the following is the most appropriate next diagnostic step?

(A) Measurement of total testosterone and dehydroepiandrosterone levels
(B) MRI of the pituitary gland
(C) Pelvic ultrasonography
(D) Progesterone challenge testing

Item 4

A 28-year-old woman is evaluated for a 1-year history of a nonpainful swelling in her neck. Her health has been otherwise excellent, with no weight loss, nervousness, or excessive tiredness. She is interested in becoming pregnant. Her mother and maternal grandmother have thyroid disease treated with levothyroxine.

On physical examination, blood pressure is 130/80 mm Hg, pulse rate is 94/min and regular, and respiration rate is 16/min; BMI is 27. Her thyroid gland is minimally enlarged bilaterally and feels firm. No specific nodules or cervical lymphadenopathy is palpated. Results of cardiac, pulmonary, abdominal, and extremity examinations are normal.

Laboratory studies:

Thyroid-stimulating hormone (TSH)	6.5 µU/mL (6.5 mU/L)
Thyroxine (T_4), free	1.2 ng/dL (15 pmol/L)
Triiodothyronine (T_3), free	4.0 ng/L (6.1 pmol/L)
Thyroid peroxidase antibodies	640 units/L (normal, <20 units/L)

Which of the following is the most appropriate next step in management?

(A) Fine-needle aspiration biopsy of the thyroid gland
(B) Levothyroxine therapy
(C) Repeat TSH measurement in 6 weeks
(D) Thyroid scan

H

Item 5

A 47-year-old man is evaluated in the emergency department for a 2-week history of a worsening productive cough associated with fever and night sweats. The patient has advanced HIV infection and has lost 8.2 kg (18.0 lb) since his last outpatient visit 3 months ago. He stopped taking all medications, including antiretroviral therapy, 4 months ago.

On physical examination, temperature is 38.2 °C (100.8 °F), blood pressure is 130/78 mm Hg, and pulse rate is 98/min; BMI is 17. The patient appears cachectic and is diaphoretic. Findings on a chest radiograph are consistent with miliary tuberculosis, and he is admitted to an isolation room.

Results of laboratory studies obtained 1 day after admission show a serum calcium level of 10.8 mg/dL (2.7 mmol/L), an albumin level of 2.4 g/dL (24 g/L), and a serum phosphorus level of 4.8 mg/dL (1.55 mmol/L). A serum parathyroid hormone (PTH) level obtained 2 days after admission is 9 pg/mL (9 ng/L).

Which of the following is the most likely underlying mechanism of this patient's hypercalcemia?

(A) Dehydration
(B) Excessive 1,25-dihydroxyvitamin D production
(C) Excessive parathyroid hormone release
(D) Presence of PTH-related protein

Item 6

A 67-year-old woman is evaluated for a 2-day history of severe muscle weakness. The patient experienced significant weight gain and developed hypertension and type 2 diabetes mellitus 2 years ago. She also reports developing muscle weakness of the lower extremities 6 month ago. Her diabetes is only partially controlled by metformin; her blood glucose measurements at home are usually greater than 250 mg/dL (13.9 mmol/L). Other medications are hydrochlorothiazide, lisinopril, amlodipine, and metoprolol.

Physical examination shows a woman who appears chronically ill. Blood pressure is 154/92 mm Hg, and other vital signs are normal; BMI is 40. Skin examination is notable for facial hirsutism. Central obesity, mild proximal muscle weakness, and 2+ peripheral edema are noted.

Results of laboratory studies show a serum creatinine level of 1.3 mg/dL (115 µmol/L), a plasma glucose level of 144 mg/dL (8.0 mmol/L), and a serum potassium level of 2.9 meq/L (2.9 mmol/L).

Which of the following tests should be performed to reveal the cause of her diabetes?

(A) Adrenal CT
(B) C-peptide measurement
(C) Glutamic acid decarboxylase antibody titer
(D) Pancreatic MRI
(E) 24-Hour urine free cortisol excretion

Item 7

A 26-year-old woman is evaluated for hyperprolactinemia after recent follow-up laboratory studies showed a serum prolactin level of 55 ng/mL (55 µg/L). Mild hyperprolactinemia (serum prolactin level of 35 ng/mL [35 µg/L]) was detected 6 years ago during an evaluation for irregular menstrual cycles; an MRI performed at that time showed a pituitary microadenoma. She was treated with a dopamine agonist, and subsequent serum prolactin measurements have shown normal levels until the most recent measurement. The patient underwent menarche at age 13 years and has had irregular menstrual cycles since that time, with multiple missed cycles. She has never been pregnant. Her family history is unremarkable, and she takes no medication.

On physical examination, blood pressure is 108/70 mm Hg, pulse rate is 82/min, and respiration rate is 12/min; BMI is 25. The patient has a normal distribution of body weight. Breast development is normal, but breast tenderness is noted on examination. No galactorrhea, acne, hirsutism, or striae are present.

Laboratory studies confirm a serum prolactin level of 55 ng/mL (55 µg/L) and show a thyroid-stimulating hormone level of 1.2 µU/mL (1.2 mU/L).

Which of the following is the most appropriate next diagnostic test?

(A) Pregnancy test
(B) Random serum growth hormone measurement
(C) Serum cortisol measurement
(D) Visual field testing

Item 8

A 28-year-old woman is reevaluated for worsening eye symptoms. The patient has a 6-month history of Graves disease. Methimazole was initiated but then discontinued when the patient became neutropenic (absolute neutrophil count, 500/µL [0.5×10^9/L]). Although treatment with methimazole abated her symptoms of thyrotoxicosis and normalized results of her thyroid function tests, her eye symptoms have progressed to severe discomfort (burning and itching) in both eyes and diplopia when she looks upward and laterally.

On physical examination, temperature is 37.2 °C (99.0 °F), blood pressure is 130/70 mm Hg, pulse rate is 90/min, and respiration rate is 16/min; BMI is 23. Examination of the thyroid gland shows an enlarged smooth gland without nodules. Examination of the eyes shows significant bilateral chemosis and erythema. Bilateral moderate proptosis and right lid and globe lag are noted. Visual acuity is normal.

Laboratory studies:

Thyroid-stimulating hormone	<0.01 µU/mL (0.01 mU/L)
Thyroxine (T_4), free	2.4 ng/dL (31 pmol/L)
Triiodothyronine (T_3)	230 ng/dL (3.5 nmol/L)
Thyroid-stimulating immunoglobins	340% (normal, <110%)

An MRI of the orbits shows bilateral proptosis and increased size of the extraocular muscles, especially the right inferior rectus muscle. Increased retro-orbital fat is seen, and the optic nerves appear normal

Which of the following is the most appropriate treatment for this patient's hyperthyroidism?

(A) Oral iodine solution
(B) Propylthiouracil
(C) Radioactive iodine therapy
(D) Thyroidectomy

Item 9

A 29-year-old woman is evaluated for recent-onset polyuria. The patient also has a 6-month history of fatigue, decreased energy, nausea, dry skin, and amenorrhea. She had pulmonary sarcoidosis 10 years ago that was successfully treated with a 2-year course of glucocorticoids and has not had any symptoms until now. She currently takes no medication and has no pertinent family history.

On physical examination, vital signs are normal; BMI is 24. Findings from examination of the heart, lungs, and thyroid gland are normal. Skin color and texture are normal, with no areas of hyperpigmentation. Diminished axillary and pubic hair and delayed relaxation of the deep tendon reflexes are noted.

Laboratory studies:

Electrolytes	
Sodium	146 meq/L (146 mmol/L)
Potassium	4.0 meq/L (4.0 mmol/L)
Chloride	96 meq/L (96 mmol/L)
Bicarbonate	28 meq/L (28 mmol/L)
Pregnancy test	Negative
Adrenocorticotropic hormone	12 pg/mL (3 pmol/L)
Cortisol (9 AM)	(Normal, 5-25 µg/dL [138-690 nmol/L])
Baseline	4.5 µg/dL (124 nmol/L)
After cosyntropin stimulation	13 µg/dL (359 nmol/L)
Follicle-stimulating hormone	3 mU/mL (3 units/L)
Luteinizing hormone	2 mU/mL (2 units/L)
Thyroid-stimulating hormone	0.5 µU/mL (0.5 mU/L)
Thyroxine (T_4), free	0.6 ng/dL (8 pmol/L)

A chest radiograph has normal findings.

Which of the following is the most appropriate diagnostic test to perform next?

(A) CT of the adrenal glands
(B) Lung biopsy
(C) Pituitary MRI
(D) Thyroid scan

Item 10

A 54-year-old woman comes to the office for advice regarding maintaining bone health. She has no history of fracture. The patient recently had a lumpectomy and radiation therapy to treat breast cancer, is currently taking tamoxifen, and will begin taking an aromatase inhibitor in 2 months. She underwent menopause at age 52 years and has persistent hot flushes. Her risk factors for osteoporosis include a slim body habitus and a mother who had a hip fracture at age 67 years.

Physical examination findings, including vital signs, are normal. BMI is 20.

Results of routine laboratory studies are normal.

A dual-energy x-ray absorptiometry scan shows T-scores of −2.1 in the lumbar spine, −2.3 in the femoral neck, and −1.9 in the total hip. Her Fracture Risk Assessment Tool (FRAX) score indicates a 22% risk of major osteoporotic fracture and a 2.4% risk of hip fracture over the next 10 years. Optimal calcium and vitamin D supplementation is recommended, and she is encouraged to begin weight-bearing exercise as tolerated.

Which of the following pharmacologic agents can be started in this patient?

(A) Alendronate
(B) Denosumab
(C) Estrogen
(D) Raloxifene
(E) Teriparatide

Item 11

A 15-year-old girl is evaluated for excessive urination and thirst. She has been drinking almost 5 liters (169 ounces) of fluid daily for the past 2 months. The patient's mother has type 2 diabetes mellitus.

On physical examination, vital signs are normal; BMI is 35. Results of general medical and neurologic examinations are unremarkable. She is not dehydrated, and no ketones are detected on her breath.

Laboratory studies:

Hemoglobin A_{1c}	8.7%
Glucose, random	324 mg/dL (18.0 mmol/L)
Electrolytes	Normal
Urine ketones	Absent

In addition to treating the patient's hyperglycemia, which of the following is the most appropriate next step in management?

(A) Measure fasting plasma C-peptide level
(B) Measure fasting plasma insulin level
(C) Measure stimulated plasma C-peptide level
(D) Obtain islet cell and glutamic acid decarboxylase antibody titers

Item 12

A 29-year-old man is evaluated for possible infertility. He and his wife have been trying to conceive for 2 years. His wife had a full anatomic evaluation with normal results. The patient reports normal libido and erectile function and had normal puberty. Family history is unremarkable. He takes no medication.

On physical examination, vital signs are normal; BMI is 22. Visual field examination findings and testicular volume are normal, as is hair distribution. All other physical examination findings are unremarkable.

Which of the following is the most appropriate next diagnostic test?

(A) Luteinizing and follicle-stimulating hormone measurements
(B) Semen analysis
(C) Testicular ultrasonography
(D) Total testosterone measurement

Item 13

A 27-year-old woman is evaluated during the fourth week of an uneventful pregnancy. She has a 3-year history of primary hypothyroidism due to Hashimoto thyroiditis that is treated with levothyroxine, 125 µg/d. She also takes prenatal vitamins and iron sulfate.

On physical examination, temperature is 37.1 °C (98.8 °F), blood pressure is 128/80 mm Hg, pulse rate is 95/min, and respiration rate is 18/min and regular; BMI is 25. She has a mild fine hand tremor. Lung, cardiac, and skin examination findings are normal. The thyroid gland is smooth and slightly enlarged without a bruit or nodules.

Laboratory studies show a serum thyroid-stimulating hormone level of 4.2 µU/mL (4.2 mU/L) and a serum free thyroxine (T_4) level of 1.6 ng/dL (21 pmol/L).

Which of the following is the most appropriate management?

(A) Increase the levothyroxine dosage by 10% now
(B) Increase the levothyroxine dosage by 30% now
(C) Repeat thyroid function tests in 5 weeks
(D) Repeat thyroid function tests in the second trimester

H

Item 14

A 67-year-old man is evaluated in the emergency department for an explosive headache and blurred vision that began 4 hours ago. He reports a 3-month history of fatigue, weight gain (total, 4.5 kg [10 lb]), and erectile dysfunction. The patient has a 2-year history of atrial fibrillation treated with warfarin and metoprolol.

Physical examination reveals a pale man who appears uncomfortable. Blood pressure is 88/56 mm Hg, pulse rate is 88/min, and respiration rate is 18/min. Visual field examination reveals bitemporal hemianopia. Except for the finding of neck stiffness, the remainder of the physical examination is unremarkable.

Results of laboratory studies are notable for a serum sodium level of 128 meq/L (128 mmol/L).

A noncontrast CT scan shows a heterogeneous sellar mass with suprasellar extension and bowing of the optic chiasm.

In addition to neurosurgical consultation, which of the following is the most appropriate initial management?

(A) Glucocorticoid administration
(B) Insulin tolerance test
(C) Lumbar puncture
(D) Serum prolactin measurement

Item 15

A 62-year-old woman is evaluated for a 1-week history of fatigue, lethargy, constipation, and nocturnal polyuria and polydipsia. The patient has advanced breast cancer, which has metastasized to her liver. Conventional therapy is no longer helpful, and she is scheduled to see her oncologist to discuss the next steps in her cancer management.

Physical examination shows a pale and somnolent woman. Blood pressure is 98/65 mm Hg and resting pulse rate is 103/min. Cardiopulmonary examination findings are normal. The mucous membranes are dry. The liver edge is palpated 3 cm below the right costal margin.

Laboratory studies:

Blood urea nitrogen	37 mg/dL (13.2 mmol/L)
Calcium	15.7 mg/dL (3.9 mmol/L)
Creatinine	1.4 mg/dL (124 µmol/L)
Sodium	151 meq/L (151 mmol/L)

A bone scan shows metastatic disease to the liver.

Which of the following is the most appropriate immediate next step in treating this patient?

(A) An intravenous bisphosphonate
(B) Intravenous furosemide
(C) Intravenous glucocorticoids
(D) Intravenous normal saline

Item 16

A 59-year-old woman is evaluated for muscle cramps and difficult-to-control hypertension. The patient reports no headaches or unexplained sweating. She started taking hydrochlorothiazide 20 months ago when hypertension was diagnosed but changed her medication after developing hypokalemia (serum potassium level, 1.9 meq/L [1.9 mmol/L]). Subsequent addition of lisinopril, atenolol, amlodipine, and potassium chloride has resulted in no improvement in blood pressure control.

Physical examination reveals a woman with normal features. Temperature is 36.5 °C (97.7 °F), blood pressure is 186/102 mm Hg with no orthostatic changes, pulse rate is 66/min with no orthostatic changes, and respiration rate is 16/min; BMI is 29. Results of examination of the lungs, heart, and thyroid gland are normal.

Laboratory studies:

Electrolytes	
Sodium	143 meq/L (143 mmol/L)
Potassium	2.9 meq/L (2.9 mmol/L)
Chloride	96 meq/L (96 mmol/L)
Bicarbonate	33 meq/L (33 mmol/L)

Which of the following is the most appropriate next diagnostic test?

(A) CT of the abdomen
(B) Dexamethasone suppression test
(C) Measurement of plasma catecholamine levels
(D) Serum aldosterone to plasma renin activity ratio determination
(E) 24-Hour measurement of urine free cortisol excretion

Item 17

A 58-year old woman is evaluated for a 3-week history of fatigue and weight loss. The patient has no significant medical history and takes no prescription medication, but she does take a daily over-the-counter multivitamin and a calcium supplement. She has a 50-pack-year smoking history.

Physical examination reveals a lethargic, ill-appearing woman. Temperature is 37.3 °C (99.1 °F), blood pressure is 136/78 mm Hg, pulse rate is 95/min, and respiration rate is 12/min. Other physical examination findings are unremarkable.

Laboratory studies:

Hemoglobin	8.3 g/dL (83 g/L)
Albumin	4.6 g/dL (46 g/L)
Blood urea nitrogen	43 mg/dL (15.4 mmol/L)
Calcium	14.5 mg/dL (3.6 mmol/L)
Creatinine	2.4 mg/dL (212 µmol/L)
Sodium	145 meq/L (145 mmol/L)

A chest radiograph shows a 5-cm mass in the right lower lobe of the lung but is otherwise unremarkable.

Which of the following is the most likely cause of her hypercalcemia?

(A) Malignancy
(B) Primary hyperparathyroidism
(C) Sarcoidosis
(D) Vitamin D intoxication

Item 18

A 42-year-old man is evaluated for a 6-month history of painful and enlarged breasts. The patient had normal puberty and has no relevant personal or family medical history. He takes no medication.

On physical examination, vital signs are normal; BMI is 25. Examination of the chest shows symmetric tender gynecomastia. Testicular volume is normal, no abdominal or testicular masses are palpated, and no lymphadenopathy is noted.

Laboratory studies show a serum human chorionic gonadotropin level of 2 mU/mL (2 units/L) (normal, <5 mU/mL [5 units/L]), a luteinizing hormone level of 5 mU/mL (5 units/L), and a total testosterone level of 400 ng/dL (14 nmol/L).

Which of the following is the most appropriate next diagnostic test?

(A) Adrenal CT
(B) Breast ultrasonography
(C) Estradiol level determination
(D) Karyotype
(E) Testicular ultrasonography

Item 19

A 33-year-old woman is evaluated after having three episodes of severe hypoglycemia, each resulting in a visit to the emergency department, in the past month. Two of the episodes occurred while she was asleep, and the most recent one happened midafternoon yesterday. The patient has a 19-year history of type 1 diabetes mellitus and has been trying to lower her hemoglobin A_{1c} level to less than 7.0% before she tries to get pregnant. She states that she no longer experiences any warning symptoms before she becomes hypoglycemic. The patient had an episode of diabetic ketoacidosis in her teens. She has mild background diabetic retinopathy, some numbness in her feet from peripheral neuropathy, and occasional orthostatic hypotension. She eats a healthy diet, counts carbohydrates, and adjusts her preprandial insulin intake. Medications are insulin glargine, 24 units at bedtime, and insulin glulisine, 6 to 10 units before breakfast, lunch, and dinner, depending on her planned carbohydrate intake and preprandial blood glucose level.

On physical examinations, vital signs are normal; BMI is 30.

Results of laboratory studies show a hemoglobin A_{1c} value of 6.6% and no evidence of microalbuminuria.

Which of the following is the most appropriate treatment for this patient?

(A) Increased carbohydrate intake at meals
(B) Insulin dose reductions
(C) α-Lipoic acid
(D) Preprandial pramlintide
(E) Substitution of insulin detemir for insulin glargine

Item 20

A 40-year-old man is evaluated after the incidental discovery of a small nodule in the right lobe of the thyroid gland on a CT scan obtained because of chest pain. The patient reports feeling well now, with no nervousness, palpitations, neck discomfort, or dysphagia. His mother has papillary thyroid cancer that was diagnosed in her 30s.

Physical examination shows a healthy-appearing, alert man. Vital signs are normal; BMI is 28. Lung, heart, and abdominal examination findings are normal. On neck examination, the thyroid gland is barely palpable, with no nodes or cervical lymphadenopathy.

Laboratory studies show a thyroid-stimulating hormone level of 1.5 µU/mL (1.5 mU/L).

A Doppler ultrasound of the thyroid gland shows a right-lobe 6-mm hypoechoic nodule with microcalcifications, blurred nodule margins, and increased central vascularity. No enlarged cervical lymph nodes are present on either side.

Which of the following is the most appropriate management?

(A) Fine-needle aspiration biopsy
(B) Repeat thyroid ultrasonography in 3 months
(C) Right thyroid lobectomy
(D) Thyroid MRI

Item 21

A 27-year-old man is evaluated for a 7-month history of loss of strength and progressive fatigue and a decreased sense of well being. The patient sustained a severe traumatic brain injury in an automobile collision 16 months ago. He has had no excessive urination, cold intolerance, constipation, or loss of libido or other symptoms of sexual dysfunction. His only medication is a daily multivitamin.

On physical examination, vital signs are normal; BMI is 30. Increased abdominal girth is noted. All other findings, including those from a neurologic examination, are normal.

Laboratory studies:

Complete blood count	Normal
Basic metabolic panel	Normal
Testosterone (8 AM)	980 ng/dL (34 nmol/L)
Thyroid-stimulating hormone	2.0 µU/mL (2.0 mU/L)
Thyroxine (T_4), free	1.4 ng/dL (18 pmol/L)

Which of the following is the most appropriate next diagnostic test?

(A) Fasting growth hormone measurement
(B) Glucose tolerance test
(C) Gonadotropin-releasing hormone test
(D) Insulin-like growth factor 1 measurement

Item 22

A 66-year-old woman comes to the office for management of osteoporosis discovered on a screening dual-energy x-ray absorptiometry (DEXA) scan. The patient has no personal history of fractures and no family history of parathyroid disease or low bone mineral density. She has hypertension treated with lisinopril but takes no other medications or supplements.

On physical examination, vital signs are normal; BMI is 22. Dentition is good. Other than mild kyphosis, physical examination findings are unremarkable.

Laboratory studies:

Albumin	4.0 g/dL (40 g/L)
Calcium	8.7 mg/dL (2.2 mmol/L)
Creatinine	0.7 mg/dL (61.9 µmol/L)
Phosphorus	2.9 mg/dL (0.94 mmol/L)
Parathyroid hormone	176 pg/mL (176 ng/L)

The DEXA scan showed T-scores of −2.1 in the lumbar spine, −3.0 in the femoral neck, and −2.5 in the total hip. Radiographs of the lateral spine show no compression fractures.

Which of the following is the most appropriate next step in management?

(A) Measurement of 1,25-dihydroxyvitamin D level
(B) Measurement of 25-hydroxyvitamin D level
(C) Parathyroidectomy
(D) Repeat DEXA scan in 1 year

Item 23

A 46-year-old woman is evaluated after undergoing a total thyroidectomy 6 weeks ago for metastatic (stage III) papillary thyroid cancer. A 4.5-cm left papillary thyroid cancer was removed. Metastatic disease was identified in a single cervical lymph node (level III). The patient has been taking levothyroxine since the surgery.

On physical examination, blood pressure is 130/70 mm Hg, pulse rate is 88/min and regular, and respiration rate is 16/min and regular. Examination of the neck shows a well-healing incision without palpable masses or lymphadenopathy. The lungs are clear to auscultation, and no murmurs, enlargement, or other abnormalities are seen on cardiac examination. No Chvostek sign is elicited.

Laboratory studies show a serum thyroid-stimulating hormone level of 0.1 µU/mL (0.1 mU/L), an undetectable serum thyroglobulin level (<0.5 ng/mL [0.5 µg/L] [normal, 1.6-59.9 ng/mL {1.6-59.9 µg/L}]), and no thyroglobulin antibodies.

Which of the following is the most appropriate next step in treatment?

(A) Chemotherapy with doxorubicin
(B) External-beam radiation therapy
(C) Radioactive iodine therapy
(D) Observation

Item 24

A 48-year-old man is evaluated during a routine examination. He has a 6-year history of hypertension treated with amlodipine and atenolol and is currently asymptomatic. His father had a myocardial infarction at age 50 years, and his mother developed type 2 diabetes mellitus at age 64 years.

On physical examination, blood pressure is 138/89 mm Hg, pulse rate is 76/min, and respiration rate is 18/min; BMI is 33. Central obesity is noted, but all other findings are unremarkable.

Results of laboratory studies show a hemoglobin A_{1c} level of 6.6% and a fasting plasma glucose level of 114 mg/dL (6.3 mmol/L)

Which of the following diagnostic tests should be performed next?

(A) Oral glucose tolerance test
(B) Repeat measurement of fasting plasma glucose level
(C) Repeat measurement of hemoglobin A_{1c} value
(D) No additional testing

Item 25

A 49-year-old woman is evaluated for a 1-week history of excessive fatigue and nausea. She has a history of hypertension, colon cancer, and unexplained anorexia. She was treated with megestrol, 320 mg/d, for almost a year before running out of her medications 2 weeks ago. She has had no palpitations, headaches, or unexplained sweating. Other medications are metoprolol and hydrochlorothiazide.

On physical examination, temperature is 36.5 °C (97.7 °F), blood pressure is 108/78 mm Hg with no orthostatic changes, pulse rate is 86/min with no orthostatic changes, and respiration rate is 16/min; BMI is 31. Results of examination of the lungs, heart, and thyroid gland are normal. A plethoric rounded face and central obesity with supraclavicular and posterior cervical fat pads are noted.

Laboratory studies:

Electrolytes	
Sodium	133 meq/L (133 mmol/L)
Potassium	3.9 meq/L (3.9 mmol/L)
Chloride	98 meq/L (98 mmol/L)
Bicarbonate	29 meq/L (29 mmol/L)
Adrenocorticotropic hormone	8 pg/mL (2 pmol/L)
Cortisol (9 AM)	2.7 µg/dL (75 nmol/L) (normal, 5-25 µg/dL [138-690 nmol/L])

Which of the following is the most appropriate management?

(A) CT of the adrenal glands
(B) Dexamethasone suppression test
(C) Fludrocortisone
(D) Oral hydrocortisone

Item 26

A 42-year-old man is evaluated for infertility. He and his wife have been trying to conceive for 1 year. They have a 4-year-old child conceived without problems. The patient reports a slightly decreased libido that he attributes to increased stress at work. Puberty was normal. He has osteoarthritis of the hands. Family history is unremarkable. His only medication is ibuprofen as needed.

On physical examination, vital signs are normal; BMI is 24. Testicular volume is decreased bilaterally. Visual field and thyroid examination findings are normal. No gynecomastia is noted.

Laboratory studies:

Alanine aminotransferase	48 units/L
Aspartate aminotransferase	25 units/L
Follicle-stimulating hormone	2 mU/mL (2 units/L)
Luteinizing hormone	2 mU/mL (2 units/L)
Prolactin	12 ng/mL (12 µg/L)
Testosterone, total (8 AM)	
Initial measurement	200 ng/dL (6.9 nmol/L)
Repeat measurement	190 ng/dL (6.5 nmol/L)
Thyroid-stimulating hormone	1.2 µU/mL (1.2 mU/L)
Thyroxine (T_4), free	1.2 ng/dL (15 pmol/L)

An MRI of the pituitary gland is normal.

Which of the following is the most appropriate next diagnostic test?

(A) Ferritin and iron saturation measurement
(B) Free testosterone measurement
(C) Karyotyping
(D) Testicular ultrasonography

Item 27

A 29-year-old woman is evaluated for a 2-day history of fever, cough, nasal congestion, myalgia, and fatigue. Addison disease was diagnosed 3 months ago. Medications are hydrocortisone (10 mg at 8 AM, 5 mg at noon, and 5 mg at 6 PM) and fludrocortisone (0.05 mg/d). She has been able to take her medications as scheduled and fluids as needed.

On physical examination, temperature is 38.2 °C (100.8 °F), blood pressure is 102/68 mm Hg without orthostatic changes, pulse rate is 88/min without orthostatic changes, and respiration rate is 21/min; BMI is 31. Erythema is noted in the posterior pharynx, and bilateral small cervical lymph nodes are present. The rest of the physical examination is unremarkable.

Which of the following is the most appropriate treatment?

(A) Hospital admission for intravenous fluids and glucocorticoid therapy
(B) Increased fludrocortisone dose
(C) Increased hydrocortisone dose for 3 days
(D) Symptomatic treatment for upper respiratory tract infection only

Item 28

A 55-year-old man is evaluated for anxiety, heat intolerance, and weight loss (2.3 kg [5 lb]) over the past 6 weeks. The patient also reports decreased visual acuity. He has no neck discomfort. He takes no medication.

Physical examination reveals a nervous man. Blood pressure is 150/70 mm Hg, pulse rate is 110/min and regular, and respiration rate is 16/min; BMI is 27. Other than tachycardia, the cardiopulmonary examination is unremarkable. Eye examination findings are normal. The thyroid gland is enlarged, smooth, and without bruits or nodules. The skin is warm. A bilateral hand tremor is noted. No pretibial myxedema is seen.

Laboratory studies:

Thyroid-stimulating hormone	1.5 µU/mL (0.5 mU/L)
Thyroxine (T_4), free	2.4 ng/dL (31 pmol/L)
Triiodothyronine (T_3)	220 ng/dL (3.4 nmol/L)
Thyroid-stimulating hormone–receptor and thyroid peroxidase antibodies	Negative

Radioactive iodine (^{123}I) uptake by the thyroid gland at 24 hours is 55% (normal, 10%-30%). A thyroid scan shows homogenous distribution.

Which of the following is the most appropriate next step in management?

(A) Methimazole
(B) Pituitary MRI
(C) Propylthiouracil
(D) Radioactive iodine therapy
(E) Thyroidectomy

Item 29

A 53-year-old man is evaluated after a pheochromocytoma is diagnosed on the basis of a 6-month history of hypertension and a 9-month history of recurrent palpitations, sweating, headaches, and weight loss (total, 4.5 kg [10 lb]) despite a good appetite. Medications are amlodipine, 10 mg/d; hydrochlorothiazide, 25 mg/d; and lisinopril.

Physical examination shows an anxious-looking man. Temperature is 36.5 °C (97.7 °F), blood pressure is 158/96 mm Hg without orthostatic changes, pulse rate is 102/min without orthostatic changes, and respiration rate is 16/min; BMI is 28.

Findings from examination of the lung, heart, and thyroid gland are normal. A mild resting tremor is noted in the upper extremities, but no myopathy or muscle weakness is detected.

Laboratory studies:

Glucose, fasting	150 mg/dL (8.3 mmol/L)
Metanephrine, free	160 pg/mL (0.8 nmol/L) (normal, 12-61 pg/mL [0.1-0.3 nmol/L])
Normetanephrine, free	740 pg/mL (4.1 nmol/L) (normal, 18-112 pg/mL [0.1-0.6 nmol/L])
Thyroid-stimulating hormone	1.2 µU/mL (1.2 mU/L)
Urine	
Creatinine	1100 mg/24 h
Epinephrine	220 µg/24 h (1201 nmol/24 h) (normal, 0-20 µg/24 h [0-109 nmol/24 h])
Metanephrine	0.85 mg/24 h (4.3 mmol/24 h)
Norepinephrine	2350 µg/24 h (13,889 nmol/24 h) (normal, 15-80 µg/24 h [89-473 nmol/24 h])
Normetanephrine	4550 µg/24 h (28,843 nmol/24 h) (normal, 128-484 µg/24 h [699-2643 nmol/24 h])
Vanillylmandelic acid	14 mg/24 h (71 µmol/24 h)

An electrocardiogram shows sinus tachycardia. A CT scan reveals a 3.5-cm left adrenal mass with an attenuation factor of 33 Hounsfield units.

Which of the following is the most appropriate initial management?

(A) Angiotensin receptor blocker therapy
(B) α-Blocker therapy
(C) β-Blocker therapy
(D) Surgery
(E) Observation

Item 30

A 78-year-old woman is evaluated for a 1-week history of diffuse constant headaches only occasionally relieved by acetaminophen. The patient has a history of hypertension and impaired fasting glucose, both of which are controlled with diet and exercise. She is up-to-date with preventive health screening.

Physical examination findings, including vital signs and results of neurologic evaluation, are normal.

Results of laboratory studies show a persistently elevated alkaline phosphatase level of 272 units/L; fractionation of the alkaline phosphatase shows an elevation in the bone isoform level. Other routine laboratory studies, including a complete blood count, are normal.

A bone scan shows uptake in the calvarium, left clavicle, two right ribs, and left acetabulum.

Which of the following is the most appropriate next step in management?

(A) Audiology testing
(B) Bone biopsy
(C) Plain radiographs
(D) Serum collagen type 1 cross-linked C-telopeptide (CTX) measurement
(E) Serum protein electrophoresis

Item 31

A 33-year old woman is evaluated for a 3-week history of fatigue, excessive sweating, and occasional headache on awakening. The patient has had type 1 diabetes mellitus since age 18 years. Her blood glucose log for the past 2 weeks shows fasting blood glucose levels ranging between 125 and 146 mg/dL (6.9-8.1 mmol/L) (average, 135 mg/dL [7.5 mmol/L]) and an average predinner level of 176 mg/dL (9.8 mmol/L). She does not check her level at other times during the day but occasionally experiences hypoglycemic symptoms around lunchtime, especially if she does not eat enough. She lives alone and usually exercises 1 hour each evening. Her diabetes regimen is premixed 70/30 insulin (neutral protamine Hagedorn [NPH] insulin/regular insulin) before breakfast and before dinner.

Physical examination shows a slim but well-appearing woman. Temperature is 36.6 °C (97.9 °F), blood pressure is 104/63 mm Hg, pulse rate is 66/min, and respiration rate is 14/min; BMI is 18. Other physical examination findings are unremarkable.

Results of laboratory studies show a hemoglobin A_{1c} value of 5.7% (estimated average plasma glucose level, 120 mg/dL [6.7 mmol/L]).

Which of the following is the most likely cause of her symptoms?

(A) Dawn phenomenon
(B) Nocturnal hypoglycemia

(C) Sleep apnea
(D) Somogyi phenomenon

Item 32

A 23-year-old woman is evaluated for a 3-month history of amenorrhea and galactorrhea. Her father has a history of recurrent kidney stones, and her brother has peptic ulcer disease.

On physical examination, vital signs are normal; BMI is 23. An expressible clear white nipple discharge is present bilaterally. All other examination findings are normal, including those from a visual field examination.

Laboratory studies:

Calcium	12 mg/dL (3.0 mmol/L)
Creatinine	0.7 mg/dL (61.9 µmol/L)
Parathyroid hormone	178 pg/mL (178 ng/L)
Prolactin	78 ng/mL (78 µg/L)
Thyroid-stimulating hormone	1.5 µU/mL (1.5 mU/L)

An MRI of the brain shows a 7-mm microadenoma of the pituitary gland.

Which of the following is the most likely diagnosis?

(A) Autoimmune polyglandular syndrome type 1
(B) Hashimoto thyroiditis
(C) Multiple endocrine neoplasia type 1 (MEN1)
(D) MEN2

Item 33

A 46-year-old man is evaluated for a 1-year history of low libido and erectile dysfunction. He underwent normal puberty and has two teenaged children. The patient has a history of hypertension. His only medication is chlorthalidone.

On physical examination, temperature is normal, blood pressure is 125/72 mm Hg, and pulse rate is 80/min; BMI is 42. No gynecomastia is present, and testicular volume is normal. A normal male distribution of body hair is noted.

Results of laboratory studies show a serum follicle-stimulating hormone level of 5 mU/mL (5 units/L), a serum luteinizing hormone level of 4 mU/mL (4 units/L), and a serum total testosterone level of 210 ng/dL (7 nmol/L); the serum thyroid-stimulating hormone and prolactin levels are normal.

Which of the following is the most appropriate next diagnostic test?

(A) Free testosterone assessment
(B) Karyotyping
(C) Pituitary MRI
(D) Sperm count

Item 34

A 35-year-old woman is evaluated for a nodule on the right side of her neck that she first noticed 2 weeks ago. The patient also reports recent flushing, diaphoresis, palpitations, and headaches. She has a history of hypertension treated with hydrochlorothiazide.

On physical examination, blood pressure is 145/95 mm Hg, pulse rate is 100/min and regular, and respiration rate is 16/min. Results of heart, lung, and abdominal examinations are normal. Examination of the thyroid gland shows a 2-cm firm right-sided nodule; all other thyroid findings are normal.

Results of laboratory studies show a serum calcium level of 10.8 mg/dL (2.7 mmol/L) and a thyroid-stimulating hormone (TSH) level of 2.0 µU/mL (2.0 mU/L).

An ultrasound of the thyroid gland shows a 2- × 2-cm solid right-sided nodule with no evidence of lymphadenopathy. Results of a fine-needle aspiration biopsy of the nodule show numerous plasmacytoid-appearing cells staining positive for calcitonin that are consistent with medullary thyroid cancer.

Which of the following is the most appropriate next step in management?

(A) Administer radioactive iodine
(B) Measure plasma free metanephrine and normetanephrine levels
(C) Perform a total lobectomy
(D) Suppress TSH secretion with levothyroxine

Item 35

A 34-year-old woman comes to the office for a routine follow-up evaluation. She has an 18-year history of type 1 diabetes mellitus. Her glycemic control has been poor, with hemoglobin A_{1c} values typically ranging from 8.0% to 10.0%; her most recent hemoglobin A_{1c} value obtained 6 months ago was 8.2%. The patient wants to get her diabetes under better control before conceiving. Her current diabetic regimen is neutral protamine Hagedorn (NPH) insulin at bedtime and before breakfast and insulin lispro before each meal. She takes 1 unit of insulin lispro for every 20 grams of carbohydrate in the meal, plus 1 unit for every 50 mg/dL (2.8 mmol/L) that her premeal blood glucose level is above 120 mg/dL (6.7 mmol/L). For the past 3 months, she has been eating a healthy, high-carbohydrate, high-fiber, and low–glycemic index diet, with consistent amounts of carbohydrate at each meal. Mean blood glucose levels derived from her current blood glucose log are shown; the preprandial (Pre) breakfast levels are fasting, and the postprandial (Post) levels are 2 hours after eating.

Glucose values:

Time	Pre (mg/dL [mmol/L])	Post (mg/dL [mmol/L])	Other (mg/dL [mmol/L])
Breakfast	124 (6.9)	197 (10.9)	—
Lunch	118 (6.5)	236 (13.1)	—
Dinner	121 (6.7)	264 (14.7)	—
Bedtime			
11 PM	—	—	131 (7.3)
3 AM	—	—	122 (6.8)

On physical examination, temperature is normal, blood pressure is 126/73 mm Hg, and pulse rate is 76/min; BMI is 18. All other physical examination findings are unremarkable.

Which of the following modifications to her treatment regimen is most appropriate?

(A) Add pramlintide before each meal
(B) Change the insulin lispro to regular insulin
(C) Change the NPH insulin to insulin glargine
(D) Decrease mealtime carbohydrate intake
(E) Increase the premeal insulin lispro dosage

H

Item 36

A 43-year-old man is evaluated in the hospital for perioral paresthesias and severe cramping of both hands. He had a total thyroidectomy yesterday because of papillary thyroid cancer. The surgery went well, and no involved lymph nodes were found.

On physical examination, vital signs are normal. Cardiopulmonary and abdominal examinations are unremarkable. Results of muscle strength testing are normal. Although the patient reports cramps, no tetany is detected.

Results of laboratory studies show a serum calcium level of 4.1 mg/dL (1.0 mmol/L), a serum magnesium level of 1.7 mg/dL (0.70 mmol/L), and a serum phosphorus level of 4.7 mg/dL (1.52 mmol/L); kidney function is normal.
A resting electrocardiogram is normal.

Which of the following is the most appropriate immediate treatment for this patient?

(A) Calcitriol
(B) Calcium
(C) Magnesium
(D) Teriparatide

Item 37

A 56-year-old man comes to the office for a follow-up evaluation. Three weeks ago, the patient had surgery to repair a bleeding duodenal ulcer. During his 7-day hospitalization, he was given six units of packed red blood cells. He was discharged 2 weeks ago with instructions to take omeprazole. The patient has a 12-year history of type 2 diabetes mellitus, and his hemoglobin A_{1c} values have ranged from 8.5% to 9.0% for the past 5 years. Since hospital discharge, his blood glucose levels have ranged from 140 to 160 mg/dL (7.8-8.9 mmol/L). He has a 40-pack-year smoking history but has not smoked since the surgery. Although work was increasingly stressful before ulcer repair, he says he has been feeling more relaxed since discharge and has been eating healthier foods. Medications are metformin, glyburide, simvastatin, and omeprazole.

On physical examination, temperature is 36.9 °C (98.4 °F), blood pressure is 142/83 mm Hg, pulse rate is 82/min, and respiration rate is 14/min; BMI is 34. Other physical examination findings are unremarkable.

Results of laboratory studies show a hematocrit of 43% and a hemoglobin A_{1c} value of 6.2% (estimated average plasma glucose level, 130 mg/dL [7.2 mmol/L]).

Which of the following best explains the reduction in his hemoglobin A_{1c} value?

(A) Blood transfusions
(B) Healthier diet
(C) Omeprazole interference with the hemoglobin A_{1c} assay
(D) Smoking cessation

Item 38

A 56-year-old man is evaluated for the gradual onset of low libido and erectile dysfunction over a 3-year period. The patient has a history of hypertension, depression, and chronic pancreatitis. He no longer drinks alcohol. Family history is unremarkable. Medications are lisinopril, methadone, and citalopram.

Physical examination reveals a thin man. Temperature is normal, blood pressure is 132/88 mm Hg, pulse rate is 72/min, and respiration rate is 10/min; BMI is 22. Visual field and thyroid examination findings are normal. The patient has a normal male distribution of body hair, and no gynecomastia or acne is noted. The testes are small and soft.

Results of laboratory studies show a serum follicle-stimulating hormone level of 1.2 mU/mL (1.2 units/L), a serum luteinizing hormone level of 1.1 mU/mL (1.1 units/L), and a serum total testosterone level of 125 ng/dL (4 nmol/L). The serum thyroid-stimulating hormone and prolactin levels are normal, as are results of iron studies.

An MRI of the pituitary gland is normal.

Which of the following is the most likely cause of this patient's hypogonadism?

(A) Anabolic steroid abuse
(B) Citalopram
(C) Lisinopril
(D) Methadone

Item 39

A 29-year-old woman is evaluated for a 3-month history of fatigue, nausea, poor appetite, and salt craving; she has lost 6 kg (13.2 lb) in this period. She has a 5-year history of hypothyroidism treated with levothyroxine and a family history of thyroid disease, scleroderma, and premature gray hair.

Physical examination shows a woman with evenly tanned skin, including non–sun-exposed skin. Temperature is 36.9 °C (98.4 °F), blood pressure is 82/64 mm Hg supine and 72/50 mm Hg sitting, pulse rate is 102/min supine and 124/min sitting, and respiration rate is 16/min; BMI is 23. Results of heart, lung, and thyroid gland examinations are normal. Hyperpigmentation of the gum line is noted. No muscle weakness is detected.

Laboratory studies:

Electrolytes	
Sodium	126 meq/L (126 mmol/L)
Potassium	5.7 meq/L (5.7 mmol/L)
Chloride	101 meq/L (101 mmol/L)

Bicarbonate	22 meq/L (22 mmol/L)
Thyroid-stimulating hormone	6.2 µU/mL (6.2 mU/L)
Adrenocorticotropic hormone (ACTH) (1 PM)	234 pg/mL (51 pmol/L)
Cortisol, random (1 PM)	2.5 µg/dL (69 nmol/L)
Dehydroepiandrosterone sulfate	0.2 µg/mL (0.54 µmol/L)

Which of the following is the most appropriate management?

(A) Hydrocortisone
(B) Increased levothyroxine dosage
(C) Morning (9 AM) measurement of serum cortisol and ACTH levels
(D) MRI of the pituitary gland

Item 40

A 29-year-old woman is evaluated for a 1-week history of new-onset severe headache and progressive fatigue, dizziness, weakness, arthralgia, and nausea. The patient is at 28 weeks' gestation (gravida 2, para 1). Before pregnancy, she had normal menses and no difficulty conceiving. She has a history of Hashimoto thyroiditis. Medications are levothyroxine and a multivitamin.

On physical examination, she is pale and appears ill. Blood pressure is 96/50 mm Hg, pulse rate is 90/min, and respiration rate is 14/min. Vision is normal. No evidence of Cushing syndrome or acromegaly is noted.

A noncontrast brain MRI obtained to evaluate her headache symptoms reveals a symmetric and homogeneous sellar mass measuring 15 mm in diameter with extension to the chiasm without compression. No cavernous sinus invasion is noted.

Laboratory studies:

Adrenocorticotropic hormone	<5 pg/mL (1 pmol/L)
Cortisol (8:00 AM)	7.9 µg/dL (218 nmol/L) (normal, 5-25 µg/dL [138-690 nmol/L])
Prolactin	55 ng/mL (55 µg/L)
Thyroid-stimulating hormone	1.9 µU/mL (1.9 mU/L)
Thyroxine (T_4), free	1.3 ng/dL (17 pmol/L)

Which of the following is the most likely diagnosis?

(A) Craniopharyngioma
(B) Lymphocytic hypophysitis
(C) Prolactinoma
(D) Sheehan syndrome

Item 41

A 48-year-old woman is evaluated after laboratory study results show a hemoglobin A_{1c} value of 8.5% (estimated average plasma glucose level of 197 mg/dL [10.9 mmol/L]). The patient has type 2 diabetes mellitus. Her blood glucose logs indicate an average fasting and preprandial blood glucose level of 132 mg/dL (7.3 mmol/L) for the past 3 months. She also has a history of iron deficiency anemia secondary to menorrhagia and has recently started iron replacement therapy. Other medications are neutral protamine Hagedorn (NPH) insulin at bedtime and metformin three times daily with meals.

On physical examination, temperature is 36.9 °C (98.4 °F), blood pressure is 127/78 mm Hg, pulse rate is 77/min, and respiration rate is 14/min; BMI is 26. All other findings from the physical examination are unremarkable.

Results of laboratory studies are normal except for a repeat hemoglobin A_{1c} value of 8.5% and a fasting plasma glucose level of 130 mg/dL (7.2 mmol/L); a blood glucose level obtained simultaneously on the patient's glucose monitor is 134 mg/dL (7.4 mmol/L).

Which of the following best explains the discrepancy between her average blood glucose levels as measured on the glucose monitor and her hemoglobin A_{1c} values?

(A) Inaccurate glucose monitor
(B) Iron therapy
(C) Nocturnal hypoglycemia
(D) Postprandial hyperglycemia

Item 42

H

A 57-year-old man develops tingling and numbness around his mouth and cramping in his feet and hands 8 hours after removal of a single enlarged parathyroid gland during minimally invasive surgery. He experienced some postoperative pain and is still hospitalized. The patient has a history of primary hyperparathyroidism and kidney stones. His only medication is a multivitamin.

On physical examination, vital signs are normal. A positive Chvostek sign and Trousseau phenomenon are noted, as is a spontaneous carpopedal spasm. The remainder of the examination is unremarkable.

Laboratory studies:

Albumin	3.9 g/dL (39 g/L)
Calcium	
Before surgery	11.6 mg/dL (2.9 mmol/L)
After surgery	7.2 mg/dL (1.8 mmol/L)
Creatinine	1.3 mg/dL (115 µmol/L)
Phosphorus	1.9 mg/dL (0.61 mmol/L)
Parathyroid hormone	
Before surgery	Elevated
After surgery	Normal
25-Hydroxyvitamin D	32 ng/mL (80 nmol/L)

Which of the following is the most likely cause of this patient's hypocalcemia?

(A) Chronic kidney disease
(B) Dilutional hypocalcemia
(C) Hungry bone syndrome
(D) Hyperventilation

Item 43

An 18-year-old woman is evaluated for a lump in her neck that she first noticed several weeks ago. She is in otherwise excellent health and has no history of radiation exposure or other medical issues. She has no family history of thyroid nodules or thyroid cancer and takes no medication.

On physical examination, vital signs are normal; BMI is 21. Examination of the thyroid gland shows a firm left-sided thyroid nodule that moves when she swallows. The rest of the gland is not palpable, with no cervical lymphadenopathy.

Laboratory studies show a thyroid-stimulating hormone level of 1.0 µU/mL (1.0 mU/L). Results of a complete blood count and comprehensive metabolic profile are normal.

A thyroid ultrasound shows a 2- × 2-cm solid hypoechoic left-sided thyroid nodule with increased intranodular vascular flow. Results of the fine-needle aspiration (FNA) biopsy are consistent with a follicular neoplasm.

Which of the following is the most appropriate next step in management?

(A) Levothyroxine suppression
(B) Radioactive iodine therapy
(C) Repeat FNA biopsy of the nodule in 6 months
(D) Thyroid lobectomy

Item 44

A 28-year-old woman is evaluated for a 5-month history of amenorrhea. She formerly had normal menses. The patient reports eating a healthy diet and having increased stress at work; she does not exercise. Personal and family medical history is unremarkable. She takes no medication.

On physical examination, temperature is 36.8 °C (98.2 °F), blood pressure is 110/70 mm Hg, pulse rate is 60/min, and respiration rate is 10/min; BMI is 23. Results of visual field, thyroid, and pelvic examinations are normal. Skin examination reveals mild facial acne. No galactorrhea is noted.

Laboratory studies show a serum follicle-stimulating hormone level of 4 mU/mL (4 units/L), a serum prolactin level of 14 ng/mL (14 µg/L), and a serum thyroid-stimulating hormone level of 1.3 µU/mL (1.3 mU/L). Human chorionic gonadotropin testing has negative results, and a progesterone challenge test produces no withdrawal bleeding.

A pituitary MRI is normal.

Which of the following is the most likely cause of this patient's amenorrhea?

(A) Functional hypothalamic amenorrhea
(B) Polycystic ovary syndrome
(C) Primary ovarian insufficiency
(D) Subclinical hypothyroidism

Item 45

A 56-year-old man comes to the office for a follow-up evaluation. Since receiving a diagnosis of type 2 diabetes mellitus 6 months ago, he has been eating a low-fat, high-fiber, high-carbohydrate diet and walking for 20 minutes at night. The patient has never smoked and drinks no alcohol. He originally took metformin to treat his diabetes but stopped because of persistent diarrhea. Current medications are glyburide and ramipril.

On physical examination, temperature is 36.8 °C (98.2 °F), blood pressure is 129/76 mm Hg, pulse rate is 76/min, and respiration rate is 15/min; BMI is 22. Other physical examination findings are normal.

Laboratory studies:

Alanine aminotransferase	102 units/L
Aspartate aminotransferase	96 units/L
Cholesterol	
Total	264 mg/dL (6.83 mmol/L)
LDL	157 mg/dL (4.07 mmol/L)
HDL	42 mg/dL (1.09 mmol/L)
Glucose, fasting	196 mg/dL (10.9 mmol/L)
Hemoglobin A_{1c}	9.8%
Iron studies	Normal
Triglycerides	437 mg/dL (4.94 mmol/L)
Hepatitis virus studies	Negative

Bedtime neutral protamine Hagedorn (NPH) insulin is initiated.

Which of the following is the most appropriate treatment of his hyperlipidemia?

(A) Begin a fibrate now
(B) Begin a statin now
(C) Begin a statin after results of liver chemistry studies normalize
(D) Begin nicotinic acid (niacin) now
(E) Begin either a fibrate or nicotinic acid after results of liver chemistry studies normalize

Item 46

A 58-year-old man is evaluated for a 1-week history of headache that started after he sustained minor head trauma with no loss of consciousness in a motor vehicle collision. A CT scan obtained in the emergency department revealed a sellar mass. The patient has a 2-year history of mild sexual dysfunction but no other symptoms. He takes no medication.

On physical examination, blood pressure is 126/78 mm Hg and pulse rate is 64/min; BMI is 32. Normal secondary sexual characteristics are noted, and no gynecomastia is present. Other examination findings also are normal.

Laboratory studies show normal insulin-like growth factor 1 and morning cortisol levels

An MRI shows a 1.7-cm sellar mass with suprasellar extension but no chiasmal compression.

In addition to assessing adrenal and thyroid function, which of the following is the most appropriate next diagnostic step?

(A) Dexamethasone suppression test
(B) Growth hormone stimulation test
(C) Serum prolactin measurement
(D) Serum sodium and urine osmolality measurements

H

Item 47

A 57-year-old woman returns to the office to discuss her laboratory results after a recent routine physical examination. She has hypertension treated with lisinopril but is otherwise healthy and takes no vitamins or supplements. At her previous evaluation, blood pressure was 129/84 mm Hg, pulse rate was 86/min, and BMI was 26; all other physical examination findings were normal.

Previous laboratory studies:

Albumin	3.8 g/dL (38 g/L)
Calcium	10.6 mg/dL (2.7 mmol/L)
Creatinine	0.9 mg/dL (79.6 µmol/L)
Parathyroid hormone	61 pg/mL (61 ng/L)

She has no history of fractures, kidney stones, or bone pain but recalls that her brother was evaluated for an elevated serum calcium level several years ago; she says he is currently healthy and has not required any treatment or surgery.

Which of the following is the most appropriate next test in this patient's evaluation?

(A) Measurement of the serum prolactin level
(B) Measurement of the serum 25-hydroxyvitamin D level
(C) Measurement of the urine calcium and urine creatinine levels
(D) Parathyroid sestamibi scan

Item 48

A 64-year-old woman is evaluated in the intensive care unit for persistent hypotension secondary to pyelonephritis-related gram-negative sepsis. The patient was admitted to the hospital 2 days ago and has received appropriate fluid and vasopressor resuscitation and antibiotic therapy. She is no longer receiving vasopressors.

Physical examination reveals a pale woman. Temperature is 37.9 °C (100.2 °F), blood pressure is 92/64 mm Hg supine, pulse rate is 102/min supine, and respiration rate is 16/min. The remaining physical examination findings are unremarkable.

Laboratory studies:

Albumin	2.1 g/dL (21 g/L)
Electrolytes	
Sodium	139 meq/L (139 mmol/L)
Potassium	3.6 meq/L (3.6 mmol/L)
Chloride	109 meq/L (109 mmol/L)
Bicarbonate	23 meq/L (23 mmol/L)
Cortisol, random	15 µg/dL (414 nmol/L)

Which of the following is the most appropriate management?

(A) Continuation of current therapy
(B) Cosyntropin stimulation test
(C) Morning (9 AM) measurement of serum cortisol level
(D) Stress doses of hydrocortisone

Item 49

A 62-year-old woman is admitted to the hospital in a coma. Her daughter says that her mother has had progressive lethargy, malaise, disorientation, and ataxia over the past 2 days. The patient received radioactive iodine therapy 10 years ago for an overactive thyroid gland and has hypertension. She does not drink alcohol or smoke. Medications are levothyroxine and hydrochlorothiazide, although the daughter reports that her mother is only intermittently adherent to her medication regimen.

Physical examination shows an ill-appearing woman who is comatose and not responding to verbal commands. Temperature is 35.9 °C (96.6 °F), blood pressure is 105/65 mm Hg, pulse rate is 75/min, and respiration rate is 10/min. Cardiac examination shows a grade 2/6 holosystolic murmur at the left lower sternal border. Lung examination reveals dependent crackles, but findings are otherwise normal. The thyroid gland is not palpable, and no cervical lymphadenopathy is noted. The skin is dry and cold, and the face, lips, and hands are mildly edematous. Abdominal examination findings are normal.

Laboratory studies:

Leukocyte count	20,000/µL (20×10^9/L), with 80% neutrophils
Electrolytes	
Sodium	132 meq/L (132 mmol/L)
Potassium	3.5 meq/L (3.5 mmol/L)
Chloride	103 meq/L (103 mmol/L)
Bicarbonate	26 meq/L (26 mmol/L)
Glucose	45 mg/dL (2.5 mmol/L)
pH	7.30
Thyroid-stimulating hormone	140 µU/mL (140 mU/L)
Thyroxine (T_4), free	0.2 ng/dL (3 pmol/L)
Triiodothyronine (T_3)	<20 ng/dL (0.3 nmol/L)

A serum cortisol level is pending.

A chest radiograph shows mild bibasilar infiltrates and an enlarged heart. A CT scan of the head without contrast is normal.

Which of the following is the most appropriate initial treatment of this patient?

(A) Intravenous levothyroxine
(B) Intravenous levothyroxine and hydrocortisone
(C) Intravenous liothyronine
(D) Intravenous liothyronine and hydrocortisone

Item 50

A 47-year-old man is evaluated for a 5-year history of sexual dysfunction and a 3-month history of headache. He reports low libido and erectile dysfunction. Personal and family medical histories are unremarkable. The patient takes no medication.

On physical examination, vital signs are normal; BMI is 24. Funduscopic, visual field, and cranial nerve examination findings are normal. Testes are small and descended bilaterally. No testicular mass is palpated.

Laboratory studies:

Comprehensive metabolic profile	Normal
Follicle-stimulating hormone	2 mU/mL (2 units/L)
Luteinizing hormone	1.3 mU/mL (1.3 units/L)
Prolactin	78 ng/mL (78 µg/L)
Thyroid-stimulating hormone	2.1 µU/mL (2.1 mU/L)
Total testosterone	132 ng/dL (4.6 nmol/L)

Which of the following is the most appropriate initial management?

(A) Cabergoline therapy
(B) Pituitary MRI
(C) Testicular ultrasonography
(D) Testosterone therapy

Item 51

A 35-year-old man is evaluated for a 2-month history of low libido. The patient had a normal puberty. Family history is unremarkable. He drinks two beers per week and takes no medication.

On physical examination, vital signs are normal; BMI is 23. Visual field examination findings are normal, as is testicular size. No gynecomastia is noted.

Laboratory studies:

Follicle-stimulating hormone	6 mU/mL (6 units/L)
Luteinizing hormone	5 mU/mL (5 units/L)
Thyroid-stimulating hormone	2.5 µU/mL (2.5 mU/L)
Total testosterone (4 PM)	200 ng/dL (7 nmol/L)

Which of the following is the most appropriate next diagnostic test?

(A) Measurement of serum ferritin and iron saturation levels
(B) Morning serum free testosterone measurement
(C) Morning serum total testosterone measurement
(D) Testicular ultrasonography

Item 52

A 24-year-old woman is evaluated for a 1-week history of neck discomfort that radiates to the jaw, palpitations, a fast heart rate, anxiety, and fever. The patient reports having a sore throat 4 weeks ago that resolved after a few days. She has no other symptoms and no personal history of thyroid or endocrine disorders. Her only medication is an oral contraceptive.

Physical examination shows an anxious-appearing woman. Temperature is 37.5 °C (99.5 °F), blood pressure is 140/60 mm Hg, pulse rate is 110/min, and respiration rate is 16/min; BMI is 23. Cardiopulmonary examination reveals tachycardia, but other findings are normal. The thyroid gland is slightly enlarged and tender with no nodules. No thyroid bruit is heard, and no cervical lymphadenopathy is palpated. No eye findings or pretibial myxedema is noted. The patient has a fine bilateral hand tremor.

Laboratory studies:

Erythrocyte sedimentation rate	45 mm/h
Thyroid-stimulating hormone	<0.01 µU/mL (0.01 mU/L)
Thyroxine (T_4), free	4.1 ng/dL (53 pmol/L)
Triiodothyronine (T_3)	300 ng/dL (4.6 nmol/L)

A Doppler thyroid ultrasound shows an enlarged thyroid gland with heterogeneous echotexture without cervical lymphadenopathy; no significant vascular flow is evident.

Which of the following is the most appropriate next step in management?

(A) Bilateral fine-needle aspiration biopsy
(B) Methimazole
(C) Serum thyroglobulin measurement
(D) 24-Hour radioactive iodine uptake test

Item 53

An 82-year-old woman is evaluated for the recent development of frequent episodes of confusion and forgetfulness. She has a 6-year history of type 2 diabetes mellitus and a 5-year history of heart failure. Medications are glyburide, furosemide, lisinopril, and potassium supplements.

On physical examination, temperature is normal, blood pressure is 142/77 mm Hg, pulse rate is 87/min, and respiration rate is 16/min; BMI is 20. All other physical examination findings are unremarkable, including those from a mental status examination.

Laboratory studies show a serum creatinine level of 1.3 mg/dL (115 µmol/L) and a hemoglobin A_{1c} value of 6.2%.

Which of the following is the most appropriate immediate next step in management?

(A) Discontinue glyburide
(B) Start glipizide
(C) Start metformin
(D) Start premixed 70/30 insulin (neutral protamine Hagedorn [NPH] insulin/regular insulin)

Item 54

A 58-year-old woman is evaluated during a routine physical examination. She reports no headache, heartburn, breast discomfort, change in energy or mood, or bone pain. The patient has osteoarthritis and a history of a distal tibia fracture sustained 1 year ago when she tripped while walking. She has never had kidney stones and has no family history of endocrinopathies, kidney stones, or bone disease. Medications are ibuprofen as needed and a daily multivitamin.

Physical examination finding, including vital signs, are unremarkable.

Laboratory findings:

Albumin	4.1 g/dL (41 g/L)
Blood urea nitrogen	20 mg/L (7.1 mmol/L)
Calcium	11.1 mg/dL (2.8 mmol/L)

Creatinine	0.7 mg/dL (61.9 µmol/L)
Estimated glomerular filtration rate	65 mL/min/1.73 m^2
Parathyroid hormone	63 pg/mL (63 ng/L)

A dual-energy x-ray absorptiometry scan shows T-scores of −1.8 in the lumbar spine, −2.0 in the total hip, −2.2 in the femoral neck, and −2.2 in the distal radius.

Which of the following is the most appropriate next step in managing this patient's disease?

(A) Bisphosphonate therapy
(B) Bone scan
(C) Parathyroidectomy
(D) Parathyroid hormone–related protein measurement
(E) Repeat serum calcium measurement in 1 year

Item 55

A 72-year-old man is hospitalized for treatment of community-acquired pneumonia. Despite 4 days of treatment with intravenous fluids and antibiotics appropriate for the bacteria cultured from sputum and blood, he remains febrile with mild tachycardia. The patient subsequently develops mild hypotension and is transferred to the intensive care unit. Results of two subsequent blood cultures are negative for bacteria. Medical history is significant for hypertension treated with amlodipine and recurrent osteoarthritis treated with intra-articular injections of triamcinolone several times a year; his last injection occurred 3 months ago.

Physical examination shows a pale and anxious man. Temperature is 38.0 °C (100.4 °F), blood pressure is 110/68 mm Hg supine and 102/64 mm Hg sitting, pulse rate is 102/min supine and 124/min sitting, and respiration rate is 21/min; BMI is 33. Lung examination reveals crackles and egophony in the right lower lobe area. Other physical examination findings are unremarkable.

Laboratory studies:

Albumin	2.7 g/dL (27 g/L)
Electrolytes	
Sodium	139 meq/L (139 mmol/L)
Potassium	3.6 meq/L (3.6 mmol/L)
Chloride	109 meq/L (109 mmol/L)
Bicarbonate	23 meq/L (23 mmol/L)
Cortisol, random	9.5 µg/dL (262 nmol/L)
Thyroid-stimulating hormone	Normal

Which of the following is the most appropriate next step in management?

(A) Adrenocorticotropic hormone stimulation test
(B) Hydrocortisone
(C) Pseudomonal antibiotic coverage
(D) Vasopressor support

Item 56

An 88-year-old man is evaluated during a routine physical examination. He reports moderate fatigue but has no other symptoms, such as nervousness, weight gain or loss, joint discomfort, constipation, palpitations, or dyspnea. The patient has a history of hypertension. Medications are daily lisinopril and daily low-dose aspirin.

Physical examination shows an alert and oriented older man. Blood pressure is 140/85 mm Hg; all other vital signs are normal. Cardiac examination shows a grade 1/6 crescendo-decrescendo systolic murmur, and pulmonary examination findings are normal. The thyroid gland is not palpable; no cervical lymphadenopathy is noted. Results of examination of the extremities, including pulses, are normal.

Laboratory studies:

Complete blood count	Normal
Comprehensive metabolic profile	Normal
Thyroid function tests (repeated and confirmed)	
Thyroid-stimulating hormone	6.8 µU/mL (6.8 mU/L)
Thyroxine (T_4), free	1.1 ng/dL (14 pmol/L)
Thyroid peroxidase antibody titer	Normal

Which of the following is the most appropriate management?

(A) Levothyroxine
(B) Liothyronine
(C) Radioactive iodine test
(D) Observation

Item 57

A 38-year-old woman reports a 3-month history of increasing fatigue and weight gain. She underwent transsphenoidal surgery 4 years ago to remove a nonfunctioning pituitary macroadenoma, followed 4 months later by radiation therapy because of residual tumor. She started taking hydrocortisone 14 months ago after adrenal insufficiency was diagnosed. The patient developed amenorrhea 1 year ago and began taking an oral contraceptive. Medications are hydrocortisone, norethindrone with ethinyl estradiol, and a multivitamin.

On physical examination, blood pressure is 102/68 mm Hg, pulse rate is 64/min, and respiration rate is 12/min. Mild periorbital edema is noted. The skin is pale.

Laboratory studies:

Hemoglobin	Normal
Sodium	134 meq/L (134 mmol/L)
Prolactin	22 ng/mL (22 µg/L)
Thyroid-stimulating hormone	1.1 µU/mL (1.1 mU/L)

Which of the following is the most appropriate next diagnostic test?

(A) Morning serum cortisol measurement
(B) Serum free thyroxine (T_4) measurement
(C) Serum growth hormone measurement
(D) Serum luteinizing hormone measurement

H

Item 58

A 40-year-old woman is evaluated in the emergency department at 1 AM for a 7-hour history of gradually worsening generalized abdominal pain, hyperventilation, and lethargy. Her husband reports difficulty awakening her on several occasions since onset of symptoms, both during the evening and at night. The patient has a 3-day history of nausea and anorexia. She has a 22-year history of type 1 diabetes mellitus treated with insulin. Because she has been unable to eat or drink for the past 3 days, she has reduced her dosage of basal insulin by half and taken no premeal rapid-acting insulin during this period. Her only other medical problem is hypertriglyceridemia. Medications before coming to the emergency department were insulin glargine, prandial insulin glulisine, gemfibrozil, niacin, and daily fish oil.

Physical examination shows a lethargic but arousable woman. Temperature is 96.8 °C (36.0 °F), blood pressure is 105/70 mm Hg, pulse rate is 118/min, and respiration rate is 28/min; BMI is 36. Deep sighing respirations are noted, but the chest is clear to auscultation. She has a sweet smell on her breath. Abdominal examination reveals generalized abdominal tenderness with guarding but no rebound tenderness. Bowel sounds are heard in all four quadrants.

Laboratory studies:

Hemoglobin	14.7 g/dL (147 g/L)
Leukocyte count	23,000/µL (23×10^9/L), with 90% polymorphonuclear leukocytes
Electrolytes	
Sodium	149 meq/L (149 mmol/L)
Potassium	5.1 meq/L (5.1 mmol/L)
Chloride	92 meq/L (92 mmol/L)
Bicarbonate	4 meq/L (4 mmol/L)
Glucose, fasting	615 mg/dL (34.1 mmol/L)
Amylase	1168 units/L
Urinalysis	4+ glucose, 4+ ketones, no bacteria or leukocytes

A chest radiograph is normal.

Besides administering intravenous fluids and insulin, which of the following is the most appropriate management?

(A) Abdominal CT
(B) Endoscopic retrograde cholangiopancreatography
(C) Imipenem
(D) Laparotomy
(E) Serial abdominal examinations

Item 59

A 55-year-old man is reevaluated during a follow-up examination for a wrist fracture and anemia. The patient is otherwise asymptomatic. He was treated in the emergency department 2 weeks ago after he slipped in his driveway and sustained a right wrist fracture; mild iron deficiency anemia was detected at that time. He had normal results of a routine screening colonoscopy 5 years ago. Since his emergency department evaluation, 3 stool samples have been negative for occult blood. He takes no medication.

On physical examination, vital signs are normal; BMI is 19. Other than a cast on his right wrist, all other findings are normal.

Hemoglobin level is 11.9 g/dL (119 g/L), and 25-hydroxyvitamin D level is 17 ng/mL (42 nmol/L). Results of a comprehensive metabolic profile and urinalysis are normal.

A dual-energy x-ray absorptiometry (DEXA) scan shows T-scores of −1.6 in the lumbar spine, −2.2 in the femoral neck, and −1.9 in the total hip.

Which of the following is the most appropriate next step in management?

(A) Begin alendronate
(B) Begin teriparatide
(C) Repeat DEXA scan in 1 year
(D) Screen for celiac disease

Item 60

A 66-year-old woman is evaluated in the emergency department for sudden onset of bilateral flank pain, hypotension, nausea, fatigue, and dizziness. The patient had knee replacement surgery 2 weeks ago and has been taking warfarin for prevention of deep venous thrombosis and oxycodone for pain.

On physical examination, temperature is 38.3 °C (100.9 °F), blood pressure is 98/66 mm Hg supine and 84/60 mm Hg sitting, pulse rate is 102/min supine and 122/min sitting, and respiration rate is 16/min; BMI is 29. Bilateral flank tenderness and dry mucous membranes are noted. The surgical wound is clean.

Laboratory studies:

Hematocrit	21% (34% 5 days ago)
INR	5.5
Leukocyte count	6500/µL (6.5×10^9/L)
Creatinine	1.0 mg/dL (88.4 µmol/L)
Electrolytes	
Sodium	129 meq/L (129 mmol/L)
Potassium	5.4 meq/L (5.4 mmol/L)
Chloride	95 meq/L (95 mmol/L)
Bicarbonate	24 meq/L (24 mmol/L)
Glucose, random	89 mg/dL (4.9 mmol/L)

Which of the following is the most likely cause of her symptoms?

(A) Adrenal hemorrhage
(B) Gastrointestinal bleeding
(C) Narcotic overdose
(D) Septic shock

Item 61

An 82-year-old man is intubated and admitted to the intensive care unit (ICU) for sepsis and hypotension from community-acquired pneumonia. According to his wife, the patient had coronary artery bypass graft surgery 2 years ago and has had intermittent atrial fibrillation since that time that is treated with amiodarone, 200 mg/d. He has no history of thyroid abnormalities. Other medications administered in the ICU are vasopressors, ceftriaxone, and azithromycin.

Physical examination shows a sedated, ill-appearing older man who is intubated and cannot respond to questions. Temperature is 37.8 °C (100.0 °F), blood pressure is 90/50 mm Hg (with vasopressors), pulse rate is 110/min and irregular, and respiration rate is 18/min while intubated; BMI is 30. Cardiac examination reveals an irregular rate without murmurs, rubs, or gallops. Examination of the lungs reveals bibasilar crackles and rhonchi. The thyroid gland is not palpable. No cervical lymphadenopathy is noted. No bowel sounds are heard on abdominal examination. The extremities show 2+ peripheral edema. A few scattered ecchymoses are present on the skin.

Laboratory studies:

Cortisol, random	28 µg/dL (773 nmol/L)
Thyroid antibodies	Pending
Thyroid-stimulating hormone (TSH)	16 µU/mL (16 mU/L)
Thyroxine (T_4), free	0.6 ng/dL (8 pmol/L)
Triiodothyronine (T_3)	45 ng/dL (0.7 nmol/L)

An electrocardiogram shows tachycardia and atrial fibrillation, and a chest radiograph shows bibasilar infiltrates.

Which of the following is the most likely underlying endocrine disorder in this patient?

(A) Adrenal insufficiency
(B) Euthyroid sick syndrome
(C) Hypothyroidism
(D) TSH-secreting pituitary tumor

Item 62

A 32-year-old woman is evaluated for increased hair growth on the face and chest and a 3-month history of irregular menses. She has a 5-year history of hypothyroidism. Her only medication is levothyroxine.

On physical examination, temperature is 37.0 °C (98.6 °F), blood pressure is 110/72 mm Hg, and pulse rate is 80/min; BMI is 26. Terminal hair growth of the upper lip, chin, sides of the face, and middle of the chest is noted. No acanthosis nigricans or galactorrhea is detected. Palpation of the abdomen reveals no masses. Pelvic examination reveals clitoromegaly.

Laboratory studies:

Dehydroepiandrosterone sulfate	2.78 µg/mL (7.5 µmol/L)
Prolactin	17 ng/mL (17 µg/L)
Total testosterone	279 ng/dL (9.7 nmol/L)
Thyroid-stimulating hormone	1.5 µU/mL (1.5 mU/L)

Which of the following is the most appropriate next diagnostic test?

(A) Adrenal CT
(B) Free testosterone measurement
(C) Pituitary MRI
(D) Transvaginal ultrasonography

Item 63

H

A 62-year-old man is admitted to the hospital for a right hip replacement. The patient has a 36-year history of type 1 diabetes mellitus. He also has proliferative diabetic retinopathy treated previously with laser therapy and peripheral and autonomic neuropathy. Before admission, the patient's diabetes was treated with premixed 70/30 insulin (neutral protamine Hagedorn [NPH] insulin/regular insulin); he took 18 units of this preparation before breakfast and 12 units before his evening meal. His most recent hemoglobin A_{1c} value indicated good glycemic control.

On physical examination, temperature is normal, blood pressure is 138/79 mm Hg, pulse rate is 88/min, and respiration rate is 16/min; BMI is 22. Other physical examination findings are consistent with the previously established diagnoses of diabetic retinopathy with laser scars, autonomic neuropathy, and osteoarthritis of the right hip.

Which of the following is the most appropriate insulin therapy after surgery?

(A) Insulin glargine once daily and insulin aspart before each meal
(B) Intravenous insulin infusion
(C) Previous schedule of 70/30 insulin
(D) Sliding scale insulin schedule with regular insulin given whenever the blood glucose level is 150 mg/dL (8.3 mmol/L) or greater
(E) Subcutaneous insulin infusion

Item 64

A 33-year-old woman is evaluated for a 5-month history of amenorrhea and a 3-month history of galactorrhea. The patient says her menstrual cycles were normal before onset of amenorrhea. She takes no medication.

On physical examination, vital signs are normal. Visual field findings are normal. Bilateral galactorrhea is noted.

Results of laboratory studies show a serum luteinizing hormone level of 2 mU/mL (2 units/L), a prolactin level of 965 ng/mL (965 µg/L), and a free thyroxine level of 1.1 ng/dL (14 pmol/L). A serum β-human chorionic gonadotropin measurement is normal.

An MRI shows a 1.5-cm sellar mass with suprasellar extension that impinges on the optic chiasm.

Which of the following is the most appropriate initial treatment?

(A) Dopamine agonist therapy
(B) Oral contraceptive
(C) Radiation therapy
(D) Transsphenoidal surgical resection

Item 65

H

A 72-year-old woman is evaluated in the emergency department for loss of consciousness. Her son, who brought her in, says she seemed confused and agitated when he spoke to her on the telephone less than 2 hours ago. The patient has an 8-year history of type 2 diabetes mellitus. She had strict

H CONT.

glycemic control (average hemoglobin A_{1c} level, 6.2%) until last month when she had an infected ulcer between the third and fourth toes of the right foot that resulted in amputation of the middle toe 1 week ago. According to her son, she has been depressed while recovering at home and is not eating or drinking much. Medications are glyburide, cephalexin, and ibuprofen as needed.

On physical examination, temperature is 37.9 °C (100.2 °F), blood pressure is 162/96 mm Hg, pulse rate is 112/min, and respiration rate is 21/min; BMI is 19. The patient remains unconscious and is unresponsive to noxious stimuli. Dense left hemiplegia, warmth, and profuse sweating are noted. No inguinal lymphadenopathy is observed. The right middle toe amputation is healing well without redness, discharge, or swelling. No ankle edema is noted.

Which of the following is the most appropriate next step in management?

(A) Addition of vancomycin and ceftriaxone to the antibiotic regimen
(B) Fingerstick measurement of the blood glucose level
(C) Intravenous infusion of recombinant tissue plasminogen activator
(D) Noncontrast CT of the head

Item 66

A 71-year-old woman is evaluated for a 3-month history of occasional hoarseness and intermittent difficulty swallowing. The patient has a 10-year history of a multinodular goiter. Results of previous fine-needle aspiration biopsies, including one 6 months ago, have been negative for cancer, showing only bland-appearing follicular cells, colloid, and macrophages. She is otherwise healthy and takes no medication.

Physical examination reveals a vigorous woman. Vital signs are normal. The patient's face is slightly flushed and becomes more flushed when she raises her arms. Examination of the neck shows an enlarged thyroid gland that contains several firm but not hard nodules. The gland moves easily with swallowing. All other physical examination findings are normal, with no evidence of thyrotoxicosis.

Results of laboratory studies show a serum thyroid-stimulating hormone level of 0.51 µU/mL (0.51 mU/L) and free thyroxine (T_4) level of 1.6 ng/dL (21 pmol/L).

Radioactive iodine uptake is 28%. A thyroid scan reveals multiple patchy areas of either increased or decreased uptake.

A CT scan without contrast shows a large multinodular goiter, with substernal extension and extrinsic moderate compression of the trachea on the right, and a patent airway.

Which of the following is the most appropriate treatment?

(A) External-beam radiation to the neck
(B) Levothyroxine
(C) Methimazole
(D) Thyroidectomy

Item 67

A 42-year-old man is evaluated for a 6-day history of severe burning and stabbing pain in both feet that is worse in the toes. The pain is more severe at night, is aggravated when the bed sheets touch his skin, and is partially relieved when he walks or massages his feet. The patient has an 8-year history of poorly controlled type 1 diabetes mellitus and a 2-year history of hypertension. He was hospitalized briefly 2 weeks ago for treatment of pneumonia and diabetic ketoacidosis. His fasting blood glucose levels have been in the range of 150 to 200 mg/dL (8.3-11.1 mmol/L) since hospital discharge. He does not drink alcohol or smoke. Medications are insulin glargine, insulin glulisine, and lisinopril.

On physical examination, vital signs are normal; BMI is 22. Both feet and ankles are exquisitely sensitive to touch and temperature, especially on the tips of the toes. Pulses are easily palpated in both feet. No fasciculations, muscle weakness, foot ulcers, or foot deformities are noted. Monofilament testing reveals insensate feet bilaterally. Ankle reflexes are absent bilaterally.

Results of laboratory studies show a hemoglobin A_{1c} value of 9.2%.

In addition to improving glycemic control, which of the following is the most appropriate next step in management?

(A) Desipramine
(B) Fluoxetine
(C) Nerve conduction studies
(D) Oxycodone
(E) Sural nerve biopsy

Item 68

A 78-year-old woman is evaluated for a rapidly enlarging neck mass that has been present for 4 weeks and is associated with neck discomfort, dysphagia, and hoarseness. The patient has had Hashimoto thyroiditis and hypothyroidism since age 24 years and has been taking levothyroxine since that time.

Physical examination reveals an older woman in severe distress. Temperature is 39.4 °C (102.9 °F), blood pressure is 145/75 mm Hg, pulse rate is 110/min, and respiration rate is 16/min; BMI is 23. Pulmonary examination reveals dyspnea with bilateral basilar rhonchi, and cardiac examination shows tachycardia without a murmur. The thyroid gland is enlarged and firm without nodules. Facial plethora and distended bilateral cervical neck veins are noted. The patient is hoarse. Bilateral cervical lymphadenopathy is palpated. Although neurologically intact, she finds it difficult to concentrate when asked questions.

A thyroid ultrasound shows an enlarged thyroid gland with heterogeneous echotexture but no specific nodularity and multiple bilateral cervical lymph nodes measuring 1 to 3 cm in diameter.

Which of the following is the most likely diagnosis?

(A) Bleeding into the thyroid gland
(B) Medullary thyroid cancer
(C) Papillary thyroid cancer
(D) Primary thyroid lymphoma

Item 69

A 33-year-old woman is evaluated for a 2-week history of progressive fatigue, dizziness, anorexia, and arthralgia in multiple joints. Six weeks ago, the patient (gravida 2, para 2) had a difficult labor and delivery requiring multiple blood transfusions; her pregnancy had been uneventful. She subsequently was unable to lactate and has had no menses. Her only medication is a daily multivitamin.

Physical examination reveals a pale, thin woman. Temperature is 37.1 °C (98.7 °F), blood pressure is 88/50 mm Hg, pulse rate is 88/min, and respiration rate is 16/min; BMI is 19. Visual field examination findings are normal. No galactorrhea is noted.

Laboratory studies:

Sodium	129 meq/L (129 mmol/L)
Adrenocorticotropic hormone	5 pg/mL (1 pmol/L)
Cortisol (8:00 AM)	2.4 µg/dL (66 nmol/L) (normal, 5-25 µg/dL [138-690 nmol/L])
Follicle-stimulating hormone	1.1 mU/mL (1.1 units/L)
Prolactin	1.3 ng/mL (1.3 µg/L)
Thyroid-stimulating hormone	1.3 µU/mL (1.3 mU/L)

Results of a pituitary MRI are pending.

Which of the following is the most appropriate initial treatment?

(A) Arginine vasopressin replacement therapy
(B) Hydrocortisone
(C) Hypertonic saline
(D) Levothyroxine

Item 70

An 18-year-old woman is evaluated for syncope. She has had three episodes in the past month that resolved after she drank fruit juice with sugar. She has a history of depression treated with citalopram and occasional insomnia treated with zolpidem as needed. Her mother has type 2 diabetes mellitus treated with neutral protamine Hagedorn (NPH) insulin and glyburide.

Several minutes into her evaluation, the patient becomes confused and agitated with tachycardia and profuse sweating. A blood specimen is drawn, and intravenous glucose is administered to resolve her symptoms.

Physical examination shows a pale, thin woman. Vital signs are normal, and other physical examination findings are unremarkable.

Laboratory studies:

C-peptide	0.4 ng/mL (0.13 nmol/L) (normal range, 0.5-2.5 ng/mL [0.16-0.82 nmol/L])
Glucose, fasting	34 mg/dL (1.9 mmol/L)
Insulin	26 µU/mL (187.6 pmol/L) (normal range, 2-20 µU/mL [14.4-144.3 pmol/L])
Sulfonylurea screen	Negative

Which of the following is the most appropriate next step in management?

(A) Abdominal CT
(B) Abdominal octreotide scanning
(C) Gastric emptying study
(D) Psychiatric evaluation

Item 71

A 66-year-old woman is evaluated after a right adrenal mass is found on a CT scan of the abdomen obtained for evaluation of severe abdominal pain, which has since resolved. She has no history of hypertension or diabetes mellitus and has noted no palpitations, headaches, sweating, or weight changes.

On physical examination, temperature is 36.6 °C (97.9 °F), blood pressure is 140/84 mm Hg, pulse rate is 78/min, and respiration rate is 16/min; BMI is 29. The skin is normal, as is the distribution of supraclavicular and posterior cervical fat pads. All other physical examination findings, including those from a neurologic examination, are normal.

Laboratory studies:

Creatinine	1.0 mg/dL (88.4 µmol/L)
Electrolytes	
Sodium	139 meq/L (139 mmol/L)
Potassium	4.1 meq/L (4.1 mmol/L)
Chloride	97 meq/L (97 mmol/L)
Bicarbonate	29 meq/L (29 mmol/L)
Glucose, random	89 mg/dL (4.9 mmol/L)
Cortisol (9 AM)	(Normal, 5-25 µg/dL [138-690 nmol/L])
Baseline	13.8 µg/dL (381 nmol/L)
After 1 mg dexamethasone the night before	1.1 µg/dL (30 nmol/L)
Dehydroepiandrosterone sulfate	0.2 µg/mL (0.54 µmol/L)
Urine metanephrine and normetanephrine	Normal

The previously obtained CT scan shows a right adrenal mass that measures 2.5 cm in its longest dimension and has an attenuation of 9 Hounsfield units.

Which of the following is the most appropriate management?

(A) Metaiodobenzylguanidine (MIBG) scan
(B) MRI
(C) Repeat testing in 6 to 12 months
(D) Right adrenalectomy

Item 72

H

A 62-year-old man is evaluated in the emergency department for recent onset of fever and severe abdominal pain. He also reports a history of anxiety, frequent palpitations, difficulty concentrating, dyspnea, diarrhea, nausea, vomiting, and weight loss (total, 9.1 kg [20 lb]) over the past few months. He has had no neck discomfort. An abdominal CT

H CONT. scan with iodine contrast obtained several weeks ago when he first experienced abdominal pain was normal. The patient also has a 6-month history of Graves disease treated with methimazole. He takes no other medication.

Physical examination shows an anxious and agitated man. Temperature is 38.9 °C (102.0 °F), blood pressure is 160/90 mm Hg, pulse rate is 130/min and regular, and respiration rate is 22/min. Cardiac examination shows a grade 2/6 holosystolic murmur, and crackles are heard on lung examination. Eye examination shows no acute inflammatory findings. Findings from an examination of the pharynx are normal. The thyroid gland is firm and enlarged bilaterally with no specific nodules palpated. A thyroid bruit is heard. No cervical lymphadenopathy is noted. The skin is warm and moist. Abdominal examination reveals a palpable liver 2 cm below the right costal margin. Examination of the extremities shows 2+ peripheral leg edema. Neurologic examination reveals that the patient is oriented to place but not time, giving the incorrect answer when asked for the year.

Results of laboratory serum studies show a thyroid-stimulating hormone level of less than 0.01 µU/mL (0.01 mU/L), a free thyroxine (T_4) level of 8.2 ng/dL (106 pmol/L), and a triiodothyronine (T_3) level of 650 ng/dL (10 nmol/L).

Which of the following is the most likely diagnosis?

(A) Euthyroid sick syndrome
(B) Myxedema coma
(C) Subacute thyroiditis
(D) Thyroid storm

Item 73

A 31-year-old woman is evaluated during a postpartum examination 6 months after giving birth to her first child. The patient was obese before becoming pregnant, developed gestational diabetes mellitus during pregnancy, and was able to maintain her weight and glucose level within the target range throughout her pregnancy with diet alone. Her infant weighed 4139 grams (146 ounces) at birth.

This patient's infant is at increased risk for which of the following disorders?

(A) Childhood obesity
(B) Maturity-onset diabetes of the young
(C) Type 1A diabetes mellitus
(D) Type 1B diabetes mellitus

Item 74

A 44-year-old man is evaluated for a 2-year history of headache and 1-year history of diabetes mellitus and hypertension. His glove and shoe sizes have increased several times over the past 3 years, and he reports painful knees and hips. The patient also has sleep apnea and carpal tunnel syndrome. Medications are metformin and lisinopril.

On physical examination, blood pressure is 152/92 mm Hg, pulse rate is 82/min, and respiration rate is 16/min. Coarse facial features, frontal bossing, accentuated nasolabial folds, a large tongue, and thick hands and feet are noted.

Which of the following is the most appropriate next diagnostic test?

(A) MRI of the pituitary gland
(B) Random serum growth hormone measurement
(C) Serum insulin-like growth factor 1 measurement
(D) Serum prolactin measurement

Item 75

A 67-year-old man is admitted to the hospital after being found unresponsive and intoxicated at home. Family members report that he has a history of hypertension treated with atenolol and a history of alcoholism. He lives alone and has been resistant to assistance with meals and chores. He takes no other medication.

On physical examination, the patient is lethargic but arousable and smells strongly of alcohol. Vital signs are normal except for a pulse rate of 105/min. Mucous membranes are dry. No pain is elicited on abdominal examination. Chvostek sign and Trousseau phenomenon are noted.

After an electrocardiogram shows tachycardia (heart rate to 105/min) and a prolonged corrected QT interval (0.49 s), the patient is given intravenous fluids with added thiamine and folate. A calcium infusion is initiated.

Laboratory studies (before administration of thiamine, folate, and calcium):

Amylase	110 units/L
Blood urea nitrogen	33 mg/L (11.8 mmol/L)
Creatinine	1.4 mg/dL (124 µmol/L)
Ethanol	249 mg/dL (0.25 g/dL) (normal, <1.0 mg/dL [0.001 g/dL])
Ionized calcium	2.9 mg/dL (0.7 mmol/L) (normal, 3.8-5.3 mg/dL [1.0-1.3 mmol/L])
Phosphorus	2.1 mg/dL (0.68 mmol/L)

In addition to the interventions already underway, measurement of which of the following serum levels is the most appropriate next diagnostic test?

(A) Calcitonin
(B) 1,25-Dihydroxyvitamin D
(C) Magnesium
(D) Parathyroid hormone

Item 76

A 32-year-old man is evaluated for significant blood glucose elevations associated with exercise. The patient has a 22-year history of type 1 diabetes mellitus. He reports that after a recent 6 AM five-mile run, his blood glucose level was 386 mg/dL (21.4 mmol/L); the level was 297 mg/dL (16.5 mmol/L) just before the run and 215 mg/dL (11.9 mmol/L) at bedtime the night before. He took no insulin and ate no food in the morning before his run. During the run, he felt slow and fatigued but was significantly better after drinking water and giving himself insulin. The patient had one episode of diabetic ketoacidosis 15 years ago. Medications are insulin detemir, 16 units/d in the morning, and insulin lispro, 4 to 6 units before each meal, depending on his preprandial blood glucose level and expected carbohydrate intake.

Physical examination findings, including vital signs, are normal.

Which of the following is the most likely cause of his postexercise hyperglycemia?

(A) Excess nocturnal carbohydrate intake
(B) Gastroparesis
(C) Inadequate insulin replacement
(D) Nocturnal hypoglycemia

Item 77

An 18-year-old woman is evaluated for amenorrhea. The patient underwent menarche at age 12 years and has never had any subsequent menses. She has no medical history of note. Family history is remarkable only for hypothyroidism. She takes no medication.

On physical examination vital signs are normal; BMI is 22 (height, 147.3 cm [58.0 in]; weight, 48.6 kg [107.0 lb]). Visual field, thyroid, and pelvic examination findings are normal.

Results of laboratory studies show an initial serum follicle-stimulating hormone level of 53 mU/mL (53 units/L) and a subsequent level of 62 mU/mL (62 units/L) on repeat testing. Serum thyroid-stimulating hormone, human chorionic gonadotropin, and prolactin levels are normal.

Which of the following is the most appropriate next diagnostic test?

(A) Karyotyping
(B) Pelvic ultrasonography
(C) Progesterone challenge test
(D) Serum estradiol measurement

Item 78

A 23-year-old woman is evaluated for a 2-week history of nervousness, palpitations, nausea, vomiting, and weight loss. She is 3 weeks pregnant and says she was previously in excellent health. The patient takes a daily prenatal multivitamin but no other prescription medication, iodine supplement, or other over-the-counter medication.

On physical examination, blood pressure is 130/70 mm Hg, pulse rate is 110/min and regular, and respiration rate is 16/min; BMI is 22. Results of cardiac and lung examinations are normal. Eye examination findings also are normal. Examination of the thyroid gland shows a significantly enlarged gland with a soft bruit but no nodules. No neck tenderness is detected. Abdominal examination reveals a 2-cm patch of vitiligo. A fine bilateral hand tremor and warm, moist skin are noted. No evidence of pretibial myxedema is seen.

Laboratory studies:

Complete blood count	Normal
Comprehensive metabolic profile	Normal
Thyroid-stimulating hormone	<0.01 µU/mL (0.01 mU/L)
Thyroxine (T_4), free	4.0 ng/dL (52 pmol/L)
Triiodothyronine (T_3), free	6 ng/L (9.2 pmol/L)
Human chorionic gonadotropin	Positive
Thyroid peroxidase antibodies	40 units/L (normal, <20 units/L)
Thyroid-stimulating antibodies	140% (normal, <130%)

A thyroid ultrasound shows an enlarged thyroid gland without nodules.

Which of the following is the most appropriate initial treatment?

(A) Methimazole
(B) Propylthiouracil
(C) Thyroidectomy
(D) Reassurance

Item 79

A 21-year-old man comes to the office for a follow-up evaluation. He has a 12-year history of type 1 diabetes mellitus and a recent hemoglobin A_{1c} value of 8.2%. Two days ago, he was brought to the emergency department after having a seizure at 3 AM in his dormitory. Earlier that day, he ate a hearty dinner, played basketball with friends for 3 hours, and then had three beers at a local microbrewery. His glucose monitor showed a blood glucose level of 163 mg/dL (9.0 mmol/L) before he went to bed at 11 PM. His initial plasma glucose level in the emergency department was 28 mg/dL (1.6 mmol/L). He was given intravenous glucose and recovered fully. His only medications are insulin detemir before breakfast and dinner and insulin aspart before all meals.

Physical examination shows a fit, muscular young man. Vital signs are normal; BMI is 19. All other physical examination findings are normal.

Laboratory studies show a hemoglobin A_{1c} value of 8.2%.

Which of the following is the most appropriate advice related to evening exercise to give this patient?

(A) Avoid evening exercise
(B) If alcohol is consumed, drink only light beer
(C) Eat complex carbohydrates at bedtime
(D) Omit the evening dose of insulin detemir and insulin aspart

Item 80

A 38-year-old man is evaluated for a 4-month history of progressive fatigue, cold intolerance, weight gain (total, 5.5 kg [12.0 lb]), occasional headaches, and loss of libido. He has no polydipsia or polyuria.

Physical examination reveals a pale, tired-looking man. Blood pressure is 102/78 mm Hg, pulse rate is 58/min, and respiration rate is 12/min. Deep tendon reflexes have a prolonged relaxation phase. All other examination findings are noncontributory.

Laboratory studies:

Cortisol (8 AM)	7 µg/dL (193 nmol/L) (normal, 5-25 µg/dL [138-690 nmol/L])
Insulin-like growth factor 1	80 ng/mL (80 µg/L) (normal range 101-270 ng/mL [101-270 µg/L])
Testosterone, total	112 ng/dL (3.9 nmol/L)
Thyroid-stimulating hormone	1.1 µU/mL (1.1 mU/L)
Thyroxine, free	0.4 ng/dL (5 pmol/L)

An MRI shows a 1.1-cm sellar mass that fills the sella, with no supra- or parasellar extension.

Levothyroxine is initiated.

Which of the following hormones must be administered simultaneously with levothyroxine?

(A) Glucocorticoid
(B) Growth hormone
(C) Testosterone
(D) Vasopressin

Item 81

A 38-year-old man is evaluated for a mass in his right neck that he first noticed 2 weeks ago while shaving. The patient also reports experiencing a pressure sensation when swallowing solid foods for the past year and daily diarrhea for the past 2 months. His personal medical history is unremarkable. His younger brother has nephrolithiasis, and his father died of a hypertensive crisis and cardiac arrest at age 62 years while undergoing anesthesia induction to repair a hip fracture.

On physical examination, vital signs are normal. A mass is palpated in the right lobe of the thyroid gland. No cervical lymphadenopathy is palpable.

Results of laboratory studies show a serum calcium level of 10.6 mg/dL (2.7 mmol/L) and a thyroid-stimulating hormone level of 1.9 µU/mL (1.9 mU/L).

A chest radiograph is normal. A thyroid ultrasound confirms a 1.4-cm mass in the right lobe of the thyroid gland.

Which of the following is the most likely diagnosis?

(A) Benign familial hypocalciuric hypercalcemia
(B) Multiple endocrine neoplasia type 2
(C) Parathyroid cancer
(D) Sarcoidosis

Item 82

A 25-year-old woman is evaluated for a 2-year history of increasing hair growth on the upper lip, chin, and sides of the face. She underwent menarche at age 12 years and has had irregular menses and some atypical hair growth since that time. She has no other medical problems and takes no medication.

On physical examination, temperature is normal, blood pressure is 128/70 mm Hg, pulse rate is 70/min, and respiration rate is 10/min; BMI is 27. Thyroid examination findings are normal. Mild acanthosis nigricans of the axillae and neck and terminal hair growth on the chin, upper lip, and sides of the face are noted. No evidence of abdominal or pelvic masses, clitoromegaly, or galactorrhea is detected.

Laboratory studies:

Glucose, fasting	85 mg/dL (4.7 mmol/L)
Dehydroepiandrosterone sulfate	1.8 µg/mL (4.9 µmol/L)
Follicle-stimulating hormone (day 3 of menstrual cycle)	6 mU/mL (6 units/L)
17-Hydroxyprogesterone	100 ng/dL (3 nmol/L) (normal, <200 ng/dL [6 nmol/L])
Prolactin	17 ng/mL (17 µg/L)
Thyroid-stimulating hormone	2.1 µU/mL (2.1 mU/L)
Total testosterone	98 ng/dL (3.4 nmol/L)

Which of the following is the most appropriate treatment for her hirsutism?

(A) Bromocriptine
(B) Dexamethasone
(C) Estrogen-progesterone oral contraceptive
(D) Metformin
(E) Spironolactone

Item 83

A 52-year-old man is seen for follow-up evaluation 12 weeks after undergoing transsphenoidal surgery to treat acromegaly associated with a 2.3-cm pituitary adenoma that had invaded the cavernous sinus. He reports continuing headache and bilateral pain in the hip, knee, and elbows. The patient has a history of type 2 diabetes mellitus, sleep apnea, and hypertension. Medications are metformin, lisinopril, metoprolol, and ibuprofen as needed.

On physical examination, blood pressure is 148/92 mm Hg and pulse rate is 88/min. Frontal bossing, prominent nasolabial folds, a large tongue, and thickened hands and feet are noted.

Laboratory study results show that the serum insulin-like growth factor 1 (IGF-1) level, which was 1030 ng/mL (1030 µg/L) (normal for age, 87-238 ng/mL [87-238 µg/L]) before surgery, is still elevated at 780 ng/mL (780 µg/L).

Which of the following is the most appropriate next step in treatment?

(A) Bromocriptine
(B) Octreotide
(C) Repeat transsphenoidal surgery
(D) Observation

Item 84

A 52-year-old man is evaluated for recent onset of fatigue and muscle weakness. The patient further reports nocturia and polyuria over the past 4 weeks and a 6-kg (13.2-lb) weight loss over the past 2 months. He has COPD and a 55-pack-year smoking history. His only medication is an albuterol inhaler.

On physical examination, temperature is 36.7 °C (98.1 °F), blood pressure is 188/102 mm Hg, pulse rate is 96/min, and respiration rate is 22/min; BMI is 23. Temporal muscle wasting and proximal muscle wasting and weakness are noted in the upper and lower extremities. Hyperpigmented mucous membranes are noted. A view of the patient's toenail beds is shown.

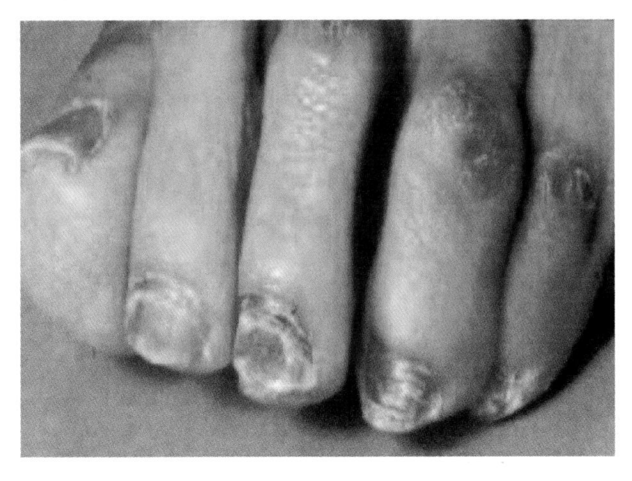

Laboratory studies:

Creatinine	0.8 mg/dL (70.7 µmol/L)
Electrolytes	
Sodium	145 meq/L (145 mmol/L)
Potassium	2.4 meq/L (2.4 mmol/L)
Chloride	101 meq/L (101 mmol/L)
Bicarbonate	33 meq/L (33 mmol/L)
Glucose, random	312 mg/dL (17.3 mmol/L)
Adrenocorticotropic hormone (ACTH)	243 pg/mL (53 pmol/L)
Urine	
Cortisol, free	460 µg/24 h (1268 nmol/24 h)
Potassium, spot test	45 meq/L (45 mmol/L) (normal, 17-164 meq/L [17-164 mmol/L])

Which of the following is the most likely cause of this patient's findings?

(A) Adrenal adenoma
(B) Adrenal carcinoma
(C) Ectopic ACTH secretion
(D) Pituitary adenoma

Answers and Critiques

Item 1 Answer: B

Educational Objective: **Predict the results of laser photocoagulation therapy for diabetic retinopathy.**

This patient will most likely have diminished peripheral and night vision but retained central vision after photocoagulation. Panretinal laser photocoagulation delivers several thousand small burns to the periphery of the retina, which results in the avascular scarring and shriveling of new vessels shown.

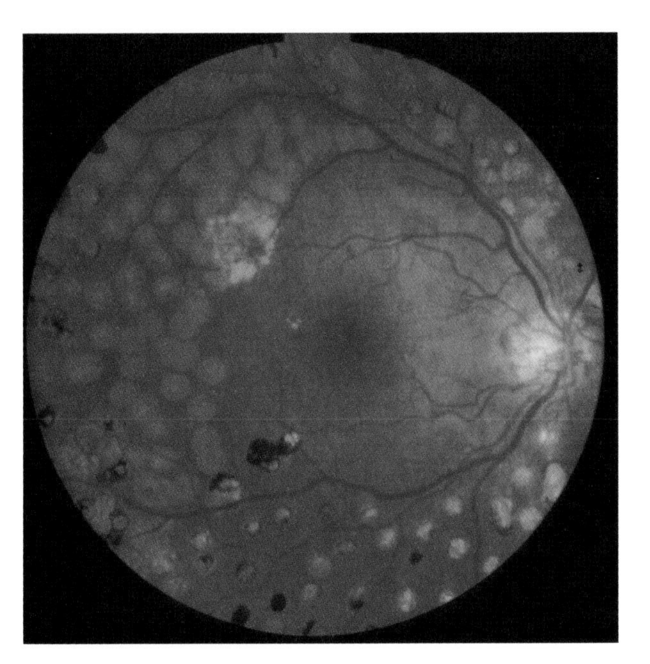

As a result, more retinal blood flow is available for the central part of the retina, which helps retain central vision. However, this procedure also causes deterioration of peripheral vision, which often is most noticeable at night.

This patient's overall visual acuity is unlikely to improve but should not get significantly worse, unless the proliferative retinopathy progresses.

Because central vision remains intact, neither binocular vision nor depth perception will be affected.

KEY POINT

- **Panretinal laser photocoagulation therapy for diabetic retinopathy typically results in retained central vision but poorer peripheral and night vision.**

Bibliography

Cheung N, Mitchell P, Wong TY. Diabetic retinopathy. Lancet. 2010;376(9735):124-136. [PMID: 20580421]

Item 2 Answer: B

Educational Objective: **Manage an adrenal incidentaloma.**

This patient should undergo right adrenalectomy. The increasing use of imaging studies has revealed many previously unrecognized, often asymptomatic adrenal masses (adrenal incidentalomas) in 2% to 3% of the scanned population older than 50 years and in up to 7% of those older than 70 years. Adrenal masses in younger patients are more clinically significant. The evaluation of adrenal masses should address the origin and nature of the mass (primary versus metastatic, benign versus malignant). For a primary tumor, whether it is functioning or not must be determined. Nearly 10% of all adrenal incidentalomas are functioning, although most do not have overt clinical manifestations. He has an incidental but large adrenal mass without any clinical or biochemical features to suggest excessive adrenocortical hormone or catecholamine secretion. The size of the mass (7 cm) and its high CT attenuation (77 Hounsfield units) are suggestive of malignancy. The risk of primary or metastatic cancer is nearly 2% for tumors less than 4 cm in diameter but increases to 25% for tumors 6 cm or larger. For masses 6 cm or larger, surgical removal of the mass is the most appropriate management option.

A biopsy of the adrenal mass is not indicated in this patient because a negative result may be a false-negative, and a positive result only confirms the need to surgically remove the mass.

In the absence of hypertension, hypokalemia, or clinical features suggestive of hypercortisolism, the possibility of hyperaldosteronism or Cushing syndrome is remote. Therefore, neither determining the serum aldosterone to plasma renin activity ratio nor measuring the 24-hour excretion of urine cortisol is likely to be useful.

KEY POINT

- **An adrenal incidentaloma that is 6 cm in size or larger and has a high CT attenuation value has a high likelihood of being malignant; surgical removal of the mass is thus the most appropriate management.**

Bibliography

Nieman LK. Approach to the patient with an adrenal incidentaloma. J Clin Endocrinol Metab. 2010;95(9):4106-4113. [PMID: 20823463]

Item 3 Answer: D

Educational Objective: **Evaluate secondary amenorrhea.**

Progesterone challenge testing is the most appropriate next diagnostic step in this patient. By definition, secondary amenorrhea is the absence of menses for 3 or more consecutive months in a woman who previously has menstruated. Oligomenorrhea (irregular and infrequent menses) is much more common than complete amenorrhea, but the diagnostic considerations are similar. To check for primary ovarian insufficiency and other common endocrinologic causes of amenorrhea, initial laboratory studies should include measurement of the follicle-stimulating hormone (FSH), prolactin, thyroxine (T_4), and thyroid-stimulating hormone levels. Serum FSH values greater than 35 milliunits/mL (35 units/L) are consistent with primary ovarian insufficiency, and values of 20 to 35 milliunits/mL (20-35 units/L) suggest a low ovarian reserve. Her laboratory evaluation has excluded pregnancy, thyroid disease, hyperprolactinemia, and primary ovarian insufficiency. Therefore, the next step is to determine whether she is making adequate estrogen, which the progesterone challenge test can help determine. If withdrawal bleeding occurs, then the patient is producing enough estrogen. If no withdrawal bleeding occurs, then the patient is in a low-estrogen state, and a hypothalamic or pituitary cause is most likely responsible, given her normal FSH level.

Measurement of her total testosterone and dehydroepiandrosterone levels is not indicated at this time because she has no clinical evidence of hyperandrogenism, such as hirsutism or the presence of virilization (voice deepening, clitoral enlargement).

An MRI of the pituitary gland also is not indicated at this time because her prolactin and FSH levels are normal.

Asherman syndrome due to endometrial scarring should be considered as the cause of secondary amenorrhea in any woman who previously had dilation and curettage or a uterine infection. The patient had normal menses until amenorrhea began and has no history of uterine procedures. Therefore, an anatomic abnormality is less likely, and pelvic ultrasonography is not needed.

KEY POINT

- **In a patient with secondary amenorrhea and normal findings of screening laboratory studies, the cornerstone of further evaluation is a progesterone withdrawal challenge.**

Bibliography

Practice Committee of American Society for Reproductive Medicine. Current evaluation of amenorrhea. Fertil Steril. 2008;90(5 Suppl):S219-S225. [PMID: 19007635]

Item 4 Answer: B

Educational Objective: **Manage subclinical hypothyroidism in a woman with multiple risk factors.**

This patient should begin receiving levothyroxine therapy because she is at high risk for overt hypothyroidism, given her positive family history, positive thyroid peroxidase antibody assay, small goiter, and desire to become pregnant. Currently, she has subclinical hypothyroidism, which is defined by the presence of an elevated serum thyroid-stimulating hormone (TSH) level with concomitant thyroxine (T_4) and triiodothyronine (T_3) levels in the reference range. Patients typically have mild or no symptoms of hypothyroidism. The potential causes of subclinical hypothyroidism are the same as for overt hypothyroidism. Evidence suggests that patients with subclinical hypothyroidism also have mild elevations in total cholesterol, LDL cholesterol, and even C-reactive protein levels, and some recent meta-analyses have shown an increased risk for atherosclerosis and cardiac events. However, no data support treatment with levothyroxine to reverse or improve outcomes for these risks. Consensus does exist for treatment of patients with serum TSH levels greater than 10 microunits/mL (10 milliunits/L). Additionally, many advocate a lower threshold for instituting levothyroxine therapy in patients (such as this patient) with anti–thyroid peroxidase antibodies, a strong family history of thyroid disease, a goiter, or pregnancy.

Avoiding hypothyroidism during pregnancy is imperative because overt hypothyroidism has been associated with low birth weight, increased risk of miscarriage, premature birth, and fetal loss. The optimal TSH normal range in a woman desirous of becoming pregnant is 0.5 to 2.5 microunits/mL (0.5-2.5 milliunits/L).

A fine-needle aspiration biopsy of the thyroid gland should be reserved for the evaluation of a thyroid nodule and thus is not indicated in this patient.

Given her high risk of progression to overt hypothyroidism and the potential risk to the fetus should she become pregnant, waiting 6 weeks and then repeating the TSH measurement is not an appropriate choice in this patient.

This patient does not have an indication for a thyroid scan. Physical examination revealed no palpable nodules on or tenderness in the thyroid gland. A thyroid scan would add little to her evaluation and would result in unnecessary radiation exposure.

KEY POINT

- **Patients with subclinical hypothyroidism should be treated with levothyroxine if they are at high risk for progression to overt hypothyroidism (thyroid-stimulating hormone level greater than 10 microunits/mL [10 milliunits/L], positive family history, goiter, presence of anti–thyroid peroxidase antibodies, or desire to become pregnant).**

Bibliography

Lazarus JH. The continuing saga of postpartum thyroiditis. J Clin Endocrinol Metab. 2011;96(3):614-616. [PMID: 21378224]

Item 5 Answer: B

Educational Objective: **Diagnose tuberculosis-induced hypercalcemia.**

The patient has disseminated tuberculosis with hypercalcemia due to excessive production of 1,25-dihydroxyvitamin D by the tuberculous granulomas. The granulomas of tuberculosis (and other granulomatous diseases, such as sarcoidosis, Crohn disease, and leprosy) are composed of macrophages that possess the 1α-hydroxylase enzyme needed to convert 25-hydroxyvitamin D to its active form, 1,25-dihydroxyvitamin D. The serum parathyroid hormone level is less than normal, which is an appropriate response to the elevated serum calcium level.

Dehydration might worsen hypercalcemia, but dehydration alone would not explain this patient's suppressed serum parathyroid hormone (PTH) level.

The low serum PTH level argues against excessive PTH release and thus excludes a parathyroid adenoma as the cause of the hypercalcemia. In addition, primary hyperparathyroidism typically is associated with a low serum phosphorus level, which makes hyperparathyroidism an unlikely cause of this patient's hypercalcemia.

Humoral hypercalcemia of malignancy results from the systemic effect of a circulating factor produced by neoplastic cells. The hormone most commonly responsible for this syndrome is PTH-related protein (PTHrP). This protein shares significant homology with PTH. PTHrP has most, if not all, of the metabolic effects of PTH, including osteoclast activation, increased renal tubular calcium reabsorption, and increased clearance of phosphorus by the kidneys. Because tumors that produce PTHrP (squamous cell carcinoma; lung, head, and neck cancer; lymphoma) do so in small quantities, patients who have associated hypercalcemia at presentation usually have an extensive tumor burden. Therefore, it is unusual for hypercalcemia to be the presenting feature of cancer. Additionally, the patient's tuberculosis is a more likely cause of his hypercalcemia.

KEY POINT

- **Hypercalcemia can be caused by the production of 1,25-dihydroxyvitamin D by granulomatous disease.**

Bibliography

Sharma OP. Hypercalcemia in granulomatous disorders: a clinical review. Curr Opin Pulm Med. 2000;6(5):442-447. [PMID: 10958237]

Item 6 Answer: E

Educational Objective: **Diagnose Cushing syndrome as a secondary cause of diabetes.**

Measurement of the 24-hour excretion of urine free cortisol is the most appropriate next test in this patient to determine the cause of her diabetes mellitus. Various secondary causes of diabetes exist, most involving other endocrinopathies, effects of medications, pancreatic diseases, or genetic conditions. Cushing syndrome is one of these secondary causes of diabetes. The most common cause of Cushing syndrome is corticosteroid therapy, followed by the secretion of adrenocorticotropic hormone (ACTH) by a pituitary adenoma (Cushing disease) and the hyperfunctioning of an adrenocortical adenoma. In this patient, the combination of diabetes, hypertension, central obesity, hypokalemia, proximal muscle weakness, and edema strongly suggests the presence of Cushing syndrome. The diagnosis can be confirmed by several tests, including measurement of 24-hour excretion of urine free cortisol, an overnight dexamethasone suppression test, or a midnight salivary cortisol measurement.

Adrenal CT is appropriate after Cushing syndrome is diagnosed, especially when it is non–ACTH dependent, to identify the type of adrenal condition responsible. This test would be premature in this patient in whom the diagnosis has not been confirmed.

Residual beta-cell function can be assessed by measuring the C-peptide level, which is often high-normal in early type 2 diabetes because of insulin resistance. Similarly, measuring the glutamic acid decarboxylase antibody titer is useful to confirm the presence of autoimmune (type 1) diabetes when no other evidence exists. However, the C-peptide level will not indicate the cause of diabetes in this patient, and measuring the glutamic acid decarboxylase level also is unlikely to be helpful because she does not have type 1 diabetes.

Pancreatic imaging could be considered when signs and symptoms (such as abdominal or back pain, jaundice, or chronic diarrhea) suggest that an underlying pancreatic disorder is the cause of diabetes. This patient has none of these signs or symptoms, and thus a pancreatic MRI is unlikely to be revealing.

KEY POINT

- **Cushing syndrome is a likely cause of diabetes mellitus in a patient with hypertension, central obesity, and hypokalemia.**

Bibliography

Reimondo G, Pia A, Allasino B, et al. Screening of Cushing's syndrome in adult patients with newly diagnosed diabetes mellitus. Clin Endocrinol (Oxf). 2007;67(2):225-229. [PMID: 17547690]

Item 7 Answer: A

Educational Objective: **Evaluate hyperprolactinemia.**

A pregnancy test is the most appropriate next test in this woman whose serum prolactin level has again increased. Although she has a history of prolactinemia and associated oligomenorrhea, it is important first to ensure that she is not currently pregnant. Prolactin levels increase during pregnancy. Therefore, an increasing prolactin level in a woman of child-bearing age should not automatically be interpreted as evidence of prolactinemia until pregnancy is excluded as a cause.

Measurement of the growth hormone (GH) level is not useful in the assessment of a woman with amenorrhea or oligomenorrhea unless acromegaly is a possible diagnosis. Even in that setting, however, a random GH value is not useful because of the pulsatile nature of GH secretion.

Clinical features of acromegaly include prognathism; enlargement of the nose, lips, and tongue; frontal bossing; dental malocclusion; increased spacing between the teeth; sleep apnea; enlargement of the hands and feet; arthritis of the hips and knees; carpal tunnel syndrome; oily skin; and skin tags. Prolactin is coproduced with GH in approximately 40% of patients with acromegaly. Some of these patients also may have amenorrhea or galactorrhea. Other than amenorrhea, this patient has no signs or symptoms of acromegaly.

Measuring this patient's serum cortisol level is unlikely to be useful because she has no evidence of Cushing syndrome. Common symptoms of Cushing syndrome include muscle weakness, ecchymosis, hypokalemia, unexplained osteoporosis, new-onset hypertension, and diabetes mellitus but not hyperprolactinemia. However, menstrual irregularities are common in Cushing syndrome.

In patients with compression of the optic chiasm, the most common symptom is diminished vision in the temporal fields. Visual field testing is inappropriate unless a finding suggests a pituitary tumor with evidence of compression of the optic chiasm.

KEY POINT

- **In a woman with a modestly elevated serum prolactin level, pregnancy must first be excluded as a cause before a diagnosis of hyperprolactinemia is made.**

Bibliography

Kreitschmann-Andermahr I, Poll EM, Reineke A, et al. Growth hormone deficient patients after traumatic brain injury—baseline characteristics and benefits after growth hormone replacement—an analysis of the German KIMS database. Growth Horm IGF Res. 2008;18(6):472-478. [PMID: 18829359]

Item 8 Answer: D

Educational Objective: Treat Graves ophthalmopathy.

This patient should undergo thyroidectomy. Clinically significant ophthalmopathy occurs in approximately 5% to 10% of patients with Graves disease. Ophthalmopathy severity varies from mild to severe and may involve lid changes, proptosis or exophthalmos, and inflammatory eye changes, such as chemosis, conjunctival injection, periorbital edema, or iritis. Extraocular muscle involvement can result in double vision, whereas optic nerve compression can result in reduced visual acuity and even blindness. The precise pathophysiology of Graves ophthalmopathy is not well understood. A primary management focus in Graves ophthalmopathy is to establish a euthyroid state because persistent hypothyroidism or hyperthyroidism exacerbates disease activity. The medical treatment for ophthalmopathy includes local measures followed by a trial of corticosteroids. In patients with Graves disease, thyroid surgery usually is reserved for those with a severe allergy or intolerance to iodine or antithyroid drugs, large or obstructive goiters, or ophthalmopathy.

Oral iodine solution may decrease levels on thyroid function testing for approximately 1 to 2 weeks in some patients, but a patient such as this one who is not taking any thiourea medication that blocks thyroid hormone synthesis may have worsening hyperthyroidism, especially after the initial 1 to 2 weeks.

The use of propylthiouracil also is not appropriate because the patient already has had a severe adverse reaction to methimazole, and the likelihood of a similar or worse reaction to propylthiouracil is high.

Radioactive iodine treatment has been associated with worsening of Graves ophthalmopathy, at least transiently. Therefore, its use as treatment of hyperthyroidism in patients with severe Graves ophthalmopathy is not recommended.

Attempts to modulate the immune response (with the monoclonal antibody rituximab, for example) have had mixed results and at present are still experimental.

KEY POINT

- **In patients with Graves ophthalmopathy, treatment includes establishing normal thyroid function, local measures, prednisone, and thyroidectomy.**

Bibliography

Bahn RS. Graves' ophthalmopathy. N Engl J Med. 2010;362(8):726-738. [PMID: 20181974]

Item 9 Answer: C

Educational Objective: Diagnose central adrenal insufficiency.

This patient with a history of pulmonary sarcoidosis should next have a pituitary MRI. She has symptoms highly suggestive of adrenal insufficiency, hypothyroidism, and hypogonadism. The biochemical findings suggest a central cause of these disorders. Her partial response to cosyntropin stimulation is consistent with partial loss of adrenocorticotropic hormone (ACTH) secretion, or central adrenal insufficiency. The hypothyroidism is also central in origin because it is associated with an inappropriately normal serum thyroid-stimulating hormone level. The polyuria and hypernatremia suggest the development of diabetes insipidus in this patient. These abnormalities are most likely caused by involvement of the hypothalamus and pituitary stalk by sarcoidosis, which led to her biochemical pituitary findings and to central diabetes insipidus, which caused her hypernatremia. Other causes that should be considered are a pituitary adenoma and any other sellar or parasellar mass. A gadolinium-enhanced MRI of the pituitary gland should be performed to exclude these causes and assess for evidence of involvement of these structures with sarcoidosis. However, definitive diagnosis requires biopsy evidence of a noncaseating granuloma in the involved areas. Hypothalamic-pituitary involvement occurs in less than 10% of patients with sarcoidosis and may be difficult to diagnose because patchy involvement of the hypothalamus and pituitary stalk may lead to various combinations of anterior and posterior pituitary hormone deficiencies.

Adrenal CT is not indicated because the cause of the adrenal insufficiency is clearly central ACTH deficiency and not a primary adrenal disease.

In the absence of pulmonary symptoms, a lung biopsy is not needed in this patient. Even if the lung biopsy were positive, imaging is still necessary to address the concerns raised about a possible anatomic abnormality in the sellar region that would explain the loss of pituitary hormone secretion.

Because the hypothyroidism is this patient is central in origin, a thyroid scan measuring radioactive iodine uptake is not indicated.

KEY POINT

- **In a patient with symptoms and biochemical findings highly suggestive of central adrenal insufficiency, a pituitary MRI is appropriate to exclude other possible causes, such as a pituitary adenoma or any other sellar or perisellar mass.**

Bibliography

Toogood AA, Stewart PM. Hypopituitarism: clinical features, diagnosis, and management. Endocrinol Metab Clin North Am. 2008;37(1):235-261. [PMID: 18226739]

Item 10 Answer: A

Educational Objective: Treat a woman with low bone mass.

The most appropriate medication for this patient is alendronate. She has osteopenia, and her major osteoporotic fracture risk by the Fracture Risk Assessment Tool (FRAX) is in a range for which the National Osteoporosis Foundation (NOF) guidelines favor treatment with antiosteoporotic therapy. The NOF recommends antiosteoporotic therapy for persons whose risk of major osteoporotic fracture over the next 10 years is 20% or greater or whose risk of hip fracture over the next 10 years is 3% or greater. Given her current FRAX score and the expectation that she will lose bone mass more rapidly after an aromatase inhibitor is started, it is reasonable to initiate therapy with alendronate now. Alendronate is approved for both osteoporosis prevention and treatment by the FDA.

Denosumab, a monoclonal antibody that inhibits osteoclast formation, is reserved for patients with a high risk of fracture, including those with multiple risk factors for fracture or a history of previous fractures. This patient does not fulfill these criteria.

Estrogen is contradicted in this patient with a new diagnosis of breast cancer.

Raloxifene, a selective estrogen receptor modulator, is also approved for osteoporosis prevention by the FDA. However, vasomotor symptoms are highly associated with its use, and it may not be well tolerated in a patient already experiencing significant hot flushes.

Teriparatide, or recombinant human parathyroid hormone (1-34), is an anabolic agent that increases bone density and decreases fracture risk. However, teriparatide carries a "black box" warning because of an increased risk of osteosarcoma and is contraindicated in this patient because of her history of radiation therapy, which increases the risk of osteosarcoma. Teriparatide is also contraindicated in persons with malignancy involving bone, Paget disease, or existing hyperparathyroidism or hypercalcemia.

KEY POINT

- **In a patient with osteopenia and a history of radiation therapy, alendronate is the most appropriate drug to use for osteoporosis prevention.**

Bibliography

Lecart MP, Reginster JY. Current options for the management of postmenopausal osteoporosis. Expert Opin Pharmacother. 2011;12(16):2533-2552. [PMID: 21916810]

Item 11 Answer: D

Educational Objective: Differentiate type 1 from type 2 diabetes mellitus.

This patient's blood should be checked for pancreatic autoantibodies, such as islet cell antibodies (ICAs) and glutamic acid decarboxylase antibodies (GADAs). Although she is obese and has a mother with type 2 diabetes mellitus, she may actually have type 1 diabetes presenting at an earlier stage of the disease process (when she still has significant endogenous insulin secretion) because of her obesity and insulin resistance. In young patients with probable diabetes, the distinction between type 1 and type 2 diabetes should be made as soon as possible. If ICAs and GADAs are found in her blood, she has type 1 diabetes and should begin receiving insulin immediately. Insulin treatment in type 1 diabetes helps preserve endogenous insulin secretion for a longer period of time, which makes it easier to achieve excellent glycemic control without hypoglycemia. If testing does not show these antibodies in her blood, she has type 2 diabetes and should be treated with lifestyle modifications and, possibly, metformin.

Checking this patient's plasma C-peptide level (whether fasting or stimulated) or fasting plasma insulin level will not help distinguish type 1 from type 2 diabetes. A person who is obese and has hyperglycemia but no ketonuria or acidosis is clearly making sufficient endogenous insulin at the moment. Therefore, this patient's plasma C-peptide and insulin levels will both be high, no matter what type of diabetes she has.

KEY POINT

- **In young patients with probable diabetes mellitus, the distinction between type 1 and type 2 diabetes should be made as soon as possible by checking for the presence of pancreatic autoantibodies, which indicate type 1 disease.**

Bibliography

Effect of intensive therapy on residual beta-cell function in patients with type 1 diabetes in the diabetes control and complications trial. A randomized, controlled trial. The Diabetes Control and Complications Trial Research Group. Ann Intern Med. 1998;128(7):517-523. [PMID: 9518395]

Item 12 Answer: B

Educational Objective: Diagnose male infertility.

Semen analysis is the single best test to assess male infertility. The patient should abstain from sexual activity for 48 to 72 hours to have an adequate sample. If semen analysis results are abnormal, the test should be repeated.

Measurement of serum gonadotropin and testosterone levels is not appropriate in the initial evaluation of infertility. If the semen analysis results are abnormal, then luteinizing hormone, follicle-stimulating hormone, and total testosterone studies would be ordered to assess Leydig and Sertoli cell function.

Testicular ultrasonography is not performed in the evaluation of infertility unless an abnormality is detected on testicular examination.

KEY POINT

- **Semen analysis is the single best test to assess male infertility.**

Bibliography

Cooper TG, Noonan E, von Eckardstein S, et al. World Health Organization reference values for human semen characteristics. Hum Reprod Update. 2010;16(3):231-245. [PMID: 19934213]

Item 13 Answer: B

Educational Objective: Manage hypothyroidism during pregnancy.

This patient's levothyroxine dosage should be increased by 30% now, and the thyroid function tests should be repeated in 2 to 4 weeks. Pregnancy is known to increase levothyroxine requirements in most patients receiving thyroid replacement therapy, and this expected increase should be anticipated by increasing her levothyroxine dosage. The levothyroxine dosage is typically increased in the first (and sometimes in the second) trimester of pregnancy, with a possible total increase of 30% to 50%. During the first trimester, the goal thyroid-stimulating hormone (TSH) level is less than 2.5 microunits/mL (2.5 milliunits/L) because first trimester serum TSH levels between approximately 0.1 and 2.5 microunits/mL (0.1-2.5 milliunits/L) are associated with fewer maternal and fetal complications. In contrast, the upper range of normal for nonpregnant patients is approximately 4.5 to 5.0 microunits/mL (4.5-5.0 milliunits/L). In pregnant women with hypothyroidism, thyroid function testing should be frequent, preferably every 4 weeks, to protect the health of mother and fetus and to avoid pregnancy complications. When serum TSH values are inappropriately elevated, the dosage of levothyroxine is increased, and free thyroxine (T_4) and TSH levels are monitored every 2 to 4 weeks. The fetus is largely dependent on transplacental transfer of maternal thyroid hormones during the first 12 weeks of gestation. The presence of maternal subclinical or overt hypothyroidism may be associated with subsequent fetal neurocognitive impairment, increased risk of premature birth, low birth weight, increased miscarriage rate, and even an increased risk of fetal death.

Continuing the current levothyroxine dosage is inappropriate in this patient because her TSH level is already too high (4.2 microunits/mL [4.2 milliunits/L]). TSH levels generally should be 0.1 to 2.5 microunits/mL (0.1-2.5 milliunits/L) in the first trimester, 0.2 to 3.0 microunits/mL (0.2-3.0 milliunits/L) in the second, and 0.3 to 3.0 microunits/mL (0.3-3.0 milliunits/L) in the third.

KEY POINT

- **Early in pregnancy, levothyroxine requirements are increased in most patients with hypothyroidism by 30% to 50%.**

Bibliography

Yassa L, Marqusee E, Fawcett R, Alexander EK. Thyroid hormone early adjustment in pregnancy (the THERAPY) trial. J Clin Endocrinol Metab. 2010;95(7):3234-3241. [PMID: 20463094]

Item 14 Answer: A

Educational Objective: Manage pituitary tumor apoplexy.

This patient with pituitary tumor apoplexy should receive glucocorticoids in addition to undergoing surgical removal of his tumor. His history of fatigue, weight gain, and erectile dysfunction and laboratory finding of hyponatremia suggest panhypopituitarism, and his acute headache and neck stiffness are consistent with hemorrhage. Pituitary tumor apoplexy usually occurs in the setting of a preexisting pituitary adenoma, and thus a neuroimaging scan was appropriately obtained to confirm the diagnosis and show the pituitary anatomy. He also has evidence of bitemporal hemianopia caused by optic chiasmal compression by the mass. The anticoagulant taken by this patient may have predisposed him to hemorrhage.

Pituitary tumor apoplexy is generally a neurosurgical emergency. On occasion, hemorrhagic infarction of a pituitary adenoma may be less urgent, especially in the absence of associated mass effects, and can be managed with conservative follow-up monitoring. In the setting of local mass effects and severe headache, however, neurosurgical decompression of the pituitary gland is necessary. Urgent glucocorticoid administration is often required because of acute adrenocorticotropic hormone deficiency. The leading cause of mortality with pituitary tumor apoplexy is adrenal insufficiency.

An insulin tolerance test usually is performed to rule out both adrenal insufficiency and growth hormone deficiency, and a serum prolactin level typically is obtained after a diagnosis of pituitary adenoma is made to exclude prolactinoma. Because this patient's disorder is a neurosurgical emergency, these tests are inappropriate before the apoplexy is addressed.

A lumbar puncture is useful in patients with suspected meningitis or in whom subarachnoid hemorrhage is suspected despite a negative imaging study. However, the imaging study already provides an explanation for the stiff neck and headache, and a lumbar puncture is not only inappropriate but contraindicated in a patient with pituitary tumor apoplexy.

KEY POINT

- **In addition to neurosurgical decompression of the pituitary gland, urgent glucocorticoid administration is often necessary in patients with pituitary tumor apoplexy because of acute adrenocorticotropic hormone deficiency.**

Bibliography

Sibal L, Ball SG, Connolly V, et al. Pituitary apoplexy: a review of clinical presentation, management and outcome in 45 cases. Pituitary. 2004;7(3):157-163. [PMID: 16010459]

Item 15 Answer: D

Educational Objective: **Treat hypercalcemia.**

This patient should be hydrated with normal (0.9%) saline as the next step in her treatment. She has severe symptomatic hypercalcemia in the setting of advanced metastatic breast cancer. The history of polyuria and polydipsia and the physical examination findings of tachycardia and dry mucous membranes suggest significant dehydration, which is confirmed by the elevated blood urea nitrogen and creatinine levels. High calcium levels impair the ability of the nephron to concentrate urine, which results in inappropriate water loss from the kidney. Therefore, the most appropriate next step in this patient's treatment is to restore euvolemia and begin to lower the serum calcium level by saline diuresis. Normalization of intravascular volume with saline will improve delivery of calcium to the renal tubule and aid in excretion of calcium. As the kidneys excrete excess sodium from the saline, excretion of calcium will follow.

Hypercalcemia of malignancy may be due to local osteolytic hypercalcemia or to humoral hypercalcemia of malignancy, in which a tumor that does not involve the skeleton secretes a circulating factor that activates bone resorption. In this patient, the liver metastases are likely secreting parathyroid hormone–related protein. Control of the tumor with chemotherapy may help the patient's hypercalcemia in the long-run.

Bisphosphonate therapy may be needed if the patient remains hypercalcemic after rehydration, and intravenous furosemide may be appropriate after the patient is adequately hydrated to maintain euvolemia. Glucocorticoid therapy could be considered if bisphosphonate treatment does not adequately lower the serum calcium level. However, none of these treatments should be attempted before the patient is rehydrated with normal saline.

KEY POINT

- **In patients with acute hypercalcemia, normalization of intravascular volume with saline will improve delivery of calcium to the renal tubule and aid in excretion of calcium.**

Bibliography

Stewart, AF. Clinical practice. Hypercalcemia associated with cancer. N Engl J Med. 2005;352(4):373-379. [PMID: 15673803]

Item 16 Answer: D

Educational Objective: **Diagnose hyperaldosteronism.**

This patient should have her serum aldosterone to plasma renin activity ratio determined. She has biochemical features indicative of excessive mineralocorticoid secretion. Although several potential mineralocorticoids could be responsible for her symptoms, excessive aldosterone is the most likely cause. Hypertension and hypokalemia are two of the main manifestations of primary hyperaldosteronism. Increases in other mineralocorticoids are seen with unusually excessive cortisol secretion (Cushing syndrome), in which the mineralocorticoid activity of cortisol becomes prominent, and in congenital adrenal hyperplasia due to an enzyme deficiency. This patient's normal findings (except for blood pressure) on physical examination make the first possibility unlikely, and her less than 2-year history of hypertension makes a congenital enzyme deficiency also unlikely. The best screening test for hyperaldosteronism is the determination of the ratio of serum aldosterone to plasma renin activity. The expected findings include an elevated serum aldosterone level and suppressed plasma renin activity. Screening tests can be performed on random blood samples, even in patients taking antihypertensive medications (except the aldosterone receptor antagonists spironolactone and eplerenone). Confirmation of the biochemical diagnosis involves showing persistent elevation (poor suppressibility) of serum aldosterone in response to a high salt load.

Imaging studies are inappropriate before a clear biochemical diagnosis is established. Therefore, CT of the abdomen is premature at this time.

This patient did not exhibit any signs or symptoms that would warrant investigating the possibility of Cushing syndrome. Therefore, neither a dexamethasone suppression test nor a 24-hour measurement of urine free cortisol excretion is likely to be useful.

Nothing in the patient's history or clinical examination findings suggests the possibility of pheochromocytoma. Therefore, measurement of the plasma catecholamine levels is inappropriate as the next diagnostic test.

KEY POINT

- **The best screening test for hyperaldosteronism is the determination of the ratio of serum aldosterone to plasma renin activity.**

Bibliography

Funder JW, Carey RM, Fardella C, et al; Endocrine Society. Case detection, diagnosis, and treatment of patients with primary aldosteronism: an Endocrine Society clinical practice guideline. J Clin Endocrinol Metab. 2008;93(9):3266-3281. [PMID: 18552288]

Item 17 Answer: A

Educational Objective: Diagnose humoral hypercalcemia of malignancy.

This patient has severe hypercalcemia in the setting of a lung mass. This scenario is highly suggestive of humoral hypercalcemia of malignancy (HHM), which results from tumor production of a circulating factor, parathyroid hormone (PTH)–related protein (PTHrP), that acts on skeletal calcium release, calcium handling by the kidney, and intestinal calcium absorption. Tumors that cause HHM by secreting PTHrP are typically squamous cell carcinomas (often of the lung). Rarely, this disorder can be caused by unregulated production of 1,25-dihydroxyvitamin D (as in B-cell lymphomas) or other mediators that interfere with calcium homeostasis. Although PTHrP assays are now available commercially, results may not be available for up to 10 days. Because endogenous PTH secretion is suppressed in the setting of hypercalcemia, a low PTH level provides indirect but strong evidence of the nature of this patient's hypercalcemia. Because HHM results in a fairly rapid rise in the serum calcium level, patients tend to be more symptomatic than patients with hypercalcemia from other, more chronic causes.

Primary hyperparathyroidism is the most common cause of hypercalcemia in the outpatient setting and typically presents at an asymptomatic stage. This disorder is usually due to a benign parathyroid adenoma and not to a lung mass.

Hypercalcemia is frequently associated with sarcoidosis, with 30% to 50% of patients with the disease demonstrating some degree of abnormal calcium metabolism. However, this patient has no history or physical examination findings suggestive of sarcoidosis, and her lung mass would be an atypical manifestation of primary pulmonary sarcoidosis.

The patient takes a daily multivitamin and calcium supplement in over-the-counter dosages. The recommended daily allowance of vitamin D is 600 units. Although the point at which toxicity occurs is not clear, the Institute of Medicine's recommended tolerable intake of vitamin D is 4000 units daily, although substantially greater amounts are usually needed for clinically significant hypervitaminosis to occur. It is unlikely that the amount of vitamin D in her daily multivitamin is enough to cause acute toxicity and hypercalcemia.

KEY POINT

- **Humoral hypercalcemia of malignancy results from tumor production of a circulating factor (parathyroid hormone–related protein [PTHrP]) that acts on skeletal calcium release, calcium handling by the kidney, or intestinal calcium absorption and often involves squamous cell carcinomas of the lung.**

Bibliography

Clines GA. Mechanisms and treatment of hypercalcemia of malignancy. Curr Opin Endocrinol Diabetes Obes. 2011;18(6):339-346. [PMID: 21897221]

Item 18 Answer: C

Educational Objective: Diagnose the cause of gynecomastia.

An estradiol level should be obtained in this patient. Gynecomastia, or the abnormal growth of large mammary glands in men causing breast enlargement, results from an imbalance in the testosterone-to-estrogen ratio in men. This imbalance can be due to either a low testosterone level or an elevated estradiol level. Because the total testosterone level is normal in this patient, an estradiol level must be obtained to check for any elevation.

Adrenal CT is inappropriate in the evaluation of gynecomastia unless the estradiol level is elevated. If the estradiol level is elevated, testicular ultrasonography still should be ordered before adrenal CT to exclude a testicular neoplasm. If the testicular ultrasound shows no neoplasms, then an adrenal CT scan should be ordered to exclude an adrenal neoplasm.

In the evaluation of gynecomastia, breast ultrasonography should be obtained only if uncertainty exists about whether the patient has gynecomastia or lipomastia or if malignancy is a concern (for example, with an asymmetric growth, a breast mass, or unilateral disease). Because these possibilities do not pertain to this patient, breast ultrasonography is not necessary.

A karyotype is not appropriate in this patient. He has normal luteinizing hormone (LH) and testosterone levels. If his LH level were elevated and his testosterone level were decreased, then a karyotype would be indicated to exclude Klinefelter syndrome as a cause of the gynecomastia and hypogonadism.

Testicular ultrasonography is only ordered when the serum estradiol level is elevated to exclude a testicular neoplasm. If the testicular ultrasound is normal, then chest CT might be indicated to exclude a β-human chorionic gonadotropin–secreting mediastinal tumor, which is a rare tumor.

KEY POINT

- **Gynecomastia results from an imbalance in the testosterone-to-estrogen ratio in men.**

Bibliography

Braunstein GD. Clinical practice. Gynecomastia. N Engl J Med. 2007;357(12):1229-1237. [PMID: 17881754]

Item 19 Answer: B

Educational Objective: **Treat hypoglycemic unawareness.**

This patient's dosages of both long-acting and rapid-acting insulin should be decreased by approximately 20%. Hypoglycemia is the major rate-limiting factor in attempting tight glycemic control, especially in patients with type 1 diabetes mellitus. For 48 to 72 hours after a severe episode of hypoglycemia, the body's ability to mount an adrenergic response is blunted, as is the strength of the counterregulatory response. This increases the likelihood of a second severe episode of hypoglycemia that will not be easily recognized (hypoglycemic unawareness), and thus a vicious cycle develops. The best treatment is to reduce the dosage of insulin and scrupulously monitor the blood glucose level for 1 week so that it does not become less than 100 mg/dL (5.6 mmol/L). This intervention allows the brain to reset its adrenergic responses.

Increasing her carbohydrate intake at meals is inappropriate because of her currently healthy diet, her anticipated pregnancy, and the potential for weight gain.

Although α-lipoic acid has shown some efficacy in management of painful diabetic neuropathy, it would have no effect on her hypoglycemic unawareness.

A preprandial injection of pramlintide, a synthetic long-acting analogue of the hormone amylin, is sometimes used in the management of type 1 diabetes to slow down stomach emptying, suppress glucagon secretion, and promote satiety. In this patient, however, pramlintide might actually increase the risk of hypoglycemia.

Switching from insulin glargine to insulin detemir without reducing the dose of insulin is unlikely to be helpful in stopping or reducing this patient's hypoglycemic episodes.

KEY POINT

- **Hypoglycemia is the major rate-limiting factor in attempting tight glycemic control, especially in patients with type 1 diabetes mellitus.**

Bibliography

Cryer PE. The barrier of hypoglycemia in diabetes. Diabetes. 2008;57(12):3169-3176. [PMID: 19033403]

Item 20 Answer: A

Educational Objective: **Evaluate thyroid nodules with fine-needle aspiration biopsy.**

This patient should have a fine-needle aspiration (FNA) biopsy of the thyroid nodule. Most thyroid nodules are benign; only approximately 5% to 15% are malignant. An FNA biopsy is the most accurate method to determine whether a nodule is benign or malignant. FNA biopsy is an outpatient procedure that allows cytologic categorization of the cells within a nodule as benign, suspicious for malignancy, follicular neoplasm, or papillary thyroid cancer. FNA biopsy is also the most sensitive and specific method to help diagnose the cause of a thyroid nodule.

Because thyroid nodules are extremely common, with an estimated 30% to 50% of healthy persons likely to have a thyroid nodule on thyroid ultrasound, guidelines have been developed by the American Thyroid Association to maximize the effectiveness of thyroid FNA biopsy in diagnosing malignancy in a cost-effective manner. These guidelines take into account personal history and risk factors, family history, and ultrasound characteristics of the nodule to help predict the likelihood of malignancy and the need for thyroid FNA biopsy. The recommended nodule size threshold for performing a thyroid FNA biopsy is at least 5 mm in a patient at high risk of thyroid cancer who also has worrisome sonographic characteristics. This patient has a first-degree relative with papillary thyroid cancer. In addition, the thyroid Doppler ultrasound showed a hypoechoic nodule with microcalcifications, blurred nodule margins, and increased central vascularity.

Close monitoring with repeat thyroid ultrasonography in 3 or 6 months is inappropriate management in this patient with significant risk factors and suspicious features on the current ultrasound that should prompt an FNA biopsy.

Thyroid lobectomy is generally appropriate treatment for cancerous thyroid nodules that are less than 1 cm in diameter but is premature in this patient in whom a diagnosis of malignancy has not been established.

MRI has limited utility in evaluating thyroid nodules. Generally less helpful than Doppler ultrasonography in characterizing intrathyroid nodules, MRI may be helpful in detecting local extension of thyroid malignancies or spread into the mediastinum or retro-thyroid regions, if suspected.

KEY POINT

- **A fine-needle aspiration biopsy is the most accurate way to determine if a thyroid nodule is benign or malignant.**

Bibliography

American Thyroid Association (ATA) Guidelines Taskforce on Thyroid Nodules and Differentiated Thyroid Cancer; Cooper DS, Doherty GM, Haugen BR, et al. Revised American Thyroid Association management guidelines for patients with thyroid nodules and differentiated thyroid cancer [errata in Thyroid. 2010;20(6):674-675; and Thyroid. 2010;20(8):942]. Thyroid. 2009;19(11):1167-1214. [PMID: 1986057]

Item 21 Answer: D

Educational Objective: **Diagnose growth hormone deficiency.**

This patient should have his insulin-like growth factor 1 (IGF-1) level measured because he is at risk for growth hormone (GH) deficiency. Up to 40% of patients with a history of traumatic brain injury, particularly when severe, are found subsequently to have hypopituitarism. The most common anterior pituitary hormone disorder after traumatic brain injury is GH deficiency. Acquired GH deficiency in adults is characterized by a change in body composition (increase in central adiposity and reduction in lean skeletal muscle mass), reduction in quality of life, and decrease in bone mineral density. Increased cardiovascular risk also may be present. This patient has had progressive reduction in lean body mass, an increase in central adiposity, and progressive deterioration in his daily performance and quality of life, all of which suggest GH deficiency. In such patients, administration of GH replacement therapy may lead to an increase in muscle mass and quality of life and a reduction in central obesity.

The initial screening test for GH deficiency is measurement of the IGF-1 level. If the IGF-1 value is low, then further testing with a stimulation test to measure GH reserve should be performed to confirm a diagnosis of GH deficiency.

Measurement of the patient's fasting GH level is unlikely to be useful because GH levels are pulsatile and undetectable for much of the day in most patients. Therefore, this test is unlikely to detect GH deficiency.

A glucose tolerance test will not be useful in this patient. The nonsuppressibility of GH during a glucose tolerance test is used to diagnose GH excess in acromegaly, not GH deficiency.

A gonadotropin-releasing hormone test is used to assess luteinizing hormone and follicle-stimulating hormone reserves in the setting of hypogonadotropic hypogonadism. Although this patient has some of the symptoms of male hypogonadism (fatigue and loss of muscle strength), he does not have the anemia, poor libido, or erectile dysfunction commonly associated with the disorder. More importantly, his 8 AM serum testosterone measurement excludes the diagnosis of hypogonadism, which makes a gonadotropin-releasing hormone test unnecessary.

KEY POINT

- **The most common anterior pituitary hormone disorder after traumatic brain injury is growth hormone deficiency, which can be suggested by a decreased serum insulin-like growth factor 1 level and is confirmed by a stimulation test measuring GH reserve.**

Bibliography

Kreitschmann-Andermahr I, Poll EM, Reineke A, et al. Growth hormone deficient patients after traumatic brain injury—baseline characteristics and benefits after growth hormone replacement—an analysis of the German KIMS database. Growth Horm IGF Res. 2008;18(6):472-478. [PMID: 18829359]

Item 22 Answer: B

Educational Objective: **Diagnose vitamin D deficiency.**

This patient's serum 25-hydroxyvitamin D level should be measured. Results of her recent bone mineral density screening showed osteoporosis of the hip, and laboratory studies showed a high parathyroid hormone (PTH) level in the setting of low serum calcium and phosphorus levels. These findings collectively suggest secondary hyperparathyroidism. In this patient with normal kidney function, secondary hyperparathyroidism is likely due to vitamin D deficiency, a common problem in older adults. Therefore, screening her for vitamin D deficiency by measuring the 25-hydroxyvitamin D level would be the most appropriate next step.

A measurement of the 25-hydroxyvitamin D level is more informative in most patients with hypocalcemia than a measurement of the 1,25-dihydroxyvitamin D level because vitamin D deficiency causes hypocalcemia and stimulates PTH secretion, which in turn stimulates conversion of 25-hydroxyvitamin D to 1,25-dihydroxyvitamin D in the kidneys. Therefore, this patient's serum 1,25-dihydroxyvitamin D level may be normal in the setting of vitamin D deficiency and is not useful to check in this setting.

Parathyroidectomy also would be inappropriate in this patient because the elevation in the PTH level is an appropriate physiologic response to the low calcium (and presumed low vitamin D) level.

Repeat dual-energy x-ray absorptiometry testing in 1 year should not be recommended because this patient already has indications for medical management of her osteoporosis after the high PTH and low calcium levels have been evaluated and treated.

KEY POINT

- **Measurement of the serum 25-hydroxyvitamin D level is an appropriate initial step in the evaluation of hypocalcemia, an elevated parathyroid hormone level, and osteoporosis.**

Bibliography

Holick MF, Binkley NC, Bischoff-Ferrari HA, et al; Endocrine Society. Evaluation, treatment, and prevention of vitamin D deficiency: an Endocrine Society clinical practice guideline [erratum in J Clin Endocrinol Metab. 2011;96(12):3908]. J Clin Endocrinol Metab. 2011;96(7):1911-1930. [PMID: 21646368]

Item 23 Answer: C

Educational Objective: **Treat stage III thyroid cancer with radioactive iodine therapy.**

The patient should receive radioactive iodine therapy. She has stage III thyroid cancer because her excised malignant thyroid nodule is greater than 4 cm with cervical lymph node involvement (T3N1MX). The American Thyroid Association Guidelines indicate that a patient older than 45 years who has had a total thyroidectomy for a papillary thyroid cancer greater than 4 cm should receive radioactive iodine (^{131}I) because this treatment will decrease the risk of recurrence and death. Decreasing the risk of recurrence is critical because relapsing disease develops in approximately 12% of patients who have no evidence of disease after primary therapy.

Tumors that are not treatable with the combination of surgery, levothyroxine therapy, and repeat doses of ^{131}I are treated with external-beam radiation therapy or chemotherapy (with traditional cytotoxic drugs, such as doxorubicin), but the response to these therapies is poor. This patient has not failed to benefit from first-line therapy, and thus treatment with external-beam radiation or chemotherapy is not yet indicated.

Observation is inadequate postsurgical therapy in this patient who underwent removal of a papillary thyroid cancer greater than 4 cm and a malignant lymph node. Radioactive iodine therapy is needed to decrease the progression of local disease and potentially increase survival in this patient with stage III disease.

KEY POINT

- **Large papillary thyroid cancer (>4 cm) is treated with thyroidectomy and then with radioactive iodine to decrease the risk of recurrence and death.**

Bibliography

American Thyroid Association (ATA) Guidelines Taskforce on Thyroid Nodules and Differentiated Thyroid Cancer; Cooper DS, Doherty GM, Haugen BR, et al. Revised American Thyroid Association management guidelines for patients with thyroid nodules and differentiated thyroid cancer [errata in Thyroid. 2010;20(6):674-675; and Thyroid. 2010;20(8):942]. Thyroid. 2009;19(11):1167-1214. [PMID: 19860577]

Item 24 Answer: C

Educational Objective: **Diagnose type 2 diabetes mellitus.**

This patient is at high risk for diabetes mellitus and should have his hemoglobin A_{1c} value remeasured. He has a family history of type 2 diabetes and coronary artery disease, is obese, and has hypertension. According to the American Diabetes Association, in the absence of unequivocal symptomatic hyperglycemia, the diagnosis of diabetes must be confirmed on a subsequent day by repeating the same test suggestive of diabetes (in this patient, the hemoglobin A_{1c} measurement). If results of two different diagnostic tests are available and both are diagnostic for diabetes, additional testing is not needed. Although this patient's hemoglobin A_{1c} value is diagnostic of diabetes, his fasting serum glucose level is only in the range of impaired fasting glucose. Because this patient had two different tests with discordant results, the test that is diagnostic of diabetes (the hemoglobin A_{1c} measurement) should be repeated to confirm the diagnosis.

In this patient without any hyperglycemic symptoms, remeasuring his hemoglobin A_{1c} level is a much simpler and less burdensome way of confirming the diagnosis of diabetes than performing an oral glucose tolerance test.

Because results of measurement of the hemoglobin A_{1c} value and fasting plasma glucose level were discordant, not performing any additional testing is inappropriate.

KEY POINT

- **If results of two different diagnostic tests for diabetes mellitus are discordant, the test that is diagnostic of diabetes should be repeated.**

Bibliography

American Diabetes Association. Standards of medical care in diabetes—2011. Diabetes Care. 2011;34(Suppl 1):S11-S61. [PMID: 21193625]

Item 25 Answer: D

Educational Objective: **Manage adrenal insufficiency.**

This patient should be treated with oral hydrocortisone. She has clinical and biochemical features of glucocorticoid deficiency 2 weeks after discontinuing megestrol, which she used continuously for 1 year. Megestrol is a progestational agent with strong glucocorticoid activity that is commonly used in patients with anorexia of different causes because it is a potent appetite stimulant. Because of this potent glucocorticoid activity, chronic use of megestrol (and other agents with similar activity) leads to suppression of the hypothalamic-pituitary-adrenal axis. With the suppression of the axis, a sudden discontinuation of the drug leads to symptoms and signs of adrenal insufficiency. This patient's physical examination findings of a plethoric rounded face and central obesity with supraclavicular and posterior cervical fat pads are consistent with prolonged exposure to exogenous agents with glucocorticoid activity, as are her low serum cortisol and plasma adrenocorticotropic hormone levels. Treatment with hydrocortisone for several weeks is necessary to reactivate the axis. The advantages of hydrocortisone are that it is identical to the natural product, has a short half life, and can be tightly titrated easily.

Because adrenal insufficiency that is central in origin indicates a cause other than intrinsic adrenal disease, obtaining a CT scan of the adrenal glands is unwarranted in this patient.

The dexamethasone suppression test is helpful when investigating conditions associated with hypercortisolemia, such as Cushing syndrome. In this patient with a low serum cortisol level and symptomatic adrenal insufficiency, the dexamethasone suppression test is of no value.

Because the patient has central adrenal insufficiency, mineralocorticoid secretion by the adrenal glands is maintained and fludrocortisone therapy is unnecessary.

KEY POINT

- **Chronic use of megestrol and similar drugs with strong glucocorticoid activity leads to suppression of the hypothalamic-pituitary-adrenal axis, and sudden discontinuation of these drugs can result in symptoms and signs of adrenal insufficiency.**

Bibliography

Leinung MC, Liporace R, Miller CH. Induction of adrenal suppression by megestrol acetate in patients with AIDS. Ann Intern Med. 1995;122(11):843-845. [PMID: 7741369]

Item 26 Answer: A

Educational Objective: Diagnose the cause of secondary hypogonadism.

This patient should have iron saturation studies to determine a possible cause of his central hypogonadism, which is indicated by the low serum testosterone, follicle-stimulating hormone, and luteinizing hormone levels. The evaluation of secondary hypogonadism includes the exclusion of hyperprolactinemia and hemochromatosis as possible causes. This patient's serum prolactin level is normal, but hemochromatosis has not yet been excluded as a cause. His history of osteoarthritis is consistent with a diagnosis of hemochromatosis, as is his slightly elevated alanine aminotransferase level.

Measuring the free testosterone level is not appropriate because this patient does not have any history or physical examination findings suggestive of abnormal sex hormone–binding globulin levels, such as obesity, insulin resistance (for example, type 2 diabetes mellitus), or older age. If he had any of these findings, his total serum testosterone levels would be suspect, and the amount of free testosterone would be a better indicator of hypogonadism.

Karyotyping and testicular ultrasonography are not useful tests in the evaluation of secondary hypogonadism. A karyotype is useful in patients with primary hypogonadism and increased gonadotropin levels to exclude Klinefelter syndrome.

KEY POINT

- **The evaluation of secondary hypogonadism includes the exclusion of hyperprolactinemia and hemochromatosis as possible causes.**

Bibliography

Bhasin S, Cunningham GR, Hayes FJ, et al; Task Force, Endocrine Society. Testosterone therapy in men with androgen deficiency syndromes: an Endocrine Society clinical practice guideline. J Clin Endocrinol Metab. 2010;95(6):2536-2559. [PMID: 20525905]

Item 27 Answer: C

Educational Objective: Adjust hydrocortisone therapy during a minor illness.

This woman should increase her dose of hydrocortisone approximately threefold for 3 days. This patient with Addison disease (primary adrenal insufficiency) has an upper respiratory tract infection. She has continued to take adequate amounts of fluids and her medications as scheduled. Except for findings related to an upper respiratory tract infection, vital signs and other physical examination findings are normal. What she has not done is adjust her hydrocortisone dose during her intercurrent illness. This step in necessary to minimize the possibility of adrenal crisis. Educating patients about the need to adjust (increase) their dose of hydrocortisone with even minor intercurrent illnesses is crucial in the successful management of adrenal insufficiency.

Because this patient is not hypotensive and is able to take fluids and her medications orally, hospitalization for intravenous administration of fluids and glucocorticoids is unnecessary.

In patients with adrenal insufficiency, fludrocortisone is typically given as mineralocorticoid therapy. The additional glucocorticoid (hydrocortisone) therapy that this patient requires because of her intercurrent illness also will result in additional mineralocorticoid activity. Therefore, adjusting mineralocorticoid dosages during intercurrent medical illnesses is unnecessary.

Symptomatic treatment of her upper respiratory tract infection without adjustment of her hydrocortisone dosage is inappropriate and likely to lead to prolongation and worsening of her symptoms of adrenal insufficiency

KEY POINT

- **Adjusting (increasing) the dosage of hydrocortisone with even minor intercurrent illnesses is crucial to avoid adrenal crisis in patients with adrenal insufficiency.**

Bibliography

Chakera AJ, Vaidya B. Addison disease in adults: diagnosis and management. Am J Med. 2010;123(5):409-413. [PMID: 20399314]

Item 28 Answer: B

Educational Objective: Diagnose a thyroid-stimulating hormone–secreting pituitary tumor.

This patient should have a pituitary MRI. He has symptoms, clinical examination findings, and laboratory study results that are consistent with hyperthyroidism. The elevated radioactive iodine (^{123}I) uptake excludes subacute or silent thyroiditis. However, he also has a detectable serum thyroid-stimulating hormone (TSH) level. The serum TSH level is typically undetectable (<0.01 microunits/mL [0.01 milliunits/L]) in all patients with thyrotoxicosis due to

Graves disease, a toxic multinodular goiter, or a solitary autonomous thyroid nodule. Thyrotoxicosis with an inappropriately elevated TSH level may be associated with a TSH-secreting pituitary tumor, antibodies that interfere in the serum TSH assay, or laboratory error. The latter two causes, however, are not associated with the clinical and biochemical evidence of hyperthyroidism seen in this patient. Therefore, the most likely diagnosis in this patient is a TSH-secreting pituitary tumor. These tumors secrete TSH that stimulates the thyroid gland to secondarily release thyroxine (T_4) and triiodothyronine (T_3). The serum TSH level in patients with a TSH-secreting pituitary tumor may be detectable (inappropriately normal, detectable, or even elevated) in the setting of elevated T_4 and T_3 levels. The diagnosis should be confirmed with a pituitary MRI, and a full evaluation of pituitary function should be performed because other pituitary hormones may be secreted in excess or be deficient. The primary therapy is neurosurgical resection of the tumor.

For residual disease after surgery, medical therapy with a somatostatin analogue is highly effective in lowering the TSH level and controlling hyperthyroidism in as many as 80% of patients with TSH-secreting tumors. However, radioactive iodine, methimazole, and propylthiouracil have no role.

Because the tumor involves the pituitary gland and not the thyroid gland, thyroidectomy is inappropriate management.

KEY POINT

- **A pituitary MRI can confirm the presence of a thyroid-stimulating hormone–secreting pituitary tumor.**

Bibliography

Bahn Chair RS, Burch HB, Cooper DS, et al; American Thyroid Association; American Association of Clinical Endocrinologists. Hyperthyroidism and other causes of thyrotoxicosis: management guidelines of the American Thyroid Association and American Association of Clinical Endocrinologists [erratum in Thyroid. 2011;21(10):1169]. Thyroid. 2011;21(6):593-646. [PMID: 21510801]

Item 29 Answer: B

Educational Objective: **Treat pheochromocytoma with α-blocker therapy.**

This patient should receive α-blocker therapy as initial treatment of his condition. He has classic clinical features of a pheochromocytoma (hypertension, palpitations, sweating, and headaches). The diagnosis is confirmed biochemically by the extreme elevation in plasma metanephrine and normetanephrine levels and 24-hour excretion of urine catecholamines (norepinephrine and epinephrine) and their metabolites (metanephrine, normetanephrine, and vanillylmandelic acid). Anatomically, these findings are associated with an adrenal mass. Although eventual laparoscopic surgical resection of the tumor is necessary, intraoperative and postoperative morbidities should first be minimized by controlling blood pressure and providing adequate α-blockade with preoperative medical therapy. Most patients with a pheochromocytoma previously were treated with the long-acting competitive α-adrenergic blocking agent phenoxybenzamine for several weeks before surgery, but this drug contributed to the hypotension commonly observed during the first day after tumor removal. More recent data show the effectiveness of short-acting specific α-antagonists, such as prazosin, doxazosin, or terazosin, without this adverse effect.

This patient most likely has a pheochromocytoma and is currently being treated with an ACE inhibitor. Adding an angiotensin receptor blocker to his antihypertensive regimen offers no additional therapeutic benefit over that achieved by ACE inhibition because it will not address the pathophysiologic basis of this secondary form of hypertension.

β-Blockers should never be used in patients with suspected or confirmed pheochromocytomas until after they are first treated with α-blockers.

Surgery is the definitive treatment for patients with a pheochromocytoma but should not be performed before therapy with α-blockers.

Although this patient currently seems stable, treatment of this type of tumor cannot be delayed indefinitely because patients can have provoked or unprovoked sudden cardiac episodes that can be fatal. Observation is thus inappropriate as initial treatment.

KEY POINT

- **In patients with a biochemically confirmed diagnosis of pheochromocytoma, α-blockade should be instituted before surgery.**

Bibliography

Pacak K. Preoperative management of the pheochromocytoma patient. J Clin Endcrinol Metab. 2007;92(11):4069-4079. [PMID: 17989126]

Item 30 Answer: C

Educational Objective: **Diagnose Paget disease of bone.**

Plain radiographs of the areas showing increased activity on the bone scan should be obtained in this patient. The increased activity may represent Paget disease of bone (osteitis deformans), a focal abnormality of bone metabolism leading to an accelerated rate of bone remodeling that results in disorganized bone matrix and compromise of bone integrity. The diagnosis of Paget disease of bone is best confirmed by plain radiographs of the areas of increased uptake seen on bone scan. Pagetic lesions will show characteristic coarsened bony trabeculae, which are pathognomonic for the disease.

Paget disease of bone may cause a range of clinical symptoms, including bone pain, traumatic and pathologic fractures, skeletal deformities, and cranial nerve impairment due to nerve impingement because of bony overgrowth. Hearing loss related to impairment of cranial nerve VIII is common in Paget disease of bone. Audiology testing to document the patient's baseline hearing status for comparison with future studies should be performed after the diagnosis of Paget disease of bone is confirmed, but not before.

Also part of the differential diagnosis of the bony lesions seen on bone scan is metastatic disease, particularly in an older patient. If plain radiographs do not confirm a diagnosis of Paget disease of bone or show findings consistent with metastatic disease, a bone biopsy can be considered.

Serum collagen type 1 cross-linked C-telopeptide (CTX) measurement may be helpful in monitoring the response of Paget disease to therapy but would not distinguish Paget disease from metastatic lesions.

Serum protein electrophoresis would help diagnose multiple myeloma but would not help distinguish Paget disease from metastases, which is the appropriate goal of the next step in this patient's evaluation.

KEY POINT

- **Plain radiographs of pagetic lesions will show characteristic coarsened bony trabeculae, which will confirm the diagnosis of Paget disease of bone.**

Bibliography

Josse RG, Hanley DA, Kendler D, Ste Marie LG, Adachi JD, Brown J. Diagnosis and treatment of Paget's disease of bone. Clin Invest Med. 2007;30(5):E210-E223. [PMID: 17892763]

Item 31 Answer: B

Educational Objective: Identify nocturnal hypoglycemia.

This patient's symptoms are most likely caused by nocturnal hypoglycemia. Her hemoglobin A_{1c} value is lower than what her blood glucose log averages suggest. Frequent episodes of significant hypoglycemia for several hours each night would explain this discrepancy. The 70/30 insulin she takes twice daily gives a single large peak 6 to 8 hours after taking it. This patient exercises every evening, which means that her muscles will continue to remove glucose from her blood to replenish their glycogen stores for several hours afterward. This occurrence could cause her blood glucose to decrease to very low levels while she sleeps. Given the duration of her diabetes mellitus, the appropriate adrenergic counterregulatory response may be adequately blunted to not cause her to awaken from sleep but can lead to fatigue, sweating, and headache when she awakens.

The dawn phenomenon is defined as an elevation in blood glucose levels during the early morning hours (4 AM-8 AM) that is thought to be related to the increased physiologic release of cortisol and growth hormone that occur during this time period. The dawn phenomenon is typically identified by persistent significant elevations of morning blood glucose levels, which were not seen in this patient.

Although sleep apnea may be a cause of fatigue and early morning headache, it is more often seen in obese patients with type 2 diabetes who have an associated high hemoglobin A_{1c} value.

The "Somogyi phenomenon" is a phrase used to describe the theoretical concept that the lower the blood glucose level decreases during the night, the higher it increases the next morning because of increasingly severe rebound hyperglycemia. This idea, however attractive on a theoretical level, has been disproven as a cause of fasting hyperglycemia.

KEY POINT

- **Frequent nocturnal hypoglycemia may cause morning fatigue, sweating, and headache in patients with type 1 diabetes mellitus.**

Bibliography

Juvenile Diabetes Research Foundation Continuous Glucose Monitoring Study Group. Prolonged nocturnal hypoglycemia is common during 12 months of continuous glucose monitoring in children and adults with type 1 diabetes. Diabetes Care. 2010;33(5):1004-1008. [PMID: 20200306]

Item 32 Answer: C

Educational Objective: Diagnose multiple endocrine neoplasia type 1.

This patient most likely has multiple endocrine neoplasia type 1 (MEN1), which is characterized by tumors of the pituitary gland, the parathyroid glands, and the pancreas (the three "P"s). She has hyperprolactinemia and a pituitary adenoma, the size of which (<1 cm) suggests a microprolactinoma. Additionally, she has primary hyperparathyroidism and a family history that suggests the presence of MEN1 in her kindred. Her father's history of kidney stones suggests that he also has hyperparathyroidism as a result of MEN1, and her brother's history of peptic ulcer disease suggests the presence of a gastrin-secreting pancreatic neuroendocrine tumor in the setting of MEN1. In MEN1, primary hyperparathyroidism most often reflects parathyroid hyperplasia rather than an adenoma. The mutation in the menin gene was most likely inherited in an autosomal dominant fashion in this family.

Autoimmune polyglandular syndrome type 1 is an inherited autosomal recessive disorder characterized by chronic mucocutaneous candidiasis, autoimmune hypoparathyroidism, and adrenal insufficiency. This patient has hyperparathyroidism, not hypoparathyroidism, and thus is unlikely to have autoimmune polyglandular syndrome type 1.

This patient's thyroid-stimulating hormone level is normal, which makes the diagnosis of Hashimoto thyroiditis unlikely.

MEN2 is characterized by primary parathyroid hyperplasia, pheochromocytoma, and medullary thyroid cancer. Although this patient has evidence of primary hyperparathyroidism, she does not have a consistent family history or clinical symptoms or signs of the other components of the genetic abnormality suggestive of this diagnosis.

KEY POINT

- **Multiple endocrine neoplasia type 1 is characterized by tumors of the pituitary gland, the parathyroid glands, and the pancreas (the three "P"s).**

Bibliography

Brandi ML, Gagel RF, Angeli A, et al. Guidelines for diagnosis and therapy of MEN type 1 and type 2. J Clin Endocrinol Metab. 2001;86(12):5658-5671. [PMID: 11739416]

Item 33 Answer: A

Educational Objective: Diagnose hypogonadism in patients with obesity.

A free testosterone assessment, preferably one using equilibrium dialysis, is the most appropriate diagnostic test to determine whether this patient truly has hypogonadism. A random serum testosterone level greater than 350 ng/dL (12 nmol/L) excludes hypogonadism. Values consistently less than 200 ng/dL (6.9 nmol/L) almost always confirm hypogonadism, but values in the 200 to 350 ng/dL (6.9-12 nmol/L) range are equivocal. Unless the total testosterone level is markedly reduced and the patient has a known pituitary or gonadal pathologic abnormality, a screening testosterone value of 350 ng/dL (12 nmol/L) or lower requires confirmation by a second measurement that includes determination of the free testosterone level. Of note, obesity can cause a decrease in sex hormone–binding globulin levels. Therefore, the free testosterone level can be normal, even when the total testosterone level appears decreased. If the free testosterone level is normal, then hypogonadism is excluded and another etiology of this patient's erectile dysfunction, such as medications, must be explored.

A karyotype is not appropriate in this patient in whom hypogonadism has not been diagnosed and who has normal follicle-stimulating hormone and luteinizing hormone levels, which exclude primary hypogonadism. A karyotype is useful in patients diagnosed with primary hypogonadism to exclude Klinefelter syndrome.

A pituitary MRI is not indicated at this time because the diagnosis of secondary hypogonadism has not been confirmed.

A sperm count is not indicated in this patient because a sperm count will not reliably indicate whether a patient has hypogonadism. Men with low sperm counts can have normal testosterone levels, and men with slightly decreased testosterone levels can have normal sperm counts. In addition, this patient is not seeking fertility at this time.

KEY POINT

- **In male patients with obesity, hypogonadism is best diagnosed by a free testosterone assessment because the total testosterone level may be affected by a decrease in the sex hormone–binding globulin level.**

Bibliography

Traish AM, Miner MM, Morgentaler A, Zitzmann M. Testosterone deficiency. Am J Med. 2011;124(7):578-587. [PMID: 21683825]

Item 34 Answer: B

Educational Objective: Manage medullary thyroid cancer.

Measurement of the plasma free metanephrine and normetanephrine levels is the most appropriate initial step in management in this patient with a thyroid nodule. She has a history of hypertension, elevated serum calcium and calcitonin levels, and multiple plasmacytoid-appearing cells on fine-needle aspiration (FNA) biopsy of the nodule. These findings are suggestive of medullary thyroid cancer. Although sporadic in greater than 80% of affected patients, medullary thyroid cancer may be associated with multiple endocrine neoplasia type 2A (MEN2A), MEN2B, or familial non-MEN. The MEN2A and MEN2B syndromes are characterized by medullary thyroid cancer and pheochromocytoma. Therefore, the presence of pheochromocytoma must be excluded.

Radioactive iodine is not taken up by parafollicular cells (C cells) and, therefore, is not an appropriate treatment in patients with medullary thyroid cancer.

Because nearly 30% of patients with sporadic medullary thyroid cancer and 100% of patients with inherited medullary thyroid cancer have bilateral disease, total thyroidectomy, not thyroid lobectomy, is always the preferred surgical treatment. After initial surgery, all patients should receive levothyroxine to prevent hypothyroidism.

The administration of levothyroxine without surgery to suppress thyroid-stimulating hormone (TSH) secretion is not indicated because C-cells are not TSH responsive.

KEY POINT

- **Although sporadic in greater than 80% of affected patients, medullary thyroid cancer also may be associated with multiple endocrine neoplasia type 2A (MEN2A), MEN2B, or familial non-MEN.**

Bibliography

American Thyroid Association Guidelines Task Force; Kloos RT, Eng C, Evans DB, et al. Medullary thyroid cancer: management guidelines of the American Thyroid Association [erratum in Thyroid. 2009;19(11):1295]. Thyroid. 2009;19(6):565-612. [PMID: 19469690]

Item 35 Answer: E

Educational Objective: **Treat type 1 diabetes mellitus.**

This patient's preprandial insulin lispro dose should be changed to 1 unit for every 10 grams of carbohydrate to be consumed. She recently has made several healthy changes to her diabetic regimen and lifestyle that have resulted in close-to-ideal fasting and preprandial glucose levels, but her 2-hour postprandial levels are still too high. Changing her insulin lispro dose from 1 unit to cover each 20 grams of carbohydrate to 1 unit to cover every 10 grams of carbohydrate will give her a larger spike of rapid-acting insulin in the first 2 hours after each meal and should lower her postprandial blood glucose levels. This change should result in a lower hemoglobin A_{1c} value after a few months.

Although adding an injection of pramlintide before meals might improve her postprandial blood glucose level, optimization of her current diabetic regimen is likely to successfully control her blood glucoses without introducing an additional and expensive treatment.

Changing from insulin lispro to regular insulin would not improve her blood glucose levels 2 hours after her meals but might cause hypoglycemia 4 to 6 hours after meals.

Changing from neutral protamine Hagedorn (NPH) insulin to insulin glargine would provide no benefit because her fasting and preprandial glucose levels are already at goal, and she is not experiencing nocturnal hypoglycemia. Additionally, insulin glargine is approximately four times more expensive than NPH insulin.

The patient is already somewhat underweight, is planning to get pregnant, and is eating a healthy diet. Therefore, restricting her carbohydrate intake is not appropriate and might lead to hypoglycemia.

KEY POINT

- **Evaluating and managing postprandial blood glucose levels can help optimize insulin therapy in patients with type 1 diabetes mellitus.**

Bibliography

Singh SR, Ahmad F, Lal A, Yu C, Bai Z, Bennett H. Efficacy and safety of insulin analogues for the management of diabetes mellitus: a meta-analysis. CMAJ. 2009;180(4):385-397. [PMID: 19221352]

H

Item 36 Answer: B

Educational Objective: **Treat hypoparathyroidism occurring after thyroidectomy.**

Calcium is most likely to diminish the acute symptoms in this patient who recently underwent thyroidectomy. Complications of thyroidectomy include the inadvertent removal of or injury to the parathyroid glands. If a substantial amount of parathyroid tissue is not left in vivo, hypoparathyroidism accompanied by hypocalcemia will result postoperatively. Symptoms are primarily neuromuscular, such as paresthesias and muscle cramps, and tend to be prominent in patients who experience a rapid drop in their serum calcium level after surgery. This patient requires an emergent rapid increase in his serum calcium level, which is best accomplished by oral calcium (carbonate or citrate) supplementation. Intravenous calcium more rapidly increases the serum calcium level and may be indicated in patients with very low (<7.5 mg/dL [1.9 mmol/L]) calcium levels or more significant clinical findings associated with the hypocalcemia, such as severe musculoskeletal weakness, tetany, or electrocardiographic conduction abnormalities. Ultimately, this patient most likely will require more prolonged calcium therapy, depending on the degree of his hypoparathyroidism after surgery.

Although this patient also may require chronic vitamin D supplementation to maintain his serum calcium levels, this would not be an initial intervention in a symptomatic individual with hypocalcemia. Calcitriol (1,25-dihydroxyvitamin D) should be used because the lack of parathyroid hormone (PTH) will diminish the endogenous conversion of 25-hydroxyvitamin D to the more potent 1,25-dihydroxyvitamin D. However, calcitriol by itself will not effectively increase serum calcium levels until several days have elapsed.

Patients with hypomagnesemia may have hypocalcemia that is refractory to correction until the low magnesium levels are repleted. This patient has no evidence of significant hypomagnesemia.

Teriparatide, a recombinant form of PTH, currently is used in the treatment of advanced osteoporosis. Although it holds promise as a potential therapy for chronic hypoparathyroidism, its safety and long-term effectiveness for this use have not been established, and it does not have FDA approval for treatment of acute hypoparathyroidism.

KEY POINT

- **In most patients with hypoparathyroidism and hypocalcemia, oral calcium is appropriate emergent therapy because it is rapidly absorbed and will increase the serum calcium level within minutes.**

Bibliography

Khan MI, Waguespack SG, Hu MI. Medical management of postsurgical hypoparathyroidism [erratum in: Endocr Pract. 2011;17(6):967]. Endocr Pract. 2011;17(Suppl 1):18-25. [PMID: 21134871]

Item 37 Answer: A

Educational Objective: **Interpret hemoglobin A_{1c} values in a patient with a recent blood transfusion.**

The six units of packed red blood cells that this patient received while hospitalized most likely are responsible for his low hemoglobin A_{1c} value. In patients receiving hemodialysis, those with hemolytic anemia or certain hemoglobinopathies, or those with recent blood transfusions, hemoglobin A_{1c} values may be falsely lowered because of the presence of erythrocytes less than 120 days old in the sample. In this patient, not enough time has elapsed since the blood was transfused for the erythrocytes to become glycosylated and reflect a true hemoglobin A_{1c} level.

Although eating a healthier diet might lower his blood glucose levels over the next few months, not enough time has passed for this lifestyle intervention to affect his hemoglobin A_{1c} value so profoundly. His blood glucose log shows premeal values of 140 to 160 mg/dL (7.8-8.9 mmol/L), which means that postprandial values are likely to be even higher and not compatible with a hemoglobin A_{1c} value of 6.2%.

Omeprazole does not interfere with hemoglobin A_{1c} assays and thus is not responsible for his dramatically lower value.

Cessation of cigarette smoking, although an inherently positive lifestyle change, will not affect the hemoglobin A_{1c} level.

KEY POINT

- **Hemoglobin A_{1c} values may be falsely lowered in patients who have received recent blood transfusions.**

Bibliography

Spencer DH, Grossman BJ, Scott MG. Red cell transfusion decreases hemoglobin A1c in patients with diabetes. Clin Chem. 2011;57(2):344-346. [PMID: 21059826]

Item 38 Answer: D

Educational Objective: **Diagnose opiate-induced secondary hypogonadism.**

This patient's use of methadone is most likely responsible for his symptoms. Chronic opiate use is an acquired cause of secondary hypogonadism. The mechanism of opiate-induced hypogonadism is thought to be central hypogonadism, with downregulation of gonadotropin-releasing hormone and subsequently luteinizing hormone (LH) and follicle-stimulating hormone (FSH). This, in turn results in decreased testosterone production.

Active or anabolic steroid abuse can decrease patients' endogenous LH, FSH, and testosterone levels. However, these patients typically seek medical attention because of infertility, usually do not have low libido, are very muscular, and may have significant pustular acne. This patient has low libido, is thin (not muscular), and has no acne, all of which make anabolic steroid abuse very unlikely.

Low libido is an adverse effect of citalopram, but the drug should not cause low testosterone levels and thus is not the cause of this patient's symptoms.

Lisinopril has not been associated with low libido or erectile dysfunction and thus also is unlikely to be the cause of this patient's symptoms.

KEY POINT

- **The mechanism of opiate-induced hypogonadism is thought to be central hypogonadism, with downregulation of gonadotropin-releasing hormone and subsequently luteinizing hormone and follicle-stimulating hormone, which results in decreased testosterone production.**

Bibliography

Bliesener N, Albrecht S, Schwager A, Weckbecker K, Lichtermann D, Kingmüller D. Plasma testosterone and sexual function in men receiving buprenorphine maintenance for opioid dependence. J Clin Endocrinol Metab. 2005;90(1):203-206. [PMID: 15483091]

Item 39 Answer: A

Educational Objective: **Manage newly diagnosed adrenal insufficiency.**

Hydrocortisone therapy is most appropriate for management of this patient's disorder. She has the classic clinical (fatigue, nausea, weight loss, salt craving) and biochemical (hyponatremia, hyperkalemia, and low cortisol and high adrenocorticotropic hormone [ACTH] levels) features of primary adrenal insufficiency. The laboratory study results also suggest decreased production of mineralocorticoids (hyponatremia and hyperkalemia) and adrenal androgens (low serum dehydroepiandrosterone sulfate level). Although the random serum cortisol level is within the accepted range for the afternoon, it is inappropriately low for the degree of hypotension experienced by this patient—especially because hypotension is a strong stimulus for ACTH and cortisol release. The plasma ACTH level, which was measured at the same time as the serum cortisol level, is extremely elevated and indicates primary adrenal failure. Therefore, all three classes of corticosteroids produced by the adrenal cortex (glucocorticoids, mineralocorticoids, and adrenal androgens) are diminished, which suggests the diagnosis of primary adrenal insufficiency. The disorder is most likely autoimmune in nature, given the patient's family history, and is best treated with hydrocortisone.

Although the serum thyroid-stimulating hormone level is minimally elevated, this patient has newly diagnosed primary adrenal insufficiency that should be addressed before any adjustment in the levothyroxine dosage is made. Increasing the levothyroxine dosage before starting glucocorticoids could accelerate the metabolic clearance of endogenously secreted cortisol and potentially worsen symptoms of adrenal insufficiency.

The abnormalities in this patient's laboratory results are quite clear and associated with clinical symptoms. Therefore, repeat testing of her serum cortisol and plasma ACTH levels at 9 AM is unnecessary.

The increased plasma ACTH level is a physiologic response to the reduction in cortisol and excludes pituitary insufficiency as the cause of the patient's hypocortisolism. An MRI of the pituitary gland is thus not indicated.

KEY POINT

- **The diagnosis of primary adrenal insufficiency is suggested when all three classes of corticosteroids produced by the adrenal cortex are diminished.**

Bibliography

Chakera AJ, Vaidya B. Addison disease in adults: diagnosis and management. Am J Med. 2010;123(5):409-413. [PMID: 20399314]

Item 40 Answer: B

Educational Objective: Diagnose lymphocytic hypophysitis.

This patient most likely has lymphocytic hypophysitis, an uncommon autoimmune disorder characterized by symmetric enlargement of the sellar contents. Lymphocytic hypophysitis is usually detected during pregnancy or in the postpartum period. Antipituitary antibodies can be detected in patients with this disorder, but these antibodies are not routinely clinically measured. Lymphocytic hypophysitis is a rare cause of hypopituitarism and can be associated with central adrenal insufficiency, as seen in this patient. Adrenocorticotropic hormone deficiency is a common finding in lymphocytic hypophysitis and is a major cause of morbidity and mortality in patients with the disorder. This patient should be treated with glucocorticoid replacement therapy and observation of the mass, which often decreases in size over time. If visual field defects develop, surgery may be necessary.

Craniopharyngioma is a rare, irregular, mixed solid-cystic lesion, often with calcifications, seen in persons of this patient's age that often is associated with panhypopituitarism and diabetes insipidus. The radiographic findings and signs and symptoms in this patient are inconsistent with craniopharyngioma.

Although prolactinomas may enlarge during pregnancy, the serum prolactin level is generally greater than 500 ng/mL (500 micrograms/L), with lesions greater than 10 mm in size (macroadenomas). Given the size of her pituitary lesion, one would expect her serum prolactin level to be much higher than measured. The hyperprolactinemia in this patient most likely reflects her recent gravid state because serum prolactin levels increase throughout pregnancy. The increased size of the normal pituitary gland during pregnancy does not result in associated clinical signs or symptoms of hypopituitarism and will not cause local mass effects.

Sheehan syndrome is defined as pituitary infarction or hemorrhage in the setting of a complicated delivery and thus is not the diagnosis in this patient.

KEY POINT

- **Adrenocorticotropic hormone deficiency is a common finding in lymphocytic hypophysitis and is a major cause of morbidity and mortality.**

Bibliography

Molitch ME, Gillam MP. Lymphocytic hypophysitis. Horm Res. 2007;68(Suppl 5):145-150. [PMID: 18174733]

Item 41 Answer: D

Educational Objective: Interpret hemoglobin A_{1c} results.

The discrepancy in this patient's glucose monitor readings and hemoglobin A_{1c} values is most likely due to postprandial hyperglycemia. She tests her blood glucose level only in a fasting state and before each meal and does not obtain postprandial or other measurements. Although her records indicate an average level that is close to the target of 130 mg/dL (7.2 mmol/L), her blood glucose level may actually exceed 200 mg/dL (11.1 mmol/L) for several hours after meals. These periods of hyperglycemia will contribute to her elevated hemoglobin A_{1c} value. The hemoglobin A_{1c} level represents the average of her fasting, preprandial, postprandial, nocturnal, and other blood glucose levels during the past 3 months.

Although blood glucose monitors occasionally may produce inaccurate readings, this occurrence is extremely rare and also is unlikely in this patient because the simultaneous laboratory plasma glucose level and glucose monitor reading are within 10% of each other.

Hemoglobin A_{1c} levels vary directly with erythrocyte survival. Levels are falsely high when erythrocyte survival is prolonged (decreased erythrocyte turnover), as occurs in patients with untreated iron, vitamin B_{12}, or folate deficiency anemia. Conversely, hemoglobin A_{1c} levels may be falsely low in patients with the shorter erythrocyte survival associated with rapid cell turnover, as occurs in patients with hemolytic anemia; those being treated for iron, folate, or vitamin B_{12} deficiency; and those being treated with erythropoietin. This patient's history of recent iron deficiency anemia treated with iron is likely to falsely lower, not elevate, her hemoglobin A_{1c} level.

If the patient were having prolonged periods of nocturnal hypoglycemia, she would have a lower-than-expected hemoglobin A_{1c} value.

KEY POINT

- **Average glucose monitor readings that do not include postprandial blood glucose levels are likely to differ from average plasma glucose levels derived from hemoglobin A_{1c} values.**

Bibliography

Nathan DM, Kuenen J, Borg R, Zheng H, Schoenfeld D, Heine RJ; A1c-Derived Average Glucose Study Group. Translating the A1C assay into estimated average glucose values [erratum in Diabetes Care. 2009;32(1):207]. Diabetes Care. 2008; 31(8):1473-1478. [PMID: 18540046]

Item 42 Answer: C

Educational Objective: Diagnose hypocalcemia due to hungry bone syndrome.

This patient's hypocalcemia is most likely caused by hungry bone syndrome. He has developed hypocalcemia after surgery to correct primary hyperparathyroidism. After parathyroidectomy, patients may experience hungry bone syndrome, in which the unmineralized bone matrix produced during the period of hyperparathyroidism begins to mineralize after the parathyroid level becomes more normal. This results in low serum calcium and phosphorus levels because these minerals are consumed by the bone in the process of mineralization.

Secondary hyperparathyroidism and bone disease affect almost all patients with chronic kidney disease (CKD). Hyperphosphatemia, hypocalcemia, and deficiency of 1,25-dihydroxyvitamin D stimulate parathyroid hormone (PTH) secretion. In patients with stage 2 and stage 3 CKD, increased PTH secretion helps maintain the serum calcium level through increased mobilization of calcium from bone and decreased urine calcium excretion. Patients with stage 3 CKD have transient postprandial hypocalcemia and hyperphosphatemia, both of which contribute to the increase in the PTH level that precedes onset of the sustained hyperphosphatemia characteristic of stage 4 and stage 5 CKD. Although this patient's kidney function is mildly impaired, the dysfunction is not serious enough to cause this severe hypocalcemia, and CKD is not consistent with the measured normal PTH level.

Dilutional hypocalcemia can result from excessive intravenous fluid administration. This patient had minimally invasive surgery and would not have required a large amount of hydration.

Alkalosis due to hyperventilation can cause a decrease in the ionized calcium level because of a shift in calcium ions to the intracellular compartment. However, alkalosis does not affect the total serum calcium level.

KEY POINT

- **After parathyroidectomy, patients may experience hungry bone syndrome, in which the unmineralized bone matrix produced during the period of hyperparathyroidism begins to mineralize after the parathyroid level becomes more normal.**

Bibliography

Mittendorf EA, Merlino JI, McHenry CR. Post-parathyroidectomy hypocalcemia: incidence, risk factors, and management. Am Surg. 2004;70(2):114-119. [PMID: 15011912]

Item 43 Answer: D

Educational Objective: **Manage a thyroid nodule.**

This patient should undergo thyroid lobectomy. According to several guidelines, biopsy of any nodule greater than 1 cm in diameter is reasonable, and biopsy of smaller nodules should be considered in patients with risk factors, such as a history of radiation exposure, a family history of thyroid cancer, cervical lymphadenopathy, or worrisome ultrasound characteristics. Therefore, it was appropriate to perform a fine-needle aspiration (FNA) biopsy in this 18-year-old woman with a 2-cm hypoechoic nodule that also has increased intranodular vascularity, regardless of whether she has a personal or family history of thyroid cancer. Results were consistent with a follicular neoplasm, which has an approximately 15% to 30% chance of harboring cancer. Unlike papillary thyroid cancer, follicular thyroid cancer cannot be diagnosed on the basis of an FNA biopsy because it is difficult to differentiate a malignant from a benign adenoma. Therefore, follicular neoplasms require pathologic examination of a surgical specimen to diagnose or exclude malignancy. Either a thyroid lobectomy or total thyroidectomy is typically recommended for these nodules to allow for complete histologic evaluation.

Thyroid hormone suppression therapy with levothyroxine is frequently used in the treatment of differentiated thyroid cancers to minimize thyroid-stimulating hormone stimulation of tumor growth. However, its use in benign nodules is controversial, and using thyroid suppression therapy in this patient who does not yet have a clear diagnosis would be inappropriate.

Because the patient does not yet have a definitive diagnosis of thyroid cancer, treatment with radioactive iodine is not appropriate. Treatment with radioactive iodine is appropriate after malignancy is established.

Because results of FNA biopsy in this patient already suggest the possibility of malignancy, repeating the study in 6 months would be inappropriate. In any case, a repeat FNA biopsy would not obviate the need for a surgical specimen for a definitive diagnosis.

KEY POINT

- **Thyroid lobectomy or total thyroidectomy is typically recommended for thyroid nodules with evidence of a follicular neoplasm.**

Bibliography

American Thyroid Association (ATA) Guidelines Taskforce on Thyroid Nodules and Differentiated Thyroid Cancer; Cooper DS, Doherty GM, Haugen BR, et al. Revised American Thyroid Association management guidelines for patients with thyroid nodules and differentiated thyroid cancer [errata in Thyroid. 2010;20(6):674-675; and Thyroid. 2010;20(8):942]. Thyroid. 2009;19(11):1167-1214. [PMID: 19860577]

Item 44 Answer: A

Educational Objective: **Diagnose functional hypothalamic amenorrhea.**

Functional hypothalamic amenorrhea is the most likely diagnosis in this patient. Hypothalamic amenorrhea may result from several causes, including a tumor or infiltrative lesion, such as a lymphoma or sarcoidosis. More commonly, hypothalamic amenorrhea is functional and due to stress, excessive loss of body weight, excessive exercise, or some combination thereof and is a diagnosis of exclusion. This patient's findings of a low follicle-stimulating hormone (FSH) level and normal thyroid-stimulating hormone

(TSH) and prolactin levels; negative human chorionic gonadotropin test results; and no withdrawal bleeding after a progesterone challenge test all suggest hypothalamic amenorrhea. The pituitary MRI excludes a tumor or infiltrative lesion. The increased stress at work is the likely cause of her functional hypothalamic amenorrhea.

Polycystic ovary syndrome (PCOS) is unlikely because the patient has no evidence of significant hyperandrogenism; only mild facial acne is detected on physical examination. In addition, the progesterone challenge test resulted in no withdrawal bleeding, which indicates that she has low estrogen levels. Patients with PCOS typically have adequate estrogen levels but anovulatory cycles; a progesterone challenge test will produce withdrawal bleeding in these patients.

Primary ovarian insufficiency is not the diagnosis because the patient's FSH level is normal. In women with primary ovarian insufficiency, FSH levels are elevated (in the menopausal range).

Subclinical hypothyroidism is unlikely in this patient because her TSH level is normal, which indicates that she is euthyroid.

KEY POINT

- **Functional hypothalamic amenorrhea is a diagnosis of exclusion characterized by a low estrogen state, psychological or physical stress, normal or low follicle-stimulating hormone levels, and negative results on progesterone challenge testing.**

Bibliography

Gordon CM. Clinical practice. Functional hypothalamic amenorrhea. N Engl J Med. 2010;363(4):365-371. [PMID: 20660404]

Item 45 Answer: B

Educational Objective: **Treat a patient who has diabetes mellitus, hyperlipidemia, and nonalcoholic fatty liver disease with a statin.**

In addition to neutral protamine Hagedorn (NPH) insulin at bedtime, a statin should be added now to this patient's diabetes regimen. He has poorly controlled type 2 diabetes mellitus, and thus adding a bedtime basal insulin to his sulfonylurea is a reasonable step to improve his fasting plasma glucose level and hemoglobin A_{1c} value. His liver chemistry studies show moderately elevated aminotransferase levels, but he has no other evidence of liver disease. This makes the diagnosis of nonalcoholic fatty liver disease most likely. In light of his diabetes and significant hypercholesterolemia, the addition of a statin is likely to be beneficial. Patients with nonalcoholic fatty liver disease are not necessarily at a higher risk of adverse outcomes from statin therapy than patients without the disease, and thus statins are a treatment option in these patients. In a study of 437 patients whose liver chemistry levels were up to three times the upper limit of normal, treatment with atorvastatin resulted in a threefold reduction in cardiovascular events (10% versus 30% in the nontreatment group) and a greater reduction in liver chemistry levels compared with patients not receiving a statin during 3 years of follow-up evaluation.

Fibrates are most effective for reducing the triglyceride level and have little impact on the LDL cholesterol level, the primary lipid target in this patient.

Starting the statin should not be delayed until after his glycemic control has improved or his liver chemistry tests normalize.

Nicotinic acid can lower the LDL cholesterol level and increase the HDL cholesterol level. Its use is typically limited by its adverse effects. Nicotinic acid can cause elevation of glucose and liver chemistry levels and may cause severe hepatocellular damage. Nicotinic acid would be relatively contraindicated in this patient with probable nonalcoholic fatty liver disease.

KEY POINT

- **Statins are a viable treatment option in patients with diabetes mellitus, hyperlipidemia, and nonalcoholic fatty liver disease.**

Bibliography

Athyros VG, Tziomalos K, Gossios TD, et al; GREACE Study Collaborative Group. Safety and efficacy of long-term statin treatment for cardiovascular events in patients with coronary heart disease and abnormal liver tests in the Greek Atorvastatin and Coronary Heart Disease Evaluation (GREACE) Study: a post-hoc analysis. Lancet. 2010;376(9756):1916-1922. [PMID: 21109302]

Item 46 Answer: C

Educational Objective: Manage a sellar mass.

In this patient with an incidental sellar mass, measuring the serum prolactin level should be part of the initial evaluation. The approach to a sellar mass includes assessment for hormone hypersecretion, including evaluation for acromegaly, Cushing syndrome, and a prolactinoma. The absence of clinical findings suggestive of acromegaly or Cushing syndrome and the normal insulin-like growth factor 1 (IGF-1) and morning cortisol levels in this patient suggest a nonfunctioning pituitary macroadenoma. However, prolactin-secreting pituitary adenomas are common, and a serum prolactin level should be obtained to evaluate for this possibility. A male patient can have a prolactinoma without gynecomastia or galactorrhea. Testosterone deficiency with associated diminished libido and erectile dysfunction may be present in the setting of hyperprolactinemia. If a prolactinoma is diagnosed, a dopamine agonist is administered to reduce both the serum prolactin level and the tumor size. Further assessment includes evaluation for hypopituitarism.

A dexamethasone suppression test can help localize the tumor source in a patient with adrenocorticotropic hormone–dependent Cushing syndrome. Because this patient does not have Cushing syndrome, this test is not indicated.

A growth hormone stimulation test can be used to evaluate for possible growth hormone deficiency, but measuring the IGF-1 level is typically the initial screening test because IGF-1 is a marker for endogenous growth hormone levels. This patient has a normal IGF-1 level.

Measurement of the serum sodium and urine osmolality levels evaluates deficiency in antidiuretic hormone (ADH) secretion, which occurs in the hypothalamic region and posterior pituitary gland. Deficiencies of ADH secretion are rarely associated with either functional or nonfunctioning pituitary adenomas, although they may be a result of surgical intervention to treat an adenoma.

KEY POINT

- **In a patient with an incidental sellar mass, measuring the serum prolactin level should be part of the initial management.**

Bibliography

Freda PU, Beckers AM, Katznelson L, et al; Endocrine Society. Pituitary incidentaloma: an Endocrine Society clinical practice guideline. J Clin Endocrinol Metab. 2011;96(4):894-904. [PMID: 21474686]

Item 47 Answer: C

Educational Objective: **Diagnose benign familial hypocalciuric hypercalcemia.**

The patient should have her urine levels of calcium and creatinine measured so that the urine calcium-to-creatinine clearance ratio can be calculated. A ratio less than 0.01 would suggest benign familial hypocalciuric hypercalcemia (FHH). Although this low ratio also is seen in as many as one third of patients with primary hyperparathyroidism, this patient has none of the expected complications of primary hyperparathyroidism and has a brother with a similar history. Confirmation of the diagnosis of FHH is often possible by genetic testing for mutations in the *CASR* gene.

Measurement of the serum prolactin level could be considered if multiple endocrine neoplasia type 1 (MEN1) was in the differential diagnosis. However, this patient has no history of other tumors, which makes MEN1 an unlikely diagnosis.

Measurement of the serum 25-hydroxyvitamin D level is unlikely to help in the evaluation of a patient with a high serum calcium level and high-normal parathyroid hormone (PTH) level. The typical pattern seen in vitamin D deficiency is a high PTH level and a normal or mildly low serum calcium level.

A parathyroid sestamibi scan is inappropriate at this point in the patient's evaluation because it is a localization study meant to be performed on patients already deemed appropriate for parathyroidectomy.

KEY POINT

- **Benign familial hypocalciuric hypercalcemia is likely in the setting of a mild elevation of the serum calcium level with a high-normal or mildly elevated serum parathyroid hormone level and a family member with similar findings.**

Bibliography

Christensen SE, Nissen PH, Vestergaard P, Mosekilde L. Familial hypocalciuric hypercalcaemia: a review. Curr Opin Endocrinol Diabetes Obes. 2011;18(6):359-370. [PMID: 21986511]

Item 48 Answer: A

H

Educational Objective: **Evaluate adrenal function during critical illness.**

This patient should continue her current therapy of antibiotics and intravenous fluids. In the setting of a critically ill patient with sepsis and hypotension, the diagnosis of adrenal insufficiency is a possibility. Available assays for measuring the serum cortisol level determine the total (protein-bound and free) hormone level. The physiologic effects of cortisol are determined by the free (or unbound) fraction of the hormone pool. Patients with hypoproteinemia have lower serum total cortisol levels but may have normal serum free cortisol levels. The latter situation becomes clinically relevant in critically ill patients with hypoproteinemia, such as this patient.

A random serum cortisol level greater than 12 micrograms/dL (331 nmol/L) in a critically ill patient who has hypoproteinemia (albumin level <2.5 g/dL [25 g/L]) makes the diagnosis of adrenal insufficiency unlikely. The most appropriate management is to order no additional studies and add no new treatment but instead continue the current therapy of antibiotics and intravenous fluids.

The diagnosis of adrenal insufficiency typically relies on demonstrating a low basal serum cortisol level that does not increase appropriately after stimulation with the adrenocorticotropic hormone analogue cosyntropin. Because the adrenal glands are constantly stimulated by stressful events, such as sepsis, obtaining a cosyntropin stimulation test is unlikely to be of value in this setting.

In most healthy persons, the serum cortisol level is highest in the morning. A low morning serum cortisol measurement is compatible with adrenal insufficiency but is neither sufficiently sensitive nor specific to be diagnostic. Additionally, critically ill patients have maximally stimulated cortisol production throughout the day. Therefore, a morning serum cortisol level will not be significantly different from a random serum cortisol level and is not indicated in this patient.

Because the diagnosis of adrenal insufficiency is unlikely in this patient, the use of hydrocortisone is unnecessary.

KEY POINT

- **A random serum cortisol level greater than 12 micrograms/dL (331 nmol/L) in a critically ill patient with hypoproteinemia (albumin level <2.5 g/dL [25 g/L]) makes the diagnosis of adrenal insufficiency unlikely and treatment with hydrocortisone unnecessary.**

Bibliography

Arafah BM. Hypothalamic pituitary adrenal function during critical illness: limitations of current assessment methods. J Clin Endocrinol Metab. 2006;91(10):3725-3745. [PMID: 16882746]

Item 49 Answer: B

Educational Objective: Treat myxedema coma.

This patient's symptoms and signs strongly suggest myxedema coma, which should be treated with intravenous levothyroxine and hydrocortisone. Patients with myxedema coma frequently are nonresponsive or poorly responsive and have hypotension, hypoglycemia, bradycardia, and hypothermia. Myxedema coma is considered a medical emergency, and appropriate supportive measures (treatment of possible sepsis and pneumonia, ventilation, and assessment and treatment of cardiac issues) are very important. No consensus exists about the most efficacious thyroid hormone replacement regimen to use for myxedema coma. Intravenous levothyroxine has traditionally been administered, with an initial bolus of 200 to 500 micrograms followed by daily doses between 50 and 100 micrograms until transition to oral administration is feasible. These relatively high doses of levothyroxine are recommended to replenish the depleted tissue stores of thyroid hormone. However, they may be associated with cardiac irregularities and should be used cautiously, especially in patients with known or suspected cardiac disorders (which this patient does not have).

Thyroid hormone replacement therapy by itself may not be sufficient treatment. Patients with secondary hypothyroidism may have a degree of hypopituitarism that can lead to secondary adrenal insufficiency. Patients with myxedema coma should be checked for possible adrenal insufficiency and treated with a stress-dose glucocorticoid, such as hydrocortisone, until adrenal insufficiency is excluded and appropriate adrenal function confirmed.

Supplementation with liothyronine (oral or intravenous) has been proposed but is controversial, especially because a definitive benefit of this therapy has not been shown. If liothyronine is used, it should be administered cautiously in lower doses and in combination with levothyroxine. All underlying precipitating conditions also must be addressed.

KEY POINT

- **Intravenous levothyroxine and a glucocorticoid (such as hydrocortisone) is appropriate initial treatment of a patient in myxedema coma.**

Bibliography

Kwaku MP, Burman KD. Myxedema coma. J Intensive Care Med. 2007;22(4):224-231. [PMID: 17712058]

Item 50 Answer: B

Educational Objective: Manage hyperprolactinemia.

A pituitary MRI should be performed in this patient to evaluate for a sellar mass. He has hypogonadotropic hypogonadism, which is the likely basis of his sexual dysfunction. His hyperprolactinemia is most likely contributing to the hypogonadism. Before treatment can begin, the cause of the hyperprolactinemia must be determined. This patient has no other disorders (such as hypothyroidism, liver disease, or kidney failure) and takes no medication that could result in hyperprolactinemia. Therefore, MRI is necessary to exclude either a prolactinoma or another sellar mass.

Cabergoline, a dopamine agonist, eventually may be necessary for management of the hyperprolactinemia. However, the cause of the hyperprolactinemia first must be determined.

A testicular ultrasound has no role in managing this patient's disorder. His hypogonadism is most likely due to a central cause (low testosterone and low gonadotropin levels), and he has no palpable mass on testicular examination.

Testosterone therapy would not be indicated in this patient because the cause of his secondary hypogonadism still must be elucidated. If the cause is a pituitary adenoma, then treatment with a dopamine agonist may be sufficient to reverse the hypogonadism.

KEY POINT

- **In patients with hypogonadotropic hypogonadism and hyperprolactinemia not caused by another disorder or a medication, a pituitary MRI is appropriate to evaluate for a sellar mass.**

Bibliography

Melmed S, Casanueva FF, Hoffman AR, et al; Endocrine Society. Diagnosis and treatment of hyperprolactinemia: an Endocrine Society clinical practice guideline. J Clin Endocrinol Metab. 2011;96(2):273-288. [PMID: 21296991]

Item 51 Answer: C

Educational Objective: Diagnose male hypogonadism.

Obtaining a morning serum total testosterone level is the most appropriate next diagnostic test. According to Endocrine Society guidelines, an initial morning measurement of a patient's total testosterone level should be performed in assessing for hypogonadism; if results are abnormal, a second confirmatory morning measurement should be obtained before testing for secondary causes is begun. This recommendation is based on numerous studies showing that variability in testosterone levels from day to day or diurnally is common, with morning total testosterone levels being the most accurate in indicating a patient's androgen status.

Iron studies to exclude hemochromatosis as a cause of central hypogonadism are not indicated in this patient because a diagnosis of hypogonadism has not been confirmed.

Many free testosterone assays are grossly inaccurate and thus are not currently recommended to diagnose hypogonadism unless the assay measures free testosterone by equilibrium dialysis. Additionally, this patient has no risk factors for altered sex hormone–binding globulin levels (obesity and older age), which would make a total testosterone level less reliable. Therefore, he has no need of a free testosterone assessment.

Testicular ultrasonography is not indicated for the diagnosis of hypogonadism. A testicular examination is adequate for assessing testicular volume.

KEY POINT

- **In evaluating a male patient for hypogonadism, a morning measurement of the total testosterone level is the most appropriate initial step.**

Bibliography

Bhasin S, Cunningham GR, Hayes FJ, et al; Task Force, Endocrine Society. Testosterone therapy in men with androgen deficiency syndromes: an Endocrine Society clinical practice guideline. J Clin Endocrinol Metab. 2010;95(6):2536-2559. [PMID: 20525905]

Item 52 Answer: D

Educational Objective: Diagnose subacute thyroiditis.

This patient should have a 24-hour radioactive iodine uptake (RAIU) test. She most likely has subacute thyroiditis, a form of destructive thyroiditis, given her neck discomfort, history of a transient possible viral infection 4 weeks ago, fever, elevated erythrocyte sedimentation rate (ESR), and biochemical findings (elevated serum free thyroxine [T_4] and triiodothyronine [T_3] levels and low serum thyroid-stimulating hormone level). The RAIU test measures thyroid gland iodine uptake over a timed period, usually 24 hours. In patients with destructive thyroiditis (or exposure to exogenous thyroid hormones), results of the RAIU test will be less than normal (<5% at 24 hours). In contrast to destructive thyroiditis, Graves disease will show an elevated (or sometimes normal) RAIU, which indicates endogenous excess synthesis and production of thyroid hormones.

Fine-needle aspiration biopsy can be useful in the evaluation of thyroid nodules, which this patient does not have.

Antithyroid agents, such as methimazole or propylthiouracil, have no role in the treatment of destructive thyroiditis because endogenous production of thyroid hormones is very low. Although many patients can be treated expectantly with only β-blocker therapy, prednisone is indicated in patients with significant hormone elevation or pain.

Measurement of the serum thyroglobulin level can help distinguish exogenous levothyroxine ingestion from subacute thyroiditis. However, this patient's history and laboratory findings (tender thyromegaly, fever, elevated ESR) are not compatible with exogenous levothyroxine use.

KEY POINT

- **In patients with destructive thyroiditis, results of the 24-hour radioactive iodine uptake test will be less than normal (<5% at 24 hours).**

Bibliography

Pearce EN, Farwell AP, Braverman LE. Thyroiditis [erratum in N Engl J Med. 2003;349(6):620]. N Engl J Med. 2003;348(26):2646-2655. [PMID: 12826640]

Item 53 Answer: A

Educational Objective: Manage hypoglycemia in a patient taking a sulfonylurea.

This patient should stop taking glyburide immediately. She has impaired kidney function and heart failure, both of which significantly impair her ability to clear glyburide and glyburide metabolites from her body. The biologic half-life of glyburide is thus prolonged. Because of this long half-life and the degree of this patient's kidney impairment (estimated glomerular filtration rate <50 mL/min/1.73 m^2), merely decreasing her glyburide dosage is insufficient to reliably decrease blood drug levels and prevent the return of hypoglycemia. A hemoglobin A_{1c} value of 6.2% is dangerously low in an older patient with diabetes mellitus and has most likely resulted in frequent episodes of hypoglycemia. These episodes, in turn, have caused her recent episodes of confusion and forgetfulness. Because it may take several days after discontinuation for the glyburide to decrease to undetectable levels, evaluating her plasma glucose level in two weeks would be appropriate as a next step in management.

Although glipizide is safer and has a shorter half-life than glyburide, it also accumulates in patients with chronic kidney disease. More importantly, no hypoglycemic agent (glipizide, metformin, or insulin) should be given to this patient until glyburide is completely cleared from her body, which would completely end the cycle of recurrent hypoglycemic episodes.

KEY POINT

- **Sulfonylureas with long half-lives, such as glyburide, should not be used in older patients with type 2 diabetes mellitus and impaired kidney function or heart failure.**

Bibliography

Greco D, Pisciotta M, Gambina F, Maggio F. Severe hypoglycaemia leading to hospital admission in type 2 diabetic patients aged 80 years or older. Exp Clin Endocrinol Diabetes. 2010;118(4):215-219. [PMID: 20072965]

Item 54 Answer: C

Educational Objective: **Manage primary hyperparathyroidism.**

This patient should undergo a parathyroidectomy. She has hypercalcemia and a high-normal parathyroid hormone (PTH) level, a pattern consistent with primary hyperparathyroidism. Although the PTH level is not above the normal range, it is inappropriately high in light of her significant hypercalcemia. Although many patients with hyperparathyroidism may be appropriately observed closely or treated nonsurgically if they are asymptomatic, symptomatic hypercalcemia (for example, with nephrolithiasis and cardiac arrhythmias) is an indication for parathyroidectomy. Additional indications for surgery are a serum calcium level greater than 1.0 mg/dL (0.3 mmol/L) more than the normal range, a creatinine clearance less than 60 mL/min (0.06 L/min) (normal, 90-140 mL/min [0.09-0.14 L/min]), bone density T-scores less than −2.5 in any area, a previous fragility fracture, and age less than 50 years, regardless of symptoms.

This patient's primary indication for parathyroidectomy is the history of a fragility fracture (a fracture sustained in a fall from a standing height). Although her dual-energy x-ray absorptiometry scan does not show osteoporosis, the history of fragility fracture portends an elevated risk of future fracture. The goal of surgery will be to prevent additional bone loss, fragility fractures, or other possible complications of primary hyperparathyroidism.

Bisphosphonate therapy could be attempted if this patient refused surgery but is not as effective as surgery.

A bone scan might be helpful to evaluate for cancer with bony metastases but would not be useful in this patient with a benign parathyroid condition.

PTH-related protein (PTHrP) secretion is commonly associated with certain malignancies. However, measurement of the PTHrP level is unnecessary in this patient whose hypercalcemia is clearly caused by primary hyperparathyroidism and not by malignancy.

Repeating the serum calcium measurement in 1 year would be appropriate for a patient with primary hyperparathyroidism who did not have indications for surgery now.

KEY POINT

- **In a patient with primary hyperparathyroidism and a history of a fragility fracture, parathyroidectomy is the most appropriate management.**

Bibliography

Bilezikian JP, Khan AA, Potts JT Jr; Third International Workshop on the Management of Asymptomatic Primary Hyperthyroidism. Guidelines for the management of asymptomatic primary hyperparathyroidism: summary statement from the Third International Workshop. J Clin Endocrinol Metab. 2009;94(2):335-339. [PMID: 19193908]

Item 55 Answer: B

Educational Objective: **Manage adrenal function during critical illness.**

This patient should be treated with stress doses of hydrocortisone as the next step in management. His pneumonia was treated appropriately with intravenous fluids and antibiotics. However, despite optimal therapy, he continues to do poorly. Although his persistent illness could indicate progression into sepsis and septic shock, it is more likely that his poor response to therapy is the result of adrenal insufficiency. The repeated injections of triamcinolone most likely have suppressed his endogenous pituitary-adrenal axis and put him at increased risk for adrenal insufficiency. The timing of the symptoms is crucial in that they occurred 3 months after the last triamcinolone injection. Although the measured serum cortisol level is within the normal range, it is inappropriately low (even for a serum albumin level of 2.7 g/dL [27 g/L]) for the degree of stress (including hypotension) that he is experiencing. If the plasma adrenocorticotropic hormone (ACTH) level had been measured, it would have been inappropriately low or low-normal as a result of chronic suppression by previous glucocorticoid administration. This subnormal response to hypotension and stress is commonly observed in patients with central adrenal insufficiency.

The most appropriate management, therefore, is to treat this patient with stress doses of hydrocortisone. Glucocorticoid deficiency is associated with increased morbidity and mortality in critically ill patients. When the diagnosis is highly suspected, especially in the proper clinical setting (including previous exposure to glucocorticoids), treatment should be instituted immediately, even if the diagnosis cannot be firmly established in a timely manner.

In a stable patient, an ACTH stimulation test would be an appropriate study to assess for adrenal suppression caused by exogenous glucocorticoids. However, in a patient with likely adrenal insufficiency and vasomotor instability, immediate treatment is indicated before further study.

Although the patient is at risk for a hospital-acquired infection, possibly with a pseudomonal infection, even adequate antibiotic treatment may not be successful without treating his possible adrenal insufficiency.

Continued therapy with intravenous fluids and antibiotics is appropriate, although adding vasopressors without addressing his potential underlying adrenal suppression is not adequate therapy.

KEY POINT

- **In a critically ill patient at high risk for adrenal insufficiency, the most appropriate management is treatment with stress doses of hydrocortisone.**

Bibliography

Arafah BM. Hypothalamic pituitary adrenal function during critical illness: limitations of current assessment methods. J Clin Endocrinol Metab. 2006;91(10):3725-3745. [PMID: 16882746]

Item 56 Answer: D

Educational Objective: Interpret thyroid function studies in an older patient.

This patient should be monitored for evidence of hypothyroidism and should receive no pharmacologic therapy at present. In older persons with abnormal results on thyroid function testing, such as are seen in this patient, the tests should be repeated several times over a period of months to ensure the stability and accuracy of the results. The normal thyroid-stimulating hormone (TSH) range for most ambulatory outpatients is 0.5-5.0 microunits/mL (0.5-5.0 milliunits/L). However, the normal range is different during pregnancy and in patients older than 80 years. Several studies have shown that an elevated serum TSH level in older patients is not associated with detrimental medical outcomes (such as depressive symptoms and impaired cognitive function) but, in fact, is associated with a lower mortality rate. Although the precise numbers are somewhat controversial, the normal reference range most likely is approximately 1 to 7 microunits/mL (1-7 milliunits/L). It is now recognized that older patients generally should not be given levothyroxine solely for an elevated TSH level. A full consideration of the patient and the clinical context is necessary.

This patient is basically asymptomatic (except for mild fatigue) and in good health. His thyroid peroxidase antibody level and clinical examination findings are basically normal and thus support the concept that he does not require exogenous levothyroxine.

Most evidence to date has shown no clinical advantage of liothyronine over levothyroxine in patients requiring thyroid replacement therapy. Additionally, liothyronine and other triiodothyronine (T_3) preparations have a short half-life and have been associated with acute spikes in serum T_3 levels, which are of particular concern in older adult patients or patients with cardiac abnormalities.

A radioactive iodine test is not useful in establishing the diagnosis of hypothyroidism and thus is inappropriate in this patient.

KEY POINT

- **Older patients generally should not be given levothyroxine solely for an elevated thyroid-stimulating hormone level.**

Bibliography

Gussekloo J, van Exel E, de Craen AJ, Meinders AE, Frölich M, Westendorp RG. Thyroid status, disability and cognitive function, and survival in old age. JAMA. 2004;292(21):2591-2599. [PMID: 15572717]

Item 57 Answer: B

Educational Objective: Diagnose central hypothyroidism after pituitary irradiation.

This patient most likely has central hypothyroidism and should have her serum free thyroxine (T_4) level measured. Her hypopituitarism is a result of the radiation therapy she received as part of her treatment of a pituitary adenoma. Her symptoms are typical of hypothyroidism, and the signs and symptoms of central hypothyroidism are similar to those of primary hypothyroidism. However, the biochemical diagnosis of central hypothyroidism is established differently because patients may have either a low-normal to overtly low serum thyroid-stimulating hormone (TSH) level. Therefore, the diagnosis is made based on measurement of a low free T_4 level in association with both a low to low-normal TSH level and clinical symptoms suggestive of hypothyroidism. This patient's mild hyponatremia may be caused by her hypothyroidism and should improve with T_4 replacement. In a patient with central hypothyroidism who takes levothyroxine replacement therapy, the goal should be achievement of a normal free T_4 level because monitoring the TSH value is not useful.

Measuring this patient's morning serum cortisol level is inappropriate management because she is receiving glucocorticoid replacement therapy for adrenal insufficiency, which guarantees that the cortisol level will be low.

A random measurement of the serum growth hormone (GH) level is not useful in the assessment of GH deficiency. A serum insulin-like growth factor 1 level would be useful for assessing GH production.

Measurement of this patient's serum luteinizing hormone level will not be useful because the oral contraceptive agent she is taking will have lowered her gonadotropin levels.

KEY POINT

- **The diagnosis of central hypothyroidism is made on the basis of the serum free thyroxine (T_4) level.**

Bibliography

Darzy KH, Shalet SM. Hypopituitarism following radiotherapy. Pituitary. 2009;12(1):40-50. [PMID: 18270844]

Item 58 Answer: E

H

Educational Objective: Manage diabetic ketoacidosis.

This patient should first be admitted to the intensive care unit for administration of intravenous fluids and insulin for management of severe diabetic ketoacidosis (DKA) and subsequently have serial abdominal examinations. She has reduced her insulin intake for the past 2 days while she was not feeling well. The insulin requirement usually is increased while a patient is under the stress imposed by illness. Her serum bicarbonate level is now substantially less than 15 meq/L (15 mmol/L), and she has generalized abdominal pain in the absence of specific intra-abdominal findings on physical examination. These findings are common in DKA, with just under half of patients reporting abdominal pain. Serial abdominal examinations are necessary to determine if her abdominal symptoms improve as her ketoacidosis resolves.

H CONT.

The severity of the abdominal pain is related to the degree of metabolic acidosis. In the absence of localized findings, imaging with CT or other invasive procedures, such as laparotomy or endoscopic retrograde cholangiopancreatography, should be considered only if the patient's abdominal pain does not resolve with correction of the acidosis.

DKA also often causes an elevated leukocyte count, an elevated amylase level, and a less-than-normal temperature, all of which this patient has. However, none of these findings reliably suggests infection, and no obvious source of infection is evident. Imipenem thus should not be started.

KEY POINT

- **Diabetic ketoacidosis can cause generalized abdominal pain, leukocytosis, and hyperamylasemia.**

Bibliography

Umpierrez G, Freire AX. Abdominal pain in patients with hyperglycemic crises. J Crit Care. 2002;17(1):63-67. [PMID: 12040551]

Item 59 Answer: D

Educational Objective: Manage secondary osteoporosis.

The most appropriate next step in management is to screen this 55-year-old man for celiac disease as part of the evaluation for secondary causes of his low bone mass and fracture. This patient has a history of fragility fracture (fracture sustained in a fall from a standing height), and his bone density results show osteopenia. In an otherwise healthy 55-year-old man, these findings raise concern for a secondary cause of his low bone mass and fragility fracture. Half of the men with osteoporosis will have an identifiable cause. Therefore, screening guided by history and physical examination findings may include testing for hypogonadism, vitamin D deficiency, primary hyperparathyroidism, calcium malabsorption, and multiple myeloma. Measurement of 24-hour urine calcium excretion while the patient consumes 1000 mg/d of calcium also may be useful. Low values for urine calcium may indicate calcium malabsorption, which can be seen in celiac disease. In light of this patient's low BMI, fragility fracture, and history of iron deficiency anemia, celiac disease is a concern, even if gastrointestinal symptoms are absent.

Initiation of alendronate or teriparatide can be considered after the evaluation for secondary causes is completed. These agents will be more effective once the secondary cause of low bone mass has been corrected.

Repeating the bone density test in 1 year without any intervention now would allow time for additional bone loss to occur and thus would not be the best management.

KEY POINT

- **Low urine calcium excretion in a patient with a fragility fracture may indicate calcium malabsorption.**

Bibliography

Bours SP, van Geel TA, Geusens PP, et al. Contributors to secondary osteoporosis and metabolic bone diseases in patients presenting with a clinical fracture. J Clin Endocrinol Metab. 2011;96(5):1360-1367. [PMID: 21411547]

Item 60 Answer: A

Educational Objective: Diagnose the cause of acute adrenal insufficiency.

This patient most likely has an adrenal hemorrhage. Acute adrenal insufficiency can result from hemorrhage (spontaneous, after trauma or anticoagulation), emboli (atrial fibrillation), and sepsis (particularly secondary to meningococcemia). Patients typically have abdominal, back, or flank pain; hypotension; fever; and nausea and vomiting. The diagnosis also is suggested by the laboratory findings of hyponatremia, hyperkalemia, and a low hematocrit. This patient developed flank pain, hypotension, nausea, fatigue, and dizziness 2 weeks after knee replacement surgery, and her physical examination and laboratory findings include orthostatic changes in her blood pressure and pulse, hyponatremia, hyperkalemia, and a low hematocrit. Of note, she has been receiving an anticoagulant since surgery, which most likely caused bleeding. After blood samples are drawn for measurement of cortisol and adrenocorticotropic hormone levels, she should be treated immediately for adrenal insufficiency with hydrocortisone and intravenous fluids. Abdominal CT and additional laboratory testing can be performed at a later stage, if necessary, to confirm the diagnosis.

Although gastrointestinal bleeding could explain the patient's hypotension, fatigue, and anemia, it does not explain the rest of her clinical and electrolyte findings.

Similarly, neither a narcotic overdose nor septic shock explains the sudden onset of flank pain, anemia, hyponatremia, and hyperkalemia.

KEY POINT

- **A decreasing hematocrit, hypotension, hyponatremia, hyperkalemia, and acute onset of abdominal, back, or flank pain suggest adrenal insufficiency secondary to an adrenal hemorrhage.**

Bibliography

Bornstein SR. Predisposing factors for adrenal insufficiency. N Engl J Med. 2009;360(22):2328-2339. [PMID: 19474430]

Item 61 Answer: C

Educational Objective: Diagnose hypothyroidism in a critically ill patient.

This patient most likely has hypothyroidism, which is strongly suggested by his exceedingly high serum thyroid-stimulating hormone (TSH) level and his low free thyroxine (T_4) and total triiodothyronine (T_3) levels. Additionally, he has been taking amiodarone, which causes hypothyroidism in approximately 10% of North Americans who take it chronically and hyperthyroidism in approximately 1%. Although the role that this patient's hypothyroidism is playing in his medical condition cannot be determined with certainty, judicious administration of exogenous levothyroxine may help his general metabolism, his ability to respond beneficially to corticosteroids, and his hypotension.

Adrenal insufficiency alone is an unlikely explanation for this patient's laboratory test results and clinical presentation. The patient's random serum cortisol level is not consistent with frank adrenal insufficiency, and his TSH level is elevated. Adrenal insufficiency is rare in critically ill patients but must be considered in those with septic shock, who may develop severe, protracted hypotension that is not responsive to standard therapy. Most of these patients have elevated serum total and free cortisol levels. A recent study showed that hydrocortisone therapy (300 mg/d) given to patients with septic shock did not influence mortality but resulted in a faster reversal of shock. Such therapy is not directed at treating an adrenal dysfunction, but rather at controlling the associated overwhelming inflammatory response.

Nonthyroidal illness can alter the results of thyroid function tests, an effect referred to as euthyroid sick syndrome, which is more common in critically ill patients. The mechanisms by which nonthyroidal illness cause thyroid function test abnormalities are unknown but could relate to the systemic release of multiple cytokines. However, the serum TSH level is not expected to increase to greater than 10 microunits/mL (10 milliunits/L) in a patient with nonthyroidal illness, except perhaps in the recovery phase of a serious illness. This patient is acutely and seriously ill, is not in the recovery phase of a serious illness, and has a TSH level of 16 microunits/mL (16 milliunits/L).

A TSH-secreting pituitary tumor is typically associated with inappropriately elevated serum free T_4 and total T_3 levels; this patient's levels are low.

KEY POINT

- **Hypothyroidism is characterized by an elevated thyroid-stimulating hormone level in the setting of low triiodothyronine (T_3) and thyroxine (T_4) levels and is a common side effect of amiodarone therapy.**

Bibliography

Adler SM, Wartofsky L. The nonthyroidal illness syndrome. Endocrinol Metab Clin North Am. 2007;36(3):657-672. [PMID: 17673123]

Item 62 Answer: D

Educational Objective: Diagnose hyperandrogenism in a patient with a neoplasm.

The most appropriate next diagnostic test is transvaginal ultrasonography to examine this patient's ovaries. Her history and physical examination findings are consistent with hyperandrogenism. Her total testosterone level is elevated, and her dehydroepiandrosterone sulfate (DHEAS) level is normal. In healthy women, the ovaries and adrenal glands contribute equally to testosterone production. However, a testosterone level greater than 200 ng/dL (6.9 nmol/L) in a woman with rapid onset of hyperandrogenic symptoms (increased hirsutism in a short period of time and clitoromegaly) suggests an ovarian neoplasm, which is best diagnosed with a transvaginal ultrasound.

Dehydroepiandrosterone is produced primarily in the adrenal glands and is sulfated in the adrenal glands, liver, and small intestine to become DHEAS. Levels greater than 7.0 micrograms/mL (18.9 micromoles/L) strongly suggest an adrenal source of androgens. In this patient, whose DHEAS level is only 2.9 micrograms/mL (7.8 micromoles/L), imaging of the adrenals would be the next step only if the transvaginal ultrasound showed no ovarian neoplasm.

A free testosterone measurement is not needed because this patient's history and physical examination findings do not suggest an abnormality in her sex hormone–binding globulin level that would make the total testosterone measurement suspect.

Because elevated androgen levels in women have either an ovarian or an adrenal source, a pituitary MRI would not be useful in this patient.

KEY POINT

- **In a woman with rapid onset of hyperandrogenic symptoms, especially if her testosterone level is greater than 200 ng/dL (6.9 nmol/L), an ovarian neoplasm is likely and is best diagnosed with a transvaginal ultrasound.**

Bibliography

Martin KA, Chang RJ, Ehrmann DA, et al. Evaluation and treatment of hirsutism in premenopausal women: an Endocrine Society clinical practice guideline. J Clin Endocrinol Metab. 2008;93(4):1105-1120. [PMID: 18252793]

Item 63 Answer: A

H

Educational Objective: Treat a hospitalized patient who has diabetes mellitus with basal insulin.

This patient should begin receiving insulin glargine (once daily) and insulin aspart (before each meal) after surgery. A patient with long-standing type 1 diabetes mellitus makes no endogenous insulin and needs a flexible insulin regimen that includes half his daily requirements as a basal insulin (such as insulin glargine) and the rest as boluses of rapid-acting insulin (such as insulin aspart) before meals.

H CONT.

Neither intravenous nor subcutaneous insulin infusions are necessary in this patient, and both would likely require his transfer to the intensive care unit for safe administration.

Given his unpredictable levels of activity and eating while in the hospital, restoring the patient's previous outpatient dosage of premixed insulin is inappropriate.

A sliding scale that does not include basal insulin and does not begin insulin administration unless the blood glucose level is at or above 150 mg/dL (8.3 mmol/L) will cause wide swings from hyperglycemia to hypoglycemia and thus is inappropriate treatment for this patient.

KEY POINT

- **A sliding scale insulin regimen that includes no basal insulin is inappropriate for a hospitalized patient with diabetes mellitus.**

Bibliography

Queale WS, Seidler AJ, Brancati FL. Glycemic control and sliding scale insulin use in medical inpatients with diabetes mellitus. Arch Intern Med. 1997;157(5):545-552. [PMID: 9066459]

Item 64 Answer: A

Educational Objective: Treat a macroprolactinoma.

This patient has a macroprolactinoma, and administration of a dopamine agonist, such as cabergoline, is indicated as the initial treatment. Hyperprolactinemia can cause galactorrhea, oligomenorrhea, and amenorrhea in premenopausal women; erectile dysfunction in men; and decreased libido, infertility, and osteopenia in both sexes. Large tumors also may cause mass effects, which are often the presenting feature in men and postmenopausal women. This patient has amenorrhea and galactorrhea in the setting of a markedly elevated serum prolactin level. The MRI shows a pituitary mass greater than 1 cm that extends to the optic chiasm. These radiographic findings are consistent with a macroprolactinoma with chiasmal compression. The visual field examination indicates that the mass is not currently compressing the chiasm to the point of visual loss. Dopamine agonists normalize prolactin levels, correct amenorrhea and galactorrhea, and decrease tumor size by more than 50% in 80% to 90% of patients. They are used as first-line therapy, unless visual field loss is significant and progressive. Even with mild visual loss, dopamine agonists are usually used as first-line treatment. Cabergoline is generally more efficacious and better tolerated, although more expensive, than bromocriptine.

An oral contraceptive agent will replace gonadal corticosteroids and lead to menstruation but will not reduce tumor size. Simple replacement of estrogen with oral contraceptives is inappropriate therapy in this patient but may be preferable treatment in women with idiopathic hyperprolactinemia or microprolactinomas who do not desire fertility but are estrogen deficient. Because prolactinomas have estrogen receptors, tumor growth resulting from estrogen replacement therapy is possible. However, with the dosages routinely used in oral contraceptives, this growth is very uncommon.

Surgery is appropriate only in patients with resistance or intolerance to dopamine agonists, with a primarily cystic tumor, or with acute and unstable deterioration of vision. Radiation therapy, including stereotactic radiosurgery, is used even less commonly for prolactinomas but is indicated for macroprolactinomas that do not respond to either medical or surgical treatment.

KEY POINT

- **In a patient with a macroprolactinoma, administration of a dopamine agonist, such as cabergoline, is indicated as the initial treatment.**

Bibliography

Melmed S, Casanueva FF, Hoffman AR, et al; Endocrine Society. Diagnosis and treatment of hyperprolactinemia: an Endocrine Society clinical practice guideline. J Clin Endocrinol Metab. 2011;96(2):273-288. [PMID: 21296991]

Item 65 Answer: B

Educational Objective: Treat profound hypoglycemia in an older patient.

This patient with probable hypoglycemia should have a fingerstick measurement of her blood glucose level. Older patients who take sulfonylureas with long half-lives can have high drug levels in their blood because of decreased clearance, which results in profound and prolonged hypoglycemia. Hypoglycemia should be suspected in any patient with diabetes who has focal neurologic signs and is sweating. The fact that her average hemoglobin A_{1c} level is well below 7.0% further indicates an increased risk for hypoglycemia. Additionally, the patient has not been eating and drinking adequately since her amputation, which also can contribute to the development of hypoglycemia. Hypoglycemia can cause various neurologic findings, including coma and hemiplegia. The most immediate step is to measure her blood glucose level and, if hypoglycemia is present, treat her with glucose to prevent permanent neurologic disability.

This patient has a slight fever but not enough evidence of septicemia to justify starting empiric antibiotic therapy with vancomycin and ceftriaxone. Additionally, septicemia is unlikely to be the cause of a left hemiplegia.

If the patient does not have hypoglycemia, alternative diagnoses can be considered, including stroke. In patients with stroke, a noncontrast head CT to exclude intracerebral hemorrhage is necessary before the administration of thrombolytic drugs, such as recombinant tissue plasminogen activator. However, hypoglycemia should first be excluded as a diagnosis before a head CT or thrombolytic administration.

KEY POINT

- **Older patients who take sulfonylureas with long half-lives can develop profound hypoglycemia, which can be reversed by an infusion of glucose.**

Bibliography

Chiniwala N, Jabbour S. Management of diabetes mellitus in the elderly. Curr Opin Endocrinol Diabetes Obes. 2011;18(2):148-152. [PMID: 21522002]

Item 66 Answer: D

Educational Objective: Treat a multinodular goiter.

This patient should undergo thyroidectomy. In iodine-sufficient areas of the world, multinodular goiter is an idiopathic condition characterized by both solid and partially cystic thyroid nodules that is more common in older persons. Over time, the goiter generally grows and may require treatment. Fine-needle aspiration biopsy is used to exclude cancer in this generally benign condition and has excluded it in this patient. However, goiter growth can lead to impingement of the goiter on the trachea, esophagus, or recurrent laryngeal nerve and result in dyspnea, stridor, chronic cough, a sensation of fullness or pressure, dysphagia, or hoarseness. Hyperthyroidism also may develop if one (or more) of the nodules becomes autonomous and large enough to produce sufficient thyroid hormone to suppress thyroid-stimulating hormone (TSH) and render the patient thyrotoxic. This patient's recent symptoms are most likely due to impingement. Therefore, thyroid surgery is indicated because the local compressive symptoms are prominent and clinically significant.

No evidence of the effectiveness of external-beam radiation therapy for benign thyroid disease has been shown, which makes the therapy inappropriate in this patient.

Levothyroxine will further suppress the TSH level and may render the patient thyrotoxic. The previous practice of giving patients levothyroxine to shrink thyroid nodules has been abandoned because of its inefficacy and the morbidities associated with iatrogenic thyrotoxicosis.

Methimazole is a thioamide drug used to treat hyperthyroidism. Although this patient has a low-normal TSH level, she is not frankly thyrotoxic. Therefore, treating her with an antithyroid medication is unnecessary and will have no effect on goiter size.

In select circumstances, radioactive iodine (^{131}I) can be used to modestly decrease the size of a multinodular goiter but is not a first-line option in the United States, except in patients with thyrotoxicosis due to autonomous function. In a patient with a suppressed TSH level, this therapy will preferentially address the hyperfunctioning areas and spare those regions not visualized on imaging. As a result, the ultimate effect on goiter size may be unpredictable.

KEY POINT

- **In patients with impingement of a multinodular goiter on the trachea, esophagus, or recurrent laryngeal nerve, a thyroidectomy is indicated if local compressive symptoms are prominent and clinically significant.**

Bibliography

Bahn RS, Castro MR. Approach to the patient with nontoxic multinodular goiter. J Clin Endocrinol Metab. 2011;96(5):1202-1212. [PMID: 21543434]

Item 67 Answer: A

Educational Objective: Treat painful diabetic neuropathy.

This patient should be treated with desipramine. He is experiencing an acute episode of painful diabetic neuropathy that developed after a period of poor glycemic control. This disorder involves acute segmental demyelination in the peripheral sensory nerves. Remyelination and recovery can occur if excellent glycemic control (hemoglobin A_{1c} level <7.0%) is established and maintained for several months. Relief of symptoms often is obtained by administering a low-dose tricyclic antidepressant, such as desipramine; topical application of capsaicin cream is also appropriate.

Fluoxetine and other selective serotonin reuptake inhibitors are ineffective for treating painful diabetic neuropathy and should not be used in this patient.

Nerve conduction studies might show marked slowing of nerve conduction, and a sural nerve biopsy would confirm the presence of segmental demyelination. These diagnostic tests, however, are unnecessary in a patient in whom the diagnosis of acute painful diabetic neuropathy is so likely, given his compatible history and physical examination findings.

Starting a potentially addictive and dangerous drug (such as oxycodone), especially when used for prolonged periods, is inappropriate therapy for a condition that may well be self-limiting.

KEY POINT

- **Symptoms of painful diabetic neuropathy can be treated with a low-dose tricyclic antidepressant and topical application of capsaicin cream.**

Bibliography

Hovaguimian A, Gibbons CH. Clinical approach to the treatment of painful diabetic neuropathy. Ther Adv Endocrinol Metab. 2011;2(1):27-38. [PMID: 21709806]

Item 68 Answer: D

Educational Objective: Diagnose thyroid lymphoma.

This patient most likely has primary thyroid lymphoma. A benign goiter would not grow this rapidly and is unlikely to be associated with local symptoms. Thyroid lymphoma occurs most frequently in older patients who have a history of Hashimoto thyroiditis. Primary thyroid lymphoma typically presents as an enlarging neck mass, often with evidence of local compression of adjacent structures (such as dysphagia, hoarseness, stridor, jugular vein distention, and facial edema) and systemic symptoms ("B" symptoms) of lymphoma (such as fever, weight loss, and night sweats). A thyroid fine-needle aspiration (FNA) biopsy can suggest the diagnosis, but a core-needle or excisional biopsy is often needed to establish the diagnosis of lymphoma. Most primary thyroid lymphomas are mucosa-associated lymphoid tumors and respond to systemic chemotherapy. This patient's distended bilateral cervical neck veins suggest obstruction at the level of the thoracic inlet (that is, the thyroid gland).

Bleeding into the thyroid gland is unlikely because the gland is firm on physical examination, without any evidence of fluctuance, and the thyroid ultrasound shows heterogeneous echotexture rather than a cystic mass. Additionally, the patient has Hashimoto thyroiditis (which can predispose to lymphoma), has no history of neck trauma, and was not taking an anticoagulant medication.

With medullary and papillary thyroid cancers, the thyroid gland most likely would contain specific thyroid nodules. These cancers generally grow relatively slowly.

KEY POINT

- **Thyroid lymphoma occurs most frequently in older patients with a history of Hashimoto thyroiditis and typically presents as an enlarging neck mass, often with local and systemic symptoms.**

Bibliography

Graff-Baker A, Sosa JA, Roman SA. Primary thyroid lymphoma: a review of recent developments in diagnosis and histology-driven treatment. Curr Opin Oncol. 2010;22(1):17-22. [PMID: 19844180]

Item 69 Answer: B

Educational Objective: Manage hypopituitarism associated with Sheehan syndrome.

This patient should receive hydrocortisone as initial treatment. Given her low morning serum cortisol level, this patient has adrenal insufficiency, which makes immediate glucocorticoid therapy with hydrocortisone the most appropriate treatment. Her history and biochemical findings are consistent with hypopituitarism due to Sheehan syndrome, which involves pituitary infarction or hemorrhage in the setting of a complicated delivery, particularly one associated with significant blood loss and hypotension. The patient has no history suggestive of a preexisting pituitary lesion, so the pituitary insult most likely occurred at delivery. Nevertheless, pituitary imaging is appropriate to assess for a sellar mass. The cardinal signs of hypopituitarism due to Sheehan syndrome are subacute, progressive hypopituitarism; an inability to lactate because of prolactin deficiency; and amenorrhea. Central adrenal insufficiency is the primary cause of mortality in Sheehan syndrome.

Although loss of anterior pituitary hormones is common, the development of diabetes insipidus is rare in Sheehan syndrome. Additionally, the patient's clinical and laboratory findings are not consistent with this diagnosis. Therefore, arginine vasopressin replacement therapy is not indicated.

The hyponatremia in this patient is likely related to the hypopituitarism, and the serum sodium level should normalize with pituitary hormone replacement. The hyponatremia is not severe enough or sufficiently symptomatic to warrant aggressive management with hypertonic saline.

This patient could have central hypothyroidism. If her serum free thyroxine level is low, despite her normal serum thyroid-stimulating hormone level, levothyroxine should be administered. However, thyroid hormone replacement is not urgent because she does not have signs of severe hypothyroidism. Therefore, the diagnosis and management of central hypothyroidism should wait until after her adrenal insufficiency is treated with glucocorticoid replacement therapy.

KEY POINT

- **Patients with Sheehan syndrome and adrenal insufficiency should receive immediate glucocorticoid therapy because central adrenal insufficiency is the primary cause of mortality in Sheehan syndrome.**

Bibliography

Kristjansdottir HL, Bodvarsdottir SP, Sigurjonsdottir HA. Sheehan's syndrome in modern times: a nationwide retrospective study in Iceland. Eur J Endocrinol. 2011;164(3):349-354. [PMID: 21183555]

Item 70 Answer: D

Educational Objective: Manage fasting hypoglycemia in a patient without diabetes mellitus.

This patient should undergo a psychiatric evaluation. In a person without diabetes mellitus who has laboratory-documented hypoglycemia, the finding of an inappropriately high serum insulin level and a suppressed serum C-peptide level suggests that the hypoglycemia is due to an exogenous injection of insulin. Some patients with psychiatric issues (such as a history of depression) engage in the use of hypoglycemic agents prescribed to others, frequently as an attention-seeking behavior. Given her mother's diabetic treatment, she has ready access to both insulin and an oral hypoglycemic agent, and her negative sulfonylurea screen indicates that glyburide is not the causative agent. A psychiatric evaluation is critical in establishing a diagnosis and developing a treatment plan to address her dangerous behavior.

Although abdominal CT is an effective means of detecting the presence of an insulinoma, her laboratory study results are inconsistent with endogenous insulin secretion from an insulinoma. If she had an insulinoma, both serum insulin and C-peptide levels would be inappropriately high in the presence of hypoglycemia.

An octreotide scan may be helpful in detecting and localizing primary and metastatic neuroendocrine tumors. Octreotide scanning is particularly useful in diagnosing specific tumors of neural crest origin, particularly neoplasms that express increased levels of somatostatin receptors, such as carcinoid tumors. This study may also have a role in localizing insulin-secreting tumors that are not visible on usual studies (MRIs or CT scans). However, in this patient with a low suspicion for insulinoma, an octreotide scan would not be an appropriate initial study.

Altered gastric emptying, particularly in persons with surgical changes in the stomach and proximal small bowel (as occur with some forms of bariatric surgery), may cause clinical symptoms consistent with relative hypoglycemia (late dumping syndrome). However, this is rarely associated with clinically significant hypoglycemia in an otherwise healthy person. Without a history of altered gastrointestinal anatomy or an underlying disease that might lead to abnormal gastric function (such as diabetes), a gastric emptying study is not indicated.

KEY POINT

- **In a person without diabetes mellitus who has laboratory-documented hypoglycemia, the finding of an inappropriately high serum insulin level and a suppressed C-peptide level suggests that the hypoglycemia is due to an exogenous injection of insulin.**

Bibliography

Cryer PE, Axelrod L, Grossman AB, et al; Endocrine Society. Evaluation and management of adult hypoglycemic disorders: an Endocrine Society clinical practice guideline. J Clin Endocrinol Metab. 2009;94(3):709-728. [PMID: 19088155]

Item 71 Answer: C

Educational Objective: Manage an asymptomatic incidental adrenal mass.

This patient should have repeat testing in 6 to 12 months. She has an incidentally discovered 2.5-cm adrenal mass with no clinical or biochemical features indicating excess hormonal secretion of glucocorticoids, mineralocorticoids, or adrenal androgens by the adrenal cortex or of catecholamines by the medulla. Neither the size (<4 cm) nor the imaging characteristics (an attenuation <20 Hounsfield units) of this adrenal mass suggest possible malignancy. Therefore, observation and repeat testing in 6 to 12 months would be the most appropriate management.

Incidentally discovered adrenal masses are a common finding on imaging obtained for other purposes. Routine evaluation is assessment of possible malignancy based on the size of the lesion and other radiographic findings (including shape, homogeneity, attenuation, and contrast washout) and of possible biochemical function. Clinical evidence of a possible functional lesion should be sought, including evidence of hypertension, electrolyte abnormalities, or glucocorticoid excess. In the early stages of their disease, some patients with pheochromocytoma or Cushing syndrome may have no obvious clinical manifestations. Thus, all patients with incidental adrenal masses should be screened for those two entities, and those who also have hypertension should be screened for hyperaldosteronism. Pheochromocytoma usually is evaluated with a 24-hour urine collection of catecholamines and Cushing syndrome with a low-dose dexamethasone suppression test. Screening for hyperaldosteronism involves determining the ratio of serum aldosterone to plasma renin activity.

Because this patient is not hypertensive and has no clinical or biochemical evidence of excess catecholamine secretion, a pheochromocytoma is unlikely. Therefore, a metaiodobenzylguanidine(MIBG) scan is neither warranted nor necessary.

Similarly, obtaining an MRI in this patient who already had a CT scan would offer no additional diagnostic information and thus would be unwarranted.

This asymptomatic patient who has a nonfunctioning 2.5-cm adrenal mass with unremarkable imaging characteristics also has no indications for surgical intervention.

KEY POINT

- **Incidentally discovered adrenal masses that are small, are associated with no clinical or biochemical features suggestive of excess hormonal secretion, and have no imaging features suggestive of possible malignancy should be followed with observation and repeat testing in 6 to 12 months.**

Bibliography

Nieman LK. Approach to the patient with an adrenal incidentaloma. J Clin Endocrinol Metab. 2010;95(9):4106-4113. [PMID: 20823463]

Item 72 Answer: D

Educational Objective: Diagnose thyroid storm.

H

This patient most likely is experiencing thyroid storm, which is an exaggerated state of thyrotoxicosis. Although some overlap exists, thyroid storm can be differentiated from other forms of thyrotoxicosis by the presence of temperature elevation, significant tachycardia, heart failure, abdominal discomfort, diarrhea, nausea, vomiting, and (sometimes) jaundice. Neurologically, agitation and disorientation can occur. Serum free thyroxine (T_4) and serum triiodothyronine (T_3) levels are elevated in both thyrotoxicosis and thyroid storm, but generally more so in thyroid storm. Thyroid storm most commonly occurs in patients

H CONT.

who have untreated hyperthyroidism or are not adherent to their treatment regimen for the disorder but may be precipitated by surgery, trauma, or administration of radiocontrast agents with significant amounts of iodine. Treatment typically consists of a combination of antithyroid drugs (propylthiouracil or methimazole), iodine solution, high-dose corticosteroids, β-blockers, and (rarely) lithium. Even with aggressive therapy and supportive measures, mortality rates are as high as 15% to 20%.

Euthyroid sick syndrome does not cause these symptoms and signs of hyperthyroidism or these elevations in free T_4 and total T_3 levels. Furthermore, this patient's history of Graves disease makes euthyroid sick syndrome an unlikely diagnosis.

Myxedema coma is another life-threatening thyroid emergency characterized by the combination of mental status changes, hypothermia, hypoventilation, and hyponatremia in a patient whose clinical picture is consistent with hypothyroidism. This patient's T_3 and T_4 levels are markedly elevated, which excludes the diagnosis of hypothyroidism, and he is hyperthermic, not hypothermic.

Subacute (de Quervain) thyroiditis entails transient destruction of thyroid tissue, which leads to disruption of follicles and release of preformed thyroid hormone into the circulation that may initially cause hyperthyroidism and eventually may result in hypothyroidism. Subacute thyroiditis is thought to occur after a viral infection and usually involves thyroid tenderness, which this patient does not have. In addition, this patient is critically ill from his hyperthyroidism, which is unusual in subacute thyroiditis.

KEY POINT

- **Thyroid storm can be differentiated from other forms of thyrotoxicosis by the presence of temperature elevation, significant tachycardia, heart failure, abdominal discomfort, diarrhea, nausea, vomiting, and (sometimes) jaundice.**

Bibliography

Nayak B, Burman K. Thyrotoxicosis and thyroid storm. Endocrinol Metab Clin North Am. 2006;35(4):663-686. [PMID: 17127140]

Item 73 Answer: A

Educational Objective: **Counsel a woman about the risks of gestational diabetes mellitus.**

This patient's infant has an increased risk of childhood obesity. Gestational diabetes mellitus is hyperglycemia occurring during pregnancy and is typically identified in the second trimester. This disorder represents the inability of a woman's beta cells to adequately compensate for the degree of insulin resistance associated with various placenta-derived factors. The diagnosis of gestational diabetes is usually made on the basis of an oral glucose tolerance test, although no consensus exists at this time on the diagnostic thresholds. It has been recently recognized that the offspring of mothers who have prepregnancy obesity and develop gestational diabetes during pregnancy are at increased risk for childhood obesity. The reason for this is not clear but may involve a combination of genetic factors and maternal imprinting of genes during intrauterine life.

Women with gestational diabetes are likely to develop the disorder during future pregnancies and are at increased risk for type 2 diabetes later in life, with some estimates placing the risk of the latter as high as 50% over 10 years.

Several genetic syndromes that are collectively known as maturity-onset diabetes of the young (MODY) develop early in life (teens to early 20s). The pattern of inheritance is autosomal dominant. Several described subtypes of MODY are associated with specific genetic defects in enzymes or transcription factors affecting beta-cell function but not with gestational diabetes.

Type 1 diabetes mellitus mainly affects lean children, teenagers, and young adults. The disorder is characterized by absolute insulin deficiency from selective autoimmune destruction of insulin-secreting pancreatic beta cells. In type 1A diabetes, one or more autoantibodies directed against the beta cells or their products (such as anti–glutamic acid decarboxylase, anti–islet cell autoantigen 512, and anti-insulin antibodies) usually can be detected. Type 1B diabetes is idiopathic, has no autoimmune markers, and occurs more commonly in persons of Asian or African descent. Neither type 1A nor type 1B diabetes is associated with gestational diabetes.

KEY POINT

- **The offspring of mothers with prepregnancy obesity and gestational diabetes mellitus are at increased risk for childhood obesity.**

Bibliography

Landon MB, Gabbe SG. Gestational diabetes mellitus. Obstet Gynecol. 2011;118(6):1379-1393. [PMID: 22105269]

Item 74 Answer: C

Educational Objective: **Diagnose acromegaly.**

This patient's historical and clinical findings suggest a diagnosis of acromegaly, and this diagnosis should be confirmed by measurement of the serum insulin-like growth factor 1 (IGF-1) level. Acromegaly is due to hypersecretion of growth hormone (GH) and is most commonly caused by a pituitary adenoma. High GH levels stimulate the liver to produce excess IGF-1, and both GH and IGF-1 circulate in the blood, causing the systemic effects of acromegaly. IGF-1 is an integrated measure of GH secretion, and thus measuring the serum IGF-1 level is the single best test for making the diagnosis of acromegaly. A normal serum IGF-1 level rules out acromegaly.

An MRI can show a pituitary adenoma but cannot diagnose acromegaly. After the diagnosis has been established, however, an MRI is necessary to determine the size and location of the pituitary adenoma.

GH is usually secreted episodically in pulses. Therefore, a single random measurement of the serum GH level is not useful in diagnosing acromegaly. GH hypersecretion is autonomous in acromegaly, and GH levels are not suppressible by hyperglycemia, as they normally would be. An oral glucose tolerance test also can be useful in establishing a diagnosis in a patient in whom the diagnosis of acromegaly is not clear.

Although prolactin often is cosecreted by GH-producing tumors, measuring the serum prolactin level is not useful in making the diagnosis of acromegaly because it is neither sensitive nor specific for the disease.

KEY POINT

- **Insulin-like growth factor 1 (IGF-1) is an integrated measure of growth hormone secretion, and thus measuring the serum IGF-1 level is the single best test for making the diagnosis of acromegaly.**

Bibliography

Katznelson L, Atkinson JL, Cook DM, Ezzat SZ, Hamrahian AH, Miller KK; American Association of Clinical Endocrinologists. American Association of Clinical Endocrinologists medical guidelines for clinical practice for the diagnosis and treatment of acromegaly—2011 update. Endocr Pract. 2011;17(Suppl 4):1-44. [PMID: 21846616]

Item 75 Answer: C

Educational Objective: **Manage hypocalcemia in a malnourished patient with alcoholism.**

This patient should next have his serum magnesium level measured. He has a history of chronic alcohol abuse and serum chemistry results that are notable for hypocalcemia. Evidence of tetany and a corrected QT interval prolongation are indications for aggressive intravenous repletion of calcium. In this patient with alcohol abuse and symptomatic hypocalcemia, hypomagnesemia should be suspected. Hypomagnesemia in the setting of severe hypocalcemia should be treated promptly with intravenous magnesium to help increase serum calcium levels and prevent ventricular arrhythmias. In addition, hypomagnesemia can impair the ability to increase serum calcium levels because low levels of magnesium inhibit parathyroid hormone (PTH) secretion and induce resistance to PTH. Therefore, in addition to increasing the patient's serum calcium level, treatment of his hypomagnesemia is essential to restore normal parathyroid function.

Measurement of the serum calcitonin level is typically not helpful in the assessment of hypocalcemia because calcitonin plays only a minor role in calcium homeostasis in humans.

This patient most likely is vitamin D deficient because of poor nutrition associated with his alcohol abuse. Measurement of the serum 1,25-dihydroxyvitamin D level is unlikely to provide useful information regarding the exact cause of his hypocalcemia, and, in any case, measurement of the serum 25-hydroxyvitamin D level would be the more appropriate test.

The serum PTH level most likely would be inappropriately low in this patient as a result of his chronic alcohol abuse and hypocalcemia. Measuring this level is thus unnecessary.

KEY POINT

- **Hypomagnesemia in the setting of severe hypocalcemia should be treated promptly with intravenous magnesium to help increase serum calcium levels and prevent ventricular arrhythmias.**

Bibliography

Iwasaki Y, Asai M, Yoshida M, Oiso Y, Hashimoto K. Impaired parathyroid hormone response to hypocalcemic stimuli in a patient with hypomagnesemic hypocalcemia. J Endocrinol Invest. 2007;30(6):513-516. [PMID: 17646727]

Item 76 Answer: C

Educational Objective: **Diagnose postexercise hyperglycemia.**

This patient's significantly increased blood glucose level after running most likely results from baseline hypoinsulinemia exacerbated by the physiologic changes associated with prolonged exercise, such as stimulation of hepatic glucose release. A patient who has had type 1 diabetes mellitus for more than 20 years, including one episode of diabetic ketoacidosis, will be completely insulin deficient. Although long-acting, the treatment effect of insulin detemir does not always last a full 24 hours. The fact that his blood glucose level was 215 mg/dL (11.9 mmol/L) at bedtime the night before his run and was even higher the next morning before exercise suggests that he had low levels of insulin present in his system during the night and before starting his run. This hypoinsulinemia most likely triggered increased hepatic gluconeogenesis. In the absence of sufficient plasma insulin, the glucose could not be absorbed by the muscles and other tissues, and his blood glucose level continued to increase. Appropriate treatment is to adjust his insulin regimen to ensure adequate insulin replacement before running to minimize the expected physiologic changes associated with exercise.

Excess carbohydrate intake in the evening would likely contribute to his noted elevated bedtime and pre-exercise blood glucose levels but would not independently account for the significant rise in his blood glucose level after exercise.

Although this patient may have some degree of gastroparesis given the duration of his diabetes, this disorder is an unlikely explanation for an increased blood glucose level 12 hours or more since he last ate.

Early morning blood glucose elevations may occur in response to the nocturnal hypoglycemia associated with diabetes therapy. Although this patient had an elevated morning blood glucose level before running, his bedtime measurement also was elevated, and he took no additional insulin beyond his single dose of long-acting insulin the morning before. Therefore, nocturnal hypoglycemia is unlikely to be the cause of this patient's exercise-associated hypoglycemia.

KEY POINT

- **Hypoinsulinemia causes increased hepatic glucose output and decreased peripheral glucose uptake, which results in a higher blood glucose level and, ultimately, a higher hemoglobin A_{1c} value; prolonged exercise, which further stimulates hepatic glucose release, exacerbates this condition.**

Bibliography

Temple MY, Bar-Or O, Riddell MC. The reliability and repeatability of the blood glucose response to prolonged exercise in adolescent boys with IDDM. Diabetes Care. 1995;18(3):326-332. [PMID: 7555475]

Item 77 Answer: A

Educational Objective: **Diagnose the cause of primary ovarian insufficiency.**

Obtaining a karyotype is the most appropriate next diagnostic test because this patient has primary ovarian insufficiency, and Turner syndrome must be excluded as the cause. Primary ovarian insufficiency can be diagnosed because she has two elevated follicle-stimulating hormone (FSH) levels in the setting of amenorrhea. If evidence of Turner syndrome is found, the associated estrogen deficiency must be treated. Turner syndrome is associated with several cardiovascular malformations, including aortic valve disease, aortic dilation, and aortic coarctation; renal malformations, most commonly horseshoe kidney; and autoimmune disorders, such as thyroid disease. Therefore, cardiac imaging and kidney ultrasonography often are recommended for patients with Turner syndrome. Patients with Turner syndrome with mosaicism may have several years of normal menses before entering menopause. Turner syndrome can be associated with a short stature, stocky build, square chest, and webbed neck. This patient's short stature is the only physical examination finding consistent with Turner syndrome.

Pelvic ultrasonography is unlikely to be useful in this patient. The elevated FSH level indicates that the amenorrhea is due to decreased estradiol production from the ovaries.

A progesterone challenge test is useful when trying to determine whether a patient is in a normal or low estrogen state. Laboratory studies and clinical symptoms already have shown that this patient is in a low estrogen state, and a progesterone challenge test would not provide any additional information.

Measuring this patient's serum estradiol level will not add any additional information because the elevated FSH level indicates a low estrogen state.

KEY POINT

- **In a woman with primary ovarian insufficiency, Turner syndrome must be excluded as the cause by obtaining the patient's karyotype.**

Bibliography

Nelson LM. Clinical practice. Primary ovarian insufficiency. N Engl J Med. 2009;360(6):606-614. [PMID: 19196677]

Item 78 Answer: B

Educational Objective: **Treat hyperthyroidism in pregnancy.**

This patient should receive propylthiouracil. The symptoms, clinical findings, and presence of vitiligo suggest that she has autoimmune Graves hyperthyroidism and not gestational thyrotoxicosis. The hyperthyroidism is more severe in Graves hyperthyroidism than in gestational thyrotoxicosis and often is associated with a significantly enlarged thyroid gland, as in this patient. Although evidence of ophthalmopathy is lacking, this finding is not uncommon in Graves hyperthyroidism. Her thyroid-stimulating antibody and thyroid peroxidase antibody levels also are elevated, albeit minimally, which is consistent with this diagnosis.

Although mild hyperthyroidism in pregnancy may not require treatment, this patient has significant signs and symptoms and moderately elevated thyroid function test results. Untreated hyperthyroidism is associated with an increased risk of miscarriage, fetal growth retardation, premature delivery, and preeclampsia. The presence of maternal thyroid-stimulating antibodies also places the fetus at increased risk for neonatal hyperthyroidism, which can be life threatening. The most appropriate treatment is an antithyroid drug. A recent consensus conference suggested that propylthiouracil should be used in the first trimester of pregnancy in patients with Graves hyperthyroidism who require treatment and that methimazole be substituted in the second and third trimesters.

Methimazole is associated with an increased risk of fetal abnormalities, such as aplasia cutis and choanal atresia, when used in the first trimester. After fetal organogenesis is complete, methimazole should be used. Methimazole is the antithyroid agent of choice except in the first trimester of pregnancy, in the presence of an allergy to methimazole, or in some cases of thyroid storm. Propylthiouracil is associated with a higher risk of severe hepatotoxicity than methimazole. Close monitoring of pregnant women treated with antithyroid agents is required, as is periodic fetal thyroid ultrasonography.

Thyroidectomy is indicated in patients with a toxic adenoma, a toxic multinodular goiter, or a large malignant thyroid nodule but is not warranted in this patient with Graves hyperthyroidism.

Because of the already cited risks of untreated hyperthyroidism in pregnancy, reassurance is inadequate as initial treatment for this patient.

KEY POINT

- **In pregnant women, untreated hyperthyroidism is associated with an increased risk of miscarriage, fetal growth retardation, premature delivery, and preeclampsia.**

Bibliography

Bahn Chair RS, Burch HB, Cooper DS, et al; American Thyroid Association; American Association of Clinical Endocrinologists. Hyperthyroidism and other causes of thyrotoxicosis: management guidelines of the American Thyroid Association and American Association of Clinical Endocrinologists [erratum in Thyroid. 2011;21(10):1169]. Thyroid. 2011;21(6):593-646. [PMID: 21510801]

Item 79 Answer: C

Educational Objective: Manage delayed hypoglycemia in a patient with type 1 diabetes mellitus.

This patient should eat complex carbohydrates (at least 45 grams) at bedtime on evenings of vigorous exercise. He developed severe hypoglycemia several hours after playing basketball for 3 hours, drinking, and not eating before bedtime. Vigorous exercise depletes the muscles' glycogen stores. Although his blood glucose level was 163 mg/dL (9.0 mmol/L) just before he went to bed, his muscles continued to extract glucose from the blood for several hours to replenish their glycogen stores. The alcohol in his system inhibited the liver's ability to release glucose into the blood, and thus his plasma glucose level decreased severely while he was asleep. A substantial snack containing complex carbohydrates before bedtime would have been absorbed over several hours and thereby prevented hypoglycemia.

It is neither reasonable nor necessary to advise a fit young man with diabetes to avoid exercising in the evening.

Even light beer contains enough alcohol to inhibit hepatic glucose output. If he is willing to make the change, he should be advised to drink no alcohol on evenings of vigorous exercise.

Although omitting the insulin aspart dose might be reasonable, stopping both forms of insulin would be a poor choice. Doing so would cause his plasma glucose level to increase because of hypoinsulinemia. His plasma glucose level most likely would be extremely high by bedtime and even higher the following morning.

KEY POINT

- **In a patient with diabetes mellitus, vigorous exercise should be followed by consumption of complex carbohydrates to avoid hypoglycemia, especially when the exercise occurs in the evening.**

Bibliography

Cryer PE. The barrier of hypoglycemia in diabetes. Diabetes. 2008;57(12):3169-3176. [PMID: 19033403]

Item 80 Answer: A

Educational Objective: Treat hypopituitarism.

Glucocorticoid therapy should be started in this patient to prevent progressive adrenal insufficiency. He has hypopituitarism, given the findings of testosterone deficiency and central hypothyroidism (low serum free thyroxine and inappropriately normal serum thyroid-stimulating hormone levels). The MRI shows a suprasellar mass. Neoplastic lesions, particularly pituitary adenomas, cause hypopituitarism by direct compression of the normal pituitary gland or by disruption of the pituitary stalk. Surgery is the primary mode of therapy for tumors that warrant intervention. This patient's serum cortisol value is low normal, which suggests tenuous adrenal reserve. After thyroid hormone replacement therapy is initiated, accelerated metabolism of endogenous cortisol occurs, with induction of progressive central adrenal insufficiency. In a patient with central hypothyroidism, adrenal reserve should be evaluated; if found to be low-normal or overtly low, a glucocorticoid should be administered.

This patient has both growth hormone deficiency (low serum insulin-like growth factor 1 level) and male hypogonadism (low serum testosterone level). However, these are not as serious as the central hypothyroidism, and hormone replacement for these deficiencies can be initiated at a future time.

The patient does not have signs or symptoms of diabetes insipidus. Therefore, vasopressin replacement is not required.

KEY POINT

- **When thyroid hormone replacement therapy is initiated to treat central hypothyroidism, concomitant glucocorticoid therapy also is necessary.**

Bibliography

Grossman AB. Clinical review: The diagnosis and management of central hypoadrenalism. J Clin Endocrinol Metab. 2010;95(11):4855-4863. [PMID: 20719838]

Item 81 Answer: B

Educational Objective: Diagnose familial hyperparathyroidism.

The most likely diagnosis is multiple endocrine neoplasia type 2 (MEN2). The finding of mild hypercalcemia in a young man whose family history includes a brother with kidney stones and a father with an anesthesia-induced hypertensive crisis raises concern for MEN2. The patient likely has hyperparathyroidism, and his neck mass is most likely a medullary thyroid cancer. His history of diarrhea suggests a high serum calcitonin level caused by the medullary thyroid cancer. Undiagnosed pheochromocytoma may have been the cause of his father's death, and the brother may have hyperparathyroidism. Together, these personal and family findings suggest that this patient may belong to a MEN2 kindred. MEN2 is caused by germline transmission of a mutant *RET* proto-oncogene. The MEN2 phenotype can include primary hyperparathyroidism, pheochromocytoma, and medullary thyroid cancer. The hyperparathyroidism of MEN2 is due to benign hyperplasia involving all parathyroid glands.

Benign familial hypocalciuric hypercalcemia is a rare familial condition caused by inactivating mutations of the calcium-sensing receptor, which has a major function in regulating calcium metabolism through parathyroid tissue and renal calcium. The disorder is autosomal dominant with high penetrance. Decreased sensitivity of the calcium-sensing receptor to calcium is typical of this disorder and thus higher calcium levels are required to suppress parathyroid hormone secretion. Fractional excretion of calcium is less than 1%, despite the hypercalcemia, and the PTH level is normal or slightly elevated. The clinical significance of this disease lies mostly in its mistaken diagnosis as hyperparathyroidism. Benign hypocalciuric hypercalcemia does not explain the patient's thyroid mass or the father's probable pheochromocytoma.

Parathyroid cancer may be palpable on physical examination, but hyperplastic parathyroid glands with benign enlargement would not. Additionally, parathyroid cancer would cause more severe hypercalcemia and does not explain the patient's personal history of diarrhea or his family history.

Sarcoidosis causes hypercalcemia by production of 1,25-dihydroxyvitamin D by granulomas. This patient's neck mass and normal chest radiograph are not typical of sarcoidosis.

KEY POINT

- **The finding of mild hypercalcemia in a young patient with a family history of related endocrinopathies raises concern for multiple endocrine neoplasia type 2.**

Bibliography

Moline J, Eng C. Multiple endocrine neoplasia type 2: an overview. Genet Med. 2011;13(9):755-764. [PMID: 21552134]

Item 82 Answer: C

Educational Objective: **Manage hirsutism in polycystic ovary syndrome.**

This patient should begin taking an oral contraceptive. She has polycystic ovary syndrome (PCOS), as indicated by her irregular menses, her clinical and biochemical hyperandrogenism, and the exclusion of other possible causes. The best initial treatment for hirsutism in this population is an oral contraceptive, which decreases luteinizing hormone release through estrogen's negative feedback, thereby decreasing testosterone production by the ovary, and increases sex hormone–binding globulin levels, thereby decreasing bioavailable testosterone levels.

Bromocriptine is a dopamine agonist indicated for medical treatment of prolactin-secreting pituitary tumors. This patient exhibits no clinical or biochemical evidence of a prolactinoma that would require treatment with a dopamine agonist.

Dexamethasone is used in the treatment of congenital adrenal hyperplasia. This patient's 17-hydroxyprogesterone level is normal, which suggests that she does not have this disorder.

Although early observational trials suggested that metformin may be effective in treating hirsutism in patients with PCOS, subsequent randomized clinical control trials have had mixed results. Therefore, metformin is not the best first-line treatment for symptoms of hyperandrogenism (such as acne, hirsutism, and alopecia) in women with PCOS.

Spironolactone can be very useful for the treatment of hyperandrogenism in PCOS but is added only if an oral contraceptive does not adequately improve symptoms. Because of the teratogenic effects of spironolactone, it is not given to women without an oral contraceptive pill.

KEY POINT

- **The best initial treatment for hirsutism in women with polycystic ovary syndrome is an oral contraceptive.**

Bibliography

Martin KA, Chang RJ, Ehrmann DA, et al. Evaluation and treatment of hirsutism in premenopausal women: an Endocrine Society clinical practice guideline. J Clin Endocrinol Metab. 2008;93(4):1105-1120. [PMID: 18252793]

Item 83 Answer: B

Educational Objective: **Treat acromegaly after transsphenoidal surgery.**

The most appropriate next step in treating this patient who has acromegaly is administration of octreotide, a somatostatin analogue. The goals of therapy for acromegaly are to normalize the insulin-like growth factor 1 (IGF-1) and growth hormone (GH) levels, reduce tumor bulk, prevent or decrease the number of comorbidities, and reduce the risk of premature death. Transsphenoidal surgery will normalize biochemical IGF-1 and GH levels in as many as 90% of patients with microadenomas and 40% of patients with macroadenomas. In patients (such as this one) whose IGF-1 and GH levels remain elevated postoperatively, somatostatin analogues are commonly used to normalize levels and shrink any residual pituitary tumor. This patient's comorbidities (sleep apnea, hypertension, type 2 diabetes mellitus, arthropathy, and headache) should continue to be monitored and treated, if needed.

Dopamine agonists generally do not work as well as somatostatin analogues in the treatment of acromegaly, and cabergoline, not bromocriptine, is the most effective dopamine agonist for this purpose.

Although this patient already underwent surgical debulking of his tumor, the continued elevation of his GH and IGF-1 levels indicates that residual disease is present, most likely in the cavernous sinus, which is not surgically accessible. Therefore, repeat surgery is unlikely to be useful.

Clinical observation is inappropriate for this patient with residual active acromegaly, which has associated comorbidities and premature mortality. Therefore, therapy is indicated.

KEY POINT

- **In patients with acromegaly whose insulin-like growth factor 1 and growth hormone levels remain elevated after transsphenoidal surgery, somatostatin analogues are commonly used to normalize levels and shrink any residual pituitary tumor.**

Bibliography

Katznelson L, Atkinson JL, Cook DM, Ezzat SZ, Hamrahian AH, Miller KK; American Association of Clinical Endocrinologists. American Association of Clinical Endocrinologists medical guidelines for clinical practice for the diagnosis and treatment of acromegaly—2011 update. Endocr Pract. 2011;17(Suppl 4):1-44. [PMID: 21846616]

Item 84 Answer: C

Educational Objective: **Diagnose ectopic adrenocorticotropic hormone secretion.**

The clinical and biochemical features of this patient with Cushing syndrome (hypercortisolism, melanonychia striata on the toenails) are most likely caused by ectopic adrenocorticotropic hormone (ACTH) secretion by a malignant tumor. Patients with these tumors typically have signs and symptoms of malignancy (weight loss, cachexia, and temporal muscle wasting) and biochemical features of mineralocorticoid activity. This patient most likely has new-onset type 2 diabetes mellitus (recent-onset polyuria and nocturia, high random glucose levels) and classic features of excess mineralocorticoid activity, including hypertension, metabolic alkalosis, and excessive urine potassium loss. He has no history of gastrointestinal fluid losses. Clinical examination shows features consistent with excessive ACTH secretion (hyperpigmented mucous membranes) and excess amounts of glucocorticoids (proximal muscle wasting and weakness). The patient's history of smoking suggests the possibility of an ACTH-producing lung cancer; approximately half of all cases of ectopic ACTH secretion are due to small-cell lung cancer.

Adrenal adenomas can be associated with hypercortisolism but the features tend to be mild, with hypertension and diabetes the most prominent. Adrenal adenomas are associated with suppressed ACTH levels.

Although adrenal carcinomas may be associated with weight loss, rapid onset of cushingoid features, and findings of hypercortisolism, they also are associated with suppressed, not elevated, levels of ACTH.

The clinical and biochemical features of hypercortisolism observed in this patient are not consistent with those seen in patients with ACTH-secreting pituitary adenomas, which generally are associated with lower ACTH levels and slow onset of cushingoid features.

KEY POINT

- **Patients with ectopic adrenocorticotropic hormone (ACTH) production typically have weight loss, rapid onset of Cushing syndrome, temporal muscle wasting, and elevated plasma ACTH levels.**

Bibliography

Neiman LK, Biller BM, Findling JW, et al. The diagnosis of Cushing's syndrome: an Endocrine Society Clinical Practice Guideline. J Clin Endocrinol Metab. 2008;93(5): 1526-1540. [PMID: 18334580]

Index

Note: Page numbers followed by f and t denote figures and tables, respectively. Test questions are indicated by Q.

Index

A NAME AND ADDRESS (Please complete.)

Last Name | First Name | Middle Initial

Address

Address cont.

City | State | ZIP Code

Country

Email address

B **Order Number**

(Use the Order Number on your MKSAP materials packing slip.)

C **ACP ID Number**

(Refer to packing slip in your MKSAP materials for your ACP ID Number.)

ACP® AMERICAN COLLEGE OF PHYSICIANS INTERNAL MEDICINE | Doctors for Adults

Medical Knowledge Self-Assessment Program® 16

TO EARN *AMA PRA CATEGORY 1 CREDITS*™ YOU MUST:

1. Answer all questions.
2. Score a minimum of 50% correct.

TO EARN *FREE* SAME-DAY *AMA PRA CATEGORY 1 CREDITS*™ ONLINE:

1. Answer all of your questions.
2. Go to **mksap.acponline.org** and access the appropriate answer sheet.
3. Transcribe your answers and submit for CME credits.
4. You can also enter your answers directly at **mksap.acponline.org** without first using this answer sheet.

To Submit Your Answer Sheet by Mail or FAX for a $10 Administrative Fee per Answer Sheet:

1. Answer all of your questions and calculate your score.
2. Complete boxes A–F.
3. Complete payment information.
4. Send the answer sheet and payment information to ACP, using the FAX number/address listed below.

COMPLETE FORM BELOW ONLY IF YOU SUBMIT BY MAIL OR FAX

Last Name | First Name | MI

Payment Information. Must remit in US funds, drawn on a US bank.

The processing fee for each paper answer sheet is $10.

☐ Check, made payable to ACP, enclosed

Charge to ☐ VISA ☐ MasterCard ☐ AMERICAN EXPRESS ☐ DISCOVER

Card Number ____________________

Expiration Date ______ / ______ (MM YY)   Security code (3 or 4 digit #s) ____________

Signature ____________________

Fax to: 215-351-2799

Questions?
Go to **mskap.acponline.org** or email **custserv@acponline.org**

Mail to:
Member and Customer Service
American College of Physicians
190 N. Independence Mall West
Philadelphia, PA 19106-1572

D

TEST TYPE	Maximum Number of CME Credits
◯ Cardiovascular Medicine	18
◯ Dermatology	10
◯ Gastroenterology and Hepatology	14
◯ Hematology and Oncology	20
◯ Neurology	14
◯ Rheumatology	14
◯ Endocrinology and Metabolism	12
◯ General Internal Medicine	24
◯ Infectious Disease	16
◯ Nephrology	16
◯ Pulmonary and Critical Care Medicine	16

E

CREDITS CLAIMED ON SECTION (1 hour = 1 credit)

Enter the number of credits earned on the test to the nearest quarter hour. Physicians should claim only the credit commensurate with the extent of their participation in the activity.

☐☐.☐☐

F

Enter your score here.

Instructions for calculating your own score are found in front of the self-assessment test in each book.

You must receive a minimum score of 50% correct.

__________ %

Credit Submission Date: __________

1 Ⓐ Ⓑ Ⓒ Ⓓ Ⓔ
2 Ⓐ Ⓑ Ⓒ Ⓓ Ⓔ
3 Ⓐ Ⓑ Ⓒ Ⓓ Ⓔ
4 Ⓐ Ⓑ Ⓒ Ⓓ Ⓔ
5 Ⓐ Ⓑ Ⓒ Ⓓ Ⓔ
6 Ⓐ Ⓑ Ⓒ Ⓓ Ⓔ
7 Ⓐ Ⓑ Ⓒ Ⓓ Ⓔ
8 Ⓐ Ⓑ Ⓒ Ⓓ Ⓔ
9 Ⓐ Ⓑ Ⓒ Ⓓ Ⓔ
10 Ⓐ Ⓑ Ⓒ Ⓓ Ⓔ
11 Ⓐ Ⓑ Ⓒ Ⓓ Ⓔ
12 Ⓐ Ⓑ Ⓒ Ⓓ Ⓔ
13 Ⓐ Ⓑ Ⓒ Ⓓ Ⓔ
14 Ⓐ Ⓑ Ⓒ Ⓓ Ⓔ
15 Ⓐ Ⓑ Ⓒ Ⓓ Ⓔ
16 Ⓐ Ⓑ Ⓒ Ⓓ Ⓔ
17 Ⓐ Ⓑ Ⓒ Ⓓ Ⓔ
18 Ⓐ Ⓑ Ⓒ Ⓓ Ⓔ
19 Ⓐ Ⓑ Ⓒ Ⓓ Ⓔ
20 Ⓐ Ⓑ Ⓒ Ⓓ Ⓔ
21 Ⓐ Ⓑ Ⓒ Ⓓ Ⓔ
22 Ⓐ Ⓑ Ⓒ Ⓓ Ⓔ
23 Ⓐ Ⓑ Ⓒ Ⓓ Ⓔ
24 Ⓐ Ⓑ Ⓒ Ⓓ Ⓔ
25 Ⓐ Ⓑ Ⓒ Ⓓ Ⓔ
26 Ⓐ Ⓑ Ⓒ Ⓓ Ⓔ
27 Ⓐ Ⓑ Ⓒ Ⓓ Ⓔ
28 Ⓐ Ⓑ Ⓒ Ⓓ Ⓔ
29 Ⓐ Ⓑ Ⓒ Ⓓ Ⓔ
30 Ⓐ Ⓑ Ⓒ Ⓓ Ⓔ
31 Ⓐ Ⓑ Ⓒ Ⓓ Ⓔ
32 Ⓐ Ⓑ Ⓒ Ⓓ Ⓔ
33 Ⓐ Ⓑ Ⓒ Ⓓ Ⓔ
34 Ⓐ Ⓑ Ⓒ Ⓓ Ⓔ
35 Ⓐ Ⓑ Ⓒ Ⓓ Ⓔ
36 Ⓐ Ⓑ Ⓒ Ⓓ Ⓔ
37 Ⓐ Ⓑ Ⓒ Ⓓ Ⓔ
38 Ⓐ Ⓑ Ⓒ Ⓓ Ⓔ
39 Ⓐ Ⓑ Ⓒ Ⓓ Ⓔ
40 Ⓐ Ⓑ Ⓒ Ⓓ Ⓔ
41 Ⓐ Ⓑ Ⓒ Ⓓ Ⓔ
42 Ⓐ Ⓑ Ⓒ Ⓓ Ⓔ
43 Ⓐ Ⓑ Ⓒ Ⓓ Ⓔ
44 Ⓐ Ⓑ Ⓒ Ⓓ Ⓔ
45 Ⓐ Ⓑ Ⓒ Ⓓ Ⓔ
46 Ⓐ Ⓑ Ⓒ Ⓓ Ⓔ
47 Ⓐ Ⓑ Ⓒ Ⓓ Ⓔ
48 Ⓐ Ⓑ Ⓒ Ⓓ Ⓔ
49 Ⓐ Ⓑ Ⓒ Ⓓ Ⓔ
50 Ⓐ Ⓑ Ⓒ Ⓓ Ⓔ
51 Ⓐ Ⓑ Ⓒ Ⓓ Ⓔ
52 Ⓐ Ⓑ Ⓒ Ⓓ Ⓔ
53 Ⓐ Ⓑ Ⓒ Ⓓ Ⓔ
54 Ⓐ Ⓑ Ⓒ Ⓓ Ⓔ
55 Ⓐ Ⓑ Ⓒ Ⓓ Ⓔ
56 Ⓐ Ⓑ Ⓒ Ⓓ Ⓔ
57 Ⓐ Ⓑ Ⓒ Ⓓ Ⓔ
58 Ⓐ Ⓑ Ⓒ Ⓓ Ⓔ
59 Ⓐ Ⓑ Ⓒ Ⓓ Ⓔ
60 Ⓐ Ⓑ Ⓒ Ⓓ Ⓔ
61 Ⓐ Ⓑ Ⓒ Ⓓ Ⓔ
62 Ⓐ Ⓑ Ⓒ Ⓓ Ⓔ
63 Ⓐ Ⓑ Ⓒ Ⓓ Ⓔ
64 Ⓐ Ⓑ Ⓒ Ⓓ Ⓔ
65 Ⓐ Ⓑ Ⓒ Ⓓ Ⓔ
66 Ⓐ Ⓑ Ⓒ Ⓓ Ⓔ
67 Ⓐ Ⓑ Ⓒ Ⓓ Ⓔ
68 Ⓐ Ⓑ Ⓒ Ⓓ Ⓔ
69 Ⓐ Ⓑ Ⓒ Ⓓ Ⓔ
70 Ⓐ Ⓑ Ⓒ Ⓓ Ⓔ
71 Ⓐ Ⓑ Ⓒ Ⓓ Ⓔ
72 Ⓐ Ⓑ Ⓒ Ⓓ Ⓔ
73 Ⓐ Ⓑ Ⓒ Ⓓ Ⓔ
74 Ⓐ Ⓑ Ⓒ Ⓓ Ⓔ
75 Ⓐ Ⓑ Ⓒ Ⓓ Ⓔ
76 Ⓐ Ⓑ Ⓒ Ⓓ Ⓔ
77 Ⓐ Ⓑ Ⓒ Ⓓ Ⓔ
78 Ⓐ Ⓑ Ⓒ Ⓓ Ⓔ
79 Ⓐ Ⓑ Ⓒ Ⓓ Ⓔ
80 Ⓐ Ⓑ Ⓒ Ⓓ Ⓔ
81 Ⓐ Ⓑ Ⓒ Ⓓ Ⓔ
82 Ⓐ Ⓑ Ⓒ Ⓓ Ⓔ
83 Ⓐ Ⓑ Ⓒ Ⓓ Ⓔ
84 Ⓐ Ⓑ Ⓒ Ⓓ Ⓔ
85 Ⓐ Ⓑ Ⓒ Ⓓ Ⓔ
86 Ⓐ Ⓑ Ⓒ Ⓓ Ⓔ
87 Ⓐ Ⓑ Ⓒ Ⓓ Ⓔ
88 Ⓐ Ⓑ Ⓒ Ⓓ Ⓔ
89 Ⓐ Ⓑ Ⓒ Ⓓ Ⓔ
90 Ⓐ Ⓑ Ⓒ Ⓓ Ⓔ
91 Ⓐ Ⓑ Ⓒ Ⓓ Ⓔ
92 Ⓐ Ⓑ Ⓒ Ⓓ Ⓔ
93 Ⓐ Ⓑ Ⓒ Ⓓ Ⓔ
94 Ⓐ Ⓑ Ⓒ Ⓓ Ⓔ
95 Ⓐ Ⓑ Ⓒ Ⓓ Ⓔ
96 Ⓐ Ⓑ Ⓒ Ⓓ Ⓔ
97 Ⓐ Ⓑ Ⓒ Ⓓ Ⓔ
98 Ⓐ Ⓑ Ⓒ Ⓓ Ⓔ
99 Ⓐ Ⓑ Ⓒ Ⓓ Ⓔ
100 Ⓐ Ⓑ Ⓒ Ⓓ Ⓔ
101 Ⓐ Ⓑ Ⓒ Ⓓ Ⓔ
102 Ⓐ Ⓑ Ⓒ Ⓓ Ⓔ
103 Ⓐ Ⓑ Ⓒ Ⓓ Ⓔ
104 Ⓐ Ⓑ Ⓒ Ⓓ Ⓔ
105 Ⓐ Ⓑ Ⓒ Ⓓ Ⓔ
106 Ⓐ Ⓑ Ⓒ Ⓓ Ⓔ
107 Ⓐ Ⓑ Ⓒ Ⓓ Ⓔ
108 Ⓐ Ⓑ Ⓒ Ⓓ Ⓔ
109 Ⓐ Ⓑ Ⓒ Ⓓ Ⓔ
110 Ⓐ Ⓑ Ⓒ Ⓓ Ⓔ
111 Ⓐ Ⓑ Ⓒ Ⓓ Ⓔ
112 Ⓐ Ⓑ Ⓒ Ⓓ Ⓔ
113 Ⓐ Ⓑ Ⓒ Ⓓ Ⓔ
114 Ⓐ Ⓑ Ⓒ Ⓓ Ⓔ
115 Ⓐ Ⓑ Ⓒ Ⓓ Ⓔ
116 Ⓐ Ⓑ Ⓒ Ⓓ Ⓔ
117 Ⓐ Ⓑ Ⓒ Ⓓ Ⓔ
118 Ⓐ Ⓑ Ⓒ Ⓓ Ⓔ
119 Ⓐ Ⓑ Ⓒ Ⓓ Ⓔ
120 Ⓐ Ⓑ Ⓒ Ⓓ Ⓔ
121 Ⓐ Ⓑ Ⓒ Ⓓ Ⓔ
122 Ⓐ Ⓑ Ⓒ Ⓓ Ⓔ
123 Ⓐ Ⓑ Ⓒ Ⓓ Ⓔ
124 Ⓐ Ⓑ Ⓒ Ⓓ Ⓔ
125 Ⓐ Ⓑ Ⓒ Ⓓ Ⓔ
126 Ⓐ Ⓑ Ⓒ Ⓓ Ⓔ
127 Ⓐ Ⓑ Ⓒ Ⓓ Ⓔ
128 Ⓐ Ⓑ Ⓒ Ⓓ Ⓔ
129 Ⓐ Ⓑ Ⓒ Ⓓ Ⓔ
130 Ⓐ Ⓑ Ⓒ Ⓓ Ⓔ
131 Ⓐ Ⓑ Ⓒ Ⓓ Ⓔ
132 Ⓐ Ⓑ Ⓒ Ⓓ Ⓔ
133 Ⓐ Ⓑ Ⓒ Ⓓ Ⓔ
134 Ⓐ Ⓑ Ⓒ Ⓓ Ⓔ
135 Ⓐ Ⓑ Ⓒ Ⓓ Ⓔ
136 Ⓐ Ⓑ Ⓒ Ⓓ Ⓔ
137 Ⓐ Ⓑ Ⓒ Ⓓ Ⓔ
138 Ⓐ Ⓑ Ⓒ Ⓓ Ⓔ
139 Ⓐ Ⓑ Ⓒ Ⓓ Ⓔ
140 Ⓐ Ⓑ Ⓒ Ⓓ Ⓔ
141 Ⓐ Ⓑ Ⓒ Ⓓ Ⓔ
142 Ⓐ Ⓑ Ⓒ Ⓓ Ⓔ
143 Ⓐ Ⓑ Ⓒ Ⓓ Ⓔ
144 Ⓐ Ⓑ Ⓒ Ⓓ Ⓔ
145 Ⓐ Ⓑ Ⓒ Ⓓ Ⓔ
146 Ⓐ Ⓑ Ⓒ Ⓓ Ⓔ
147 Ⓐ Ⓑ Ⓒ Ⓓ Ⓔ
148 Ⓐ Ⓑ Ⓒ Ⓓ Ⓔ
149 Ⓐ Ⓑ Ⓒ Ⓓ Ⓔ
150 Ⓐ Ⓑ Ⓒ Ⓓ Ⓔ
151 Ⓐ Ⓑ Ⓒ Ⓓ Ⓔ
152 Ⓐ Ⓑ Ⓒ Ⓓ Ⓔ
153 Ⓐ Ⓑ Ⓒ Ⓓ Ⓔ
154 Ⓐ Ⓑ Ⓒ Ⓓ Ⓔ
155 Ⓐ Ⓑ Ⓒ Ⓓ Ⓔ
156 Ⓐ Ⓑ Ⓒ Ⓓ Ⓔ
157 Ⓐ Ⓑ Ⓒ Ⓓ Ⓔ
158 Ⓐ Ⓑ Ⓒ Ⓓ Ⓔ
159 Ⓐ Ⓑ Ⓒ Ⓓ Ⓔ
160 Ⓐ Ⓑ Ⓒ Ⓓ Ⓔ
161 Ⓐ Ⓑ Ⓒ Ⓓ Ⓔ
162 Ⓐ Ⓑ Ⓒ Ⓓ Ⓔ
163 Ⓐ Ⓑ Ⓒ Ⓓ Ⓔ
164 Ⓐ Ⓑ Ⓒ Ⓓ Ⓔ
165 Ⓐ Ⓑ Ⓒ Ⓓ Ⓔ
166 Ⓐ Ⓑ Ⓒ Ⓓ Ⓔ
167 Ⓐ Ⓑ Ⓒ Ⓓ Ⓔ
168 Ⓐ Ⓑ Ⓒ Ⓓ Ⓔ
169 Ⓐ Ⓑ Ⓒ Ⓓ Ⓔ
170 Ⓐ Ⓑ Ⓒ Ⓓ Ⓔ
171 Ⓐ Ⓑ Ⓒ Ⓓ Ⓔ
172 Ⓐ Ⓑ Ⓒ Ⓓ Ⓔ
173 Ⓐ Ⓑ Ⓒ Ⓓ Ⓔ
174 Ⓐ Ⓑ Ⓒ Ⓓ Ⓔ
175 Ⓐ Ⓑ Ⓒ Ⓓ Ⓔ
176 Ⓐ Ⓑ Ⓒ Ⓓ Ⓔ
177 Ⓐ Ⓑ Ⓒ Ⓓ Ⓔ
178 Ⓐ Ⓑ Ⓒ Ⓓ Ⓔ
179 Ⓐ Ⓑ Ⓒ Ⓓ Ⓔ
180 Ⓐ Ⓑ Ⓒ Ⓓ Ⓔ